Could It Be the CONGOS?

Could It Be the CONGOS?

British Military Doctors and the Diagnosis and Treatment of Yellow Fever in the Eighteenth- and Nineteenth-Century Caribbean

Edited and Annotated by
Pedro L.V. Welch

The University of the West Indies Press
Mona • St Augustine • Cave Hill • Global • Five Islands

The University of the West Indies Press
7A Gibraltar Hall Road, Mona
Kingston 7, Jamaica
www.uwipress.com

© 2026, Pedro L.V. Welch
ISBN: 978-976-640-984-5 (paperback)
ISBN: 978-976-640-985-2 (ePUB)

All rights reserved. Published 2026

A catalogue record of this book is available from the National

Library of Jamaica.

The University of the West Indies Press has no responsibility for the persistence or accuracy of URLs for external or third-party internet websites referred to in this publication and does not guarantee that any content on such websites is, or will remain, accurate or appropriate.

Cover and text design by Christina Moore Fuller

Cover image: Daniel Vierge, Public domain, *1878 illustration of soldiers returning from Cuba being fumigated to protect against yellow fever*

Printed in the United States of America

Contents

List of Tables vii

Acknowledgements xi

1. Introductory Comments on the Scourge of Yellow Fever in the British Caribbean   1
2. Considering a Miscellaneous Report   27
3. Reports from Antigua   38
4. Reports from Barbados   68
5. Reports from British Guiana   195
6. Reports from Dominica   224
7. Reports from Grenada   270
8. Reports from Montserrat   299
9. Reports from St Christopher (St Kitts)   307
10. Reports from St Lucia   344
11. Reports from St Vincent   351
12. Reports from Tobago   366
13. Reports from Trinidad   451
14. Reflections and Epilogue   491

Notes 497

Bibliography 535

Index 539

List of Tables

Table 1.1:	Mortality Rates among Troops	12
Table 4.1:	Return of the Storekeeper General's Department, Showing the Dates of Their Arrival at Barbados, Sickness, Deaths, Recoveries	119
Table 4.2:	Return of Convalescents of Fever Treated in the Naval Hospital, Barbados, from 20 October to 18 December 1821	121
Table 4.3:	White Employees at Naval Hospital Who Escaped Sickness, 20 June 1821–20 February 1822	134
Table 4.4:	Fatality Rate in Coloured Personnel Employed at Naval Hospital	137
Table 4.5:	Schedule for Horatio Warder and John Calometi	152
Table 4.6:	Onset of Yellow Fever among Military Personnel by Age, Rank and Arrival Date	165
Table 4.7:	Sickness Outcomes and Residence of Affected Military Personnel	166
Table 4.8:	Admissions, Deaths and Mortality Ratios by Type of Resident	182
Table 4.9:	Yellow Fever Admissions and Deaths by Period of Residence and Class Strength	190
Table 5.1:	Summary of Strength, Admissions, and Deaths of Military Ranks by Period of Residence	208
Table 5.2:	Ages of the Fatal Cases	208
Table 5.3:	Yellow Fever Cases and Fatalities among Military Units	209
Table 5.4:	Incidence and Mortality of Yellow Fever by Military Unit Strength	219
Table 6.1:	Attacks with Fever and Deaths in the Queens, June–August by Mr Ralph	226
Table 6.2:	Incident Report: Cases and Outcomes	227

Table 6.3:	Return of Hospital Servants Who Were Successively Taken Ill of Fever between 18 September 1816 and 7 February 1817	232
Table 6.4:	Strength, Cases, and Mortality Report, May–September 1838	264
Table 9.1:	Admissions of Cases at Brimstone Hill, Each Month, Noting Weather Conditions	311
Table 9.2:	Number Treated between 1 May and 18 December, Exclusive of Blacks	316
Table 9.3:	Monthly Admissions and Mortality from This Disease Category among White Troops	322
Table 9.4:	Mortality by Age, Strength and Service Duration	323
Table 9.5:	Acclimatization to Disease	323
Table 9.6:	Diseases Treated during the Year	338
Table 9.7:	Deaths of Races by Month	339
Table 11.1:	The Prevalence of a Fatality from Epidemic Fever in the Garrison of St Vincent from 1 April to 30 September 1839	357
Table 11.2:	Attacks and Deaths, 1831–42	358
Table 11.3:	Cases of Fever Treated by Two Doctors, 1841–42	361
Table 12.1:	Sick at Tobago	383
Table 12.2:	List of Persons Employed about the Sick in the Garrison or Hospital, Tobago, between November 1818 and March 1819	388
Table 12.3:	Deaths of Non-commissioned Officers and Privates in the Army Serving in the Windward and Leeward Colonies for 12 Years, from 1 January 1796 to 31 December 1807	396
Table 12.4:	Return of a Detachment of the 4th Regiment Stationed in the Island of Tobago – with the Deaths during the Time of Remaining there, from 6 April 1819 to 9 September 1820 When They Embarked for Barbados	426

List of Tables

Table 12.5: A Return of the Number of Cases and Deaths from the Epidemic Remittent Fever at Tobago from 1 April to 31 July 1841 446

Table 12.6: Military Unit Strength and Mortality Report by Age .. 446

Table 12.7: Military Unit Strength and Mortality Report by Period of Residence 447

Table 13.1: Quarterly Medical Statistics 486

Acknowledgements

The contribution of Alan Humphries, former librarian of the Thackray Medical Museum in Leeds, UK, is hereby acknowledged. He read the prescriptions which were in a few reports that are transcribed in this manuscript and translated some of these from Latin into English for me. I also acknowledge the assistance of David Michael, a former student at the University of the West Indies (Cave Hill), who assisted in typing some of the manuscript and in researching the origins of some of the British military doctors who authored the reports. My daughter, Gem Bonnett, and my son, Dr Pedro André Welch, a doctor, now resident in the United Kingdom, offered valuable help in identifying research sources and in making valuable comments on early drafts of the manuscript.

1. Introductory Comments on the Scourge of Yellow Fever in the British Caribbean

The following investigation looks at issues connected with the treatment of yellow fever by British military doctors who served in the Caribbean in the eighteenth and nineteenth centuries. In particular, it notes medical treatment in Barbados, since the data appears more voluminous for that island. Additionally, we survey several treatises published by medical practitioners in the Caribbean, with special reference to the treatment of yellow fever and other ailments, during the eighteenth to the nineteenth centuries. It must be observed, however, that in discussing the medical practice of British military doctors in the Caribbean theatre, the method used here is to let these practitioners speak. That is, we will transcribe the documentary vignettes left by these practitioners after our initial analysis and then use them to offer some informed commentary on their medical practice. Moreover, while the data from which the research is lifted is voluminous, it is not intended to answer all questions related to medical practice in the period surveyed.

It is important, also, to note that no claim is made here to any special medical competence on the part of the author. Nevertheless, use is made of commentary by medical experts or medical historians, where these could help resolve any problems that may surface in the use of the data. Our analysis begins by surveying the historical literature on yellow fever and other ailments, firstly in the writings of contemporary researchers and then in writings that date from the eighteenth century onwards. It might be useful, however, before focusing on the core of the data, to offer some brief comments on the symptoms of yellow fever and the reasons why the appearance of this disease caused so much fear to those who had the misfortune to be struck by it and to the doctors who treated them.

Factors in Outbreaks of Yellow Fever and Its Symptoms

In a few cases, yellow fever infections are mild enough to be mistaken for other classes of disease. However, in its severe attacks, results can be life-threatening, with such symptoms as a very high fever, chills, severe headache, muscle aches, vomiting and backache. The patient may often vomit a black-coloured liquid, which signals the onset of internal haemorrhage. In some cases, despite some promise of recovery, the patient may exhibit symptoms of further internal bleeding, bleeding from body orifices and the gums, and kidney and liver failure. Liver failure leads to jaundice, with its concomitant yellowing of the skin and the whites of the eyes. In most cases, the afflicted patient will pass black tarry stools (melena). Indeed, it is the yellowing of the skin that gives the fever its name, although in some eighteenth- and nineteenth-century texts, it was sometimes called "the black vomit" because of the characteristic vomiting of blood.

There are two basic kinds of yellow fever. One of these is termed jungle yellow fever, while the other is called urban yellow fever. Jungle yellow fever is spread to humans from infected monkeys via the bite of an infected female mosquito. After the ingestion of the virus from an infected monkey, it takes between one and four weeks for the mosquito to become infective. Jungle yellow fever usually occurs in people who reside and operate in tropical rainforest environments. Urban yellow fever is passed from humans to other humans through the bite of an infected female mosquito. The *Aedes aegypti* mosquito is usually indicated in this mode of transmission. In addition to the mosquito, other vectors have been identified as hosts for the virus, including some species of tick and the horsefly of Brazil.

The extreme fear of yellow fever felt by European visitors to the Caribbean and South America in the early period of European settlement into the late nineteenth century had to do with ignorance of the causes of the disease and the malignance of the yellow fever attack. Additionally, there was a high mortality rate, with people often dying within a few days, if not hours, of the appearance of the disease.

The fear and horror attached to the disease are captured in Dr

Pinckard's account of his voyage to the West Indies in 1795. He wrote,

> a degree of horror [seemed] to have overspread the nation, from the late disastrous effects of the seasoning fever or what the multitude denominate the West India Plague; insomuch that a sense of terror attaches to it the very name of the West Indies. As persons looked on, they were overheard to exclaim, "Ah, poor fellows! You are going to your last home! What a pity that such brave men shall go to that West India grave – to that hateful climate to be killed by the plague! Poor fellows, Goodbye, farewell: We shall never see you back again...."[1]

With this background, our attention is now turned to an overview of the historical events that brought yellow fever to the attention of European colonists of the New World.

Tracking the Historical Debate

Discussions on the causes and effects of yellow fever began almost with the first wave of colonization in the Caribbean. In 1648, an epidemic broke out in the Yucatan Peninsula.[2] It was there that the Spanish began to refer to the fever as *el vómito prieto* (black vomit). It seems also that this outbreak began simultaneously with an outbreak in Guadeloupe. The report of the outbreak in Guadeloupe was given by Père Jean-Baptiste Du Tertre, a French priest of the Dominican order and historian who chronicled much of the history of the early French enterprise in the Antilles. His report suggested the epidemic had begun in St Christopher (St Kitts), where it had killed about one-third of the inhabitants. In turn, a French ship, *Le Boeuf*, calling from Rochelle, France, had picked up some of the sick and dying (not to omit some of the St Kitts flora and fauna, including some of the mosquitoes that had infected them), and had taken them to Guadeloupe. The epidemic ran for about twenty months on the latter island.[3]

The outbreak in St Kitts and Guadeloupe may have also extended to Barbados. Indeed, the fact that the epidemic broke out in the same year in these Caribbean locations might suggest it had begun at one of them and been carried throughout the region from this first port of call. G.M. Findlay has noted that an ordinance issued in Massachusetts in 1648 stated inter alia that:

> All vessels which should come from the West Indies should stay at the castle and not come to shore … forasmuch as this court is credibly informed that the plague or like grievous infectious disease hath … exceedingly raged in ye Barbados, St Christophers, and other islands of ye West Indies to ye great depopulation of those. It is, therefore, ordered that all our own or other ships coming from any ports of ye West Indies to Boston Harbor, shall stop and come to ye anchor before they come at ye castle.[4]

Findlay also cites Richard Vine, who had written to Governor Winthrop of Massachusetts on 20 April 1648, reporting that sickness had caused the death of as many as twenty people in a parish in one week. Another letter, sent by Lucy Downing of Boston to the governor in December 1648, reported that she had just returned from Barbados. Still, her two sons, Jo and Robin, had since gone to the island, apparently grieving over the loss of a close friend during the Barbados epidemic. Based on the data surveyed, Findlay argues that the epidemic had started in Barbados in September of 1647, and yellow fever was still present on the island in December 1648 and might still have been present on the island when the Boston regulations were issued in 1649.

The assertion that a yellow fever epidemic had started in Barbados in 1647 is disputed in a 1931 survey by Henry Rose Carter.[5] He opposes this dating, based on observations recorded by Richard Ligon[6] that an epidemic was sweeping Barbados in 1647. The basis of Carter's doubt is that one would have to exclude the possibility of malaria and also consider the views expressed by both of these reporters that mortality was ten times greater among men than women. However, one also needs to note that Findlay's analysis finds some support in the Boston document. Moreover, malaria was not endemic in Barbados and, therefore, must be discounted as an explanation of the disease recorded by Ligon. Additionally, it may be borne in mind that a much later scholarship supports Findlay's findings and, significantly, that of one modern medical practitioner.

Kenneth Kiple has identified a yellow fever epidemic in Barbados between 1647 and 1649. He reports the epidemic may have killed as many as six thousand people. In fact, as he informs us, the disease was so severe and so connected with Barbados that it was referred to as the "Barbados Distemper".[7] In further corroboration of Ligon's description, J. Edward Hutson, a doctor who has edited a recent republication of Ligon's *A True and Exact History of the Island of Barbadoes*, has reported that "the plague rampant in Barbados at the time of Ligon's arrival was yellow fever".[8] Moreover, as Hutson informs us, "The mortality associated with yellow fever was high, particularly among whites newly arrived from England who, unlike African blacks, had no natural immunity to the virus. As a result, yellow fever also came to be known as *stranger's fever*."

Findlay's findings also echo the assertions of Sir Macfarlane Burnet and David White's study, which observes that each disease has "its own emotional colour", not necessarily connected to the real importance of the disease. As they tell us, of the various diseases labelled, for example, "the plague", "leprosy" and "influenza":

> Yellow fever is the most vividly coloured by associations [not to omit its association with Black Vomit], quite apart from the image conjured up by the name itself of an intensely jaundiced patient dying in delirium. There has been something grimly romantic about the story of its first appearance, when it seemed to rise like a miasma, from the overcrowded stinking holds of slave ships in Barbados in 1647.[9]

In short, there seems to be some consensus among many researchers that yellow fever was certainly an epidemic in Barbados in 1647. In that case, even if the epidemic at the Yucatan Peninsula in 1647 is better documented, Barbados might have been the seat of the epidemic in the wider Caribbean. Our discussion will follow up on this lead and establish the basis for considering the Barbados epidemic the source of the other epidemics.

As several historians have observed, yellow fever was virtually unknown in the pre-Columbian New World, and the native Caribbean residents showed the same susceptibility as European colonists.[10] Correspondingly, enslaved Africans generally had significantly lower incidences of the disease compared to European colonists and, for that matter, considerably lower mortality and vastly more moderate symptoms than those exhibited in the European and the native populations in the Caribbean. In that context, David Clyde notes that among British forces in the Caribbean, mortality figures for white troops for the period 1796–1802 hovered around 22 per cent, while that for black troops was about 6 per cent. These calculations were done by a British medical practitioner, Dr Robert Jackson, who was attached to the British forces in the region. However, Clyde's follow-up calculations showed that for 1804, one of every two white sailors and soldiers hospitalized died, while the comparative mortality for black troops was one in forty-three.[11]

In this context, the Barbados connection is based on the fact that the epidemic of the late 1640s coincided with the beginning of the sugar revolution and the beginning of the large-scale importation of enslaved Africans. Prior to this period, the island's economy was based on the small-scale production of tobacco and cotton, and the labour force was predominantly European. However, the use of some Amerindian labour was noted. Although the newly arrived European population was exposed to a tropical environment with potentially dangerous pathogens, it was not until the expansion of the slave trade and the increase in the African component of the population that we recorded the first major epidemic in Barbados. As we have noted earlier, we can virtually rule out malaria as the source of Ligon's plague. Further, the conditions in Barbados are described by Hutson thus:

> African blacks, as a result of many generations of exposure to yellow fever, developed a strong natural immunity to the disease, while English Whites had no resistance to it whatever. Hence, in 1647, in Barbados, a reservoir of infection (blacks), the vector necessary for transmission of the disease (the *Aedes aegypti* mosquito), and a reservoir of non-resistant subjects (whites) all came together in a crowded area (Bridgetown) and set the scene for an outbreak of yellow fever of major proportions.[12]

While we have posited that there was a general immunity to the disease among the enslaved and free African population, we take cognizance of the critique Sheldon Watts offers to Kiple's discussion of this issue.[13] Watts observes that the 1691 epidemic in Barbados swept away "great numbers of masters, servants, and slaves". The implication, of course, is that not all Africans were immune to yellow fever. Watts also points to the fact that enslaved Africans were exposed, by way of harsher living conditions, to conditions that whites did not experience. In this way, African children might have had "the opportunity to acquire immunity to the disease, through suffering a light case of what no White [medical] authority [of that period] would describe as yellow fever". In short, Watts suggests that the immunity of Africans was not an immunity conferred by superior genetic adaptation. Instead, it was an immunity conferred through an earlier encounter. The problem with this scenario is that it is difficult to see how whites, even if they lived in relative isolation from the slave quarters, could have avoided contracting the very disease African children had contracted, particularly if the vector (the mosquito) was also present. Furthermore, if blacks who had not contracted the disease in childhood were also present, they too were likely to have suffered the mortalities experienced by whites.

In sum, with or without any claim to natural genetic immunity, the enslaved were more than likely to have come from areas where yellow fever was endemic and to have descended from forebears who had come from such areas. In that case, it is not unreasonable to assume that real differences did exist in the aetiology of the disease, as it related to mortality differentials between whites and blacks. These differences appear time and time again and point to the importation of enslaved Africans and mosquitoes as a major source of the disease. In 1647, Barbados was one of the few places in the Caribbean where conditions converged to facilitate the spread of the disease. Whatever the origins of the disease, the first outbreaks of yellow fever in the Caribbean led us from the late 1640s up until the early twentieth century, when the vectors were identified and preventive measures introduced. Yellow fever epidemics were so frequent that almost every medical treatise written by various doctors who practised medicine in the Caribbean devoted some attention to the scourge.

Our attention now turns to a consideration of some of these works.

Tracking the Doctors and Their Views on Medical Treatment from the Eighteenth Century

In 1741, Henry Warren, a medical practitioner who had worked in Barbados, published a work entitled *A Treatise Concerning the Malignant Fever in Barbados and the Neighbouring Islands, with an Account There from the Year 1733 to 1738*. Warren begins his discussion by asserting that there was no "malignant distemper" indigenous to the island. Moreover, he observed that when the island was visited by what he termed variously, "the Malignant and Ardent fever of Barbados, and the *Febris Ardens Biliosa,* it was certain that "such have always been brought among us from some infected place". As far as Warren was concerned, yellow fever, which he noted the French had called *La Maladie de Siam* or *La Fièvre Malchiltli*, and the Spanish *vómito prieto* or the black vomiting", was imported to Barbados from some "Asiatic" origin.

Warren's views on the origin of yellow fever epidemics are corroborated in his eyes when one noted that "lands which abounded in woods, lakes, and marshes produced epidemical malignant diseases". However, it was clear that Barbados was not so affected. In fact, the air "was remarkably fresh and pure, and probably more salubrious than any other sugar colony". Additionally, as he further observed, "the land here, in respect of the other islands, is the best cultivated and entirely free from lakes or marshes. To add to these advantages, the island stood to the windward of the island chain, far from any other major land mass, and its weather patterns, far from contributing to epidemic conditions, actually acted against them." He informs us, "Even at the time that this malignity is actually harboured among us, a continuation of dry sultry weather has been so far from giving any aggravation to it, that it has rather seemed to repress it; and make it lie more lulled and dormant". Warren's descriptions place him firmly within the "miasmic" school. That is, the belief that somehow bad air spread fevers, mostly emanating from swamps, bogs and marshes. The fact that Barbados had few of these natural features clearly perplexed him. The only alternative that seemed plausible to him was that the fevers that ravaged Barbados so often had to be of an imported variety.

It is clear, then, that Warren is a keen observer of the conditions under which the disease spread and of variations in the effect of the disease on various social and ethnic groups. He asks, "How come it that strangers and newcomers whose blood is purest and least impregnated with exalted oils and salts should be most liable to this disease?" "How come it that the negroes whose food is mostly rancid fish or flesh, nay often the flesh of dogs, cats, asses, horses, rats, etc. – who mostly lead intemperate lives, and who are always sore clad, and most exposed to surfeits, heats, colds, and all the injuries of the air, are so little subjected to this danger?" Warren had clearly missed the implications of his own evidence. As he had observed, the fact that the deplorable conditions under which the enslaved had lived could have led to increased exposure to various disease strains. It might have given some of them immunity to various tropical diseases – an immunity not so much caused by any genetic conferment but rather by repeated exposure to milder strains, which granted subsequent immunity in a more virulent attack. But, then again, it would be several generations before the knowledge would be acquired that germs and microbes caused some diseases. Warren could not be expected to move above the collective medical wisdom of his age.

Warren comes closer, perhaps, than any of his medical contemporaries to touching on the real cause of yellow fever. It seems that he considered that yellow fever was caused not only by some "miasmatic influence" but also by some more visible material cause. He observed that the bites of animals and some insects created "different distempers", but unfortunately, he dismisses this possibility in the case of yellow fever. Additionally, it appears that, unlike his contemporaries, and certainly those who would follow them over the next hundred years, he was a moderate in advocating the traditional modes of treatment. He warns, "I do, in a great measure, forbid the ordinary evacuations, by bloodletting, emetics, *vesicatories* or purgatives in this pestilential fever, in which from long and attentive observation, I declare them to be equally pernicious and destructive in their consequences...."

Warren was equally appalled at the widespread use of calomel (a mercury-based compound) by local practitioners, whom he termed "plantation practitioners". If they understood "the true nature of the use and inward operation of mercury, [he was] persuaded [that] they would be more cautious of playing with so dangerous a weapon ...." In the place of these dangerous medicines, he advocated the use of "lenitive purges" such as "manna, cassia, lenitive electuary, or the like". Additionally, great care was to be taken to "keep up nature's strength and spirits by giving now and then a little warm Madeira wine, canary, or such cardiacs as are not too inflaming". In these prescriptions, Warren was way ahead of his contemporaries.

The medicines prescribed by Warren were generally mild compared to those often prescribed at that time. Manna refers to a secretion from the flowering ash of Southern Europe. Sap-sucking insects feed on this plant and secrete a liquid, somewhat like honeydew. When dried, the secretion has a sweet taste. When eaten in large quantities, it is mildly laxative and was used as a medicine for that purpose. Lenitive purges were mild purges with a laxative action. Cassia was a plant related to cinnamon. Even in modern usage, it is known for its medicinal use in relieving nausea, flatulence and diarrhoea and lowering the temperature of the body during a fever. Unlike many of his contemporaries and some of the doctors of later vintage, Warren had hit on a therapeutic regime that was significantly less harmful. Well into the nineteenth century, doctors would prescribe mercury-based compounds, which, if they did not kill the patient, certainly did nothing to alleviate their symptoms if they did not, in fact, make recovery more difficult. Certainly, Warren's patients would have been relieved of considerable agony by his decision to avoid totally the use of *vesicatories*. This term refers to the use of blistering agents, which were in common use at the time Warren wrote his treatise and, indeed, remained in common use throughout the eighteenth and nineteenth centuries.

Warren's indictment of the local "practitioners of chirurgery" is still a recurring theme in the literature some seventy-five years later. Dr George Pinckard, who served with the British Navy in the Caribbean theatre, observed that local practitioners "were pre-eminent in their ignorance". Indeed, "some practitioners in medicine [could] be found in the colony (Barbados) who in learning and manners [were] not far removed from the slaves. They [were] more illiterate than you can believe; and the very Negro doctors of the estates too justly vie with them in medical knowledge". Pinckard was particularly distressed "to see among them men who, instead of having the care of the health and lives of their fellow subjects, ought not to be entrusted to compound a pill, or a bolus...."[14]

Another medical practitioner, Dr John Tennent, offers valuable insights into the perceptions of medical practitioners in the Caribbean. His pamphlet, entitled "A Reprieve from Death in Two Physical Chapters", was published in 1741. Tennent felt that the principal causes of yellow fever were to be found in marshes and rivers. Like his European contemporaries, he did not consider mosquitoes or other insects as disease vectors, but his focus on rivers and marshes was logically sound. Since mosquitoes tend to live near human habitation in places where adequate moisture is available, it was well enough to consider keeping people away from such environments. However, Tennent's mode of treatment followed a familiar regime. He advocated the use of "blisters", "bleeding sometimes" and "cooling medicines such as juice of lemons, spirit of sulphur, nitre, sugar of lead, *sal prindla* (possibly prunella), with sweats of several kinds, now and then".

Additionally, he proposed the use of "snake root". Snake root or "Seneca" was a medicine first popularized in colonial North America and later extensively used by doctors in the Caribbean. It induces sweating and increases salivation, thus possibly having some effect on the high temperatures associated with yellow fever. The use of bleeding, sweats and purging was entirely consistent with a "miasmic" view of disease, which placed the cause as lying in the putrefaction of vegetable matter and subsequent contamination of the air. This contamination, doctors felt, affected the blood, and the best way to deal with the disease was to stimulate vomiting, sweating and salivating, thus eliminating the poison from the system.

Another commentary on the treatment of yellow fever was published in 1781 by John Rollo, who informs us in the preface to his book that his observations were made on the disease that broke out among British troops in St Lucia between 1778 and 1789.[15] Rollo followed up this first publication with another, published in 1783, which commented on conditions leading to yellow fever and possible treatments for this and other diseases. The first book was addressed to the Hon. John Vaughan, "General and Commander of His Majesty's Forces in the West Indies". The value of Rollo's contribution lies in the statistics he offers on the mortality rates among the troops and in his presentation of various treatments. The table that follows, as well as his descriptions of the medical regime he followed, illustrates that usefulness.

Table 1.1: Mortality Rates among Troops

The Situation in the Island in Which the Men Were Fixed	No. of Men in Health, Originally in Each Situation	No. of Sick from Each	No. of Relapses	No. of Deaths
Morne Fortune	86	18	10	1
South Side of Grand Cul-de-Sac	17	16	11	1
Low Battery North Side Cul-de-Sac	16	16	8	2
High Ground; North Side Cul-de-Sac	13	6	5	2
Carenage Town	4	4	1	1
Ridge of Hills to Windward of Town and Vigie	42	28	13	1
South Side of Carenage Bay	23	17	17	8
Rock Battery, Situated at the Extremity of Carenage Bay	7	3	1	--

Rollo's statistics show a variable picture of mortality, which ranged from just over 1 per cent in the area of Morne Fortune to 35 per cent in the south side of Carenage Bay. In part, the difference in the statistics he presents may be due to marked environmental differences. Morne Fortune is an area of high elevation, and although mosquito attacks are not unknown at high elevations, they are rarer. In the case of Morne Fortune, the absence of any standing body of water might also have diminished the threat. On the other hand, the south side of Carenage Bay was the site of an extensive mangrove swamp – an ideal habitat for the breeding of mosquitoes.[16] If we take Rollo's figures for the sick as a ratio to the strength of the garrison at each location, the picture of infirmity is even more striking. In two cases, the entire force was infirm. It is not surprising, given such profiles of infirmity, that some medical practitioners felt hopeless when confronted with yellow fever. Indeed, for troops embarking for the Caribbean, as well as their families and fellow countrymen, the trip was viewed as akin to a death sentence.

Rollo's prescription shows that the treatment of yellow fever had not advanced since Warren's time. Indeed, it might well have retrogressed. He did not refer specifically to bleeding as a remedy, although it might be assumed that in common with his fellows, this would have been one of his first approaches. He tells us, "The more effectual means for this purpose, we found to be nauseating doses of tartar emetic; and at the time of the usual exacerbation of the fever, an opiate by itself or combined with an antimonial, according to the state of the stomach." Tartar emetic was a drug containing antimony, which is a metal usually found in association with lead. It induced severe vomiting. Although drugs containing antimony are still used today, they are used in more enlightened pharmacology to treat diseases of tropical parasites, such as leishmaniasis and schistosomiasis. Additionally, Rollo proposed the use of blisters, particularly if delirium was present, and the use of ipecacuanha, which was a root discovered in Brazil and used as an emetic/purgative/diaphoretic for the treatment of fevers. All in all, his patients were in for a torrid time. If they survived the disease, they also had to survive a vigorous regime of induced vomiting, urination and defecation, not to omit bloodletting. Apart from this survey of the medical literature of the seventeenth and eighteenth centuries, we will now focus on an overview of some contemporary sources that will also help guide our investigation.

Sampling a More Recent Historiography

Thus far, we have focused on historiography more contemporaneous with the period covering our investigation. Following the suggestions of reviewers of this manuscript, our attention is directed to a few modern sources that have engaged with the history of yellow fever in the Caribbean and in the Americas. These sources are of relatively recent publication and are recommended to anyone studying epidemic diseases in the eighteenth- and nineteenth-century Caribbean. Our first source is *Medicalizing Blackness: Making Racial Difference in the Atlantic World, 1780–1840*, authored by Lana Hogarth. This manuscript is a fairly comprehensive study of questions of race in the healthcare history of the Atlantic world. Of particular interest to our investigation is Hogarth's examination of perceptions held by medical and non-medical officials of differences between enslaved and free Africans and the white colonial inhabitants. In her own words, we are informed that her study tells "how physicians in the English-speaking Greater Caribbean engaged in this process, not for the sake of justifying slavery but for their own intellectual, professional and pecuniary gain …."[17] In that context, Hogarth looks at how British military officials routinely recruited African enslaved militia on the basis that "Black people…were less susceptible to tropical fevers and thus more likely to survive military service in the region …." When blacks succumbed to the ravages of yellow fever, it surprised medical and military commentators, who then were forced to look for an explanation for this departure. Thus British physician James Clark, who was serving on the island of Dominica in the 1790s, is cited as observing that "new negroes who had lately been imported from the coast of Africa, fell ill with fever, while those who had been acclimatized, escaped". As Hogarth notes, "For Clark, immunity was not an innate trait but acquired through being adapted to a new climate." As a capstone to Clark's assumption, Hogarth further notes that when British military physicians stationed in Barbados were confronted with scores of black troops falling ill to yellow fever, they looked to local factors to explain this departure. As we have already noted, some enslaved arrivals may have already acquired some immunity through an early encounter with yellow fever in Africa, and it is clear from the available data that blacks had lower mortality rates than whites. In any case, Hogarth's study represents an essential contribution to the historiography of yellow fever epidemics in the Americas. Another valuable resource for studying epidemics, including yellow fever, in the anglophone New

World, is Erica Charters's work *Disease, War, and the Imperial State: The Welfare of the British Armed Forces During the Seven Years' War*.

As in the case of Hogarth's study, when it came to the question of mortality profiles, Charters observes that yellow fever "fatally struck only large groups of newcomers ...." One of the key contributions of Charters's investigation is her analysis of the medical philosophies held by British military practitioners in the eighteenth century. Of particular interest are the views held by such practitioners on the contribution of the social habits of yellow fever sufferers. Thus, we note Charters's citation of Dr James Lind's eighteenth-century publication "An Essay on Disease Incidental to Europeans in Hot Climates".[18] Lind had observed that the key approach to health care in such circumstances was the avoidance of hard labour, especially in the sun, abstinence from spirits and debauchery. Some military leaders' views were also noted. Charters cites a British captain, Richard Gardiner, who pointed to a lack of acclimatization as a primary factor in attacks of fever. Other British military leaders, probably following the lead of James Lind, attributed the cause of many of the debilitating illnesses that afflicted the troops as being largely due "to excessive drinking and indiscipline".[19] Given the prevailing views held by military leaders, generally in line with the prevailing opinions held by medical practitioners, it is not surprising that as "the British campaigns of 1759 and 1762 demonstrate, [military tactics and strategy] ... consisted of trying to batter defensive forces before disease incapacitated too many unseasoned troops".[20] Again, we find useful commentary on the British military and medical approaches to the scourge of yellow fever in this source.

Another significant study of yellow fever outbreaks in the late eighteenth century is Billy G. Smith's *Ship of Death: A Voyage that Changed the Atlantic World*. This book provides a compelling account of a yellow fever epidemic that traced the path of the *Hankey*, a ship whose voyages across the Atlantic between 1792 and 1793 played a pivotal role in spreading the disease.

As Smith informs us, "The *Hankey* crisscrossed the Atlantic for six months, disgorging sick passengers and infected mosquitoes wherever it went...[the] result was a pandemic that killed hundreds of thousands of people around the Atlantic Ocean ... the ship of death's terrible endowment returned annually for the two decades following its 1792–93 voyages ...."[21] Quite apart from the general chronicling of the *Hankey's* voyages, Smith also tracks these voyages to specific destinations. Thus, the voyage of the ship to Barbados, then to St Vincent and later to Grenada, began on 14 February 1793. At each stop, outbreaks of yellow fever followed. In Grenada, the impact on the port town at St George's was particularly troubling. Smith cites Dr John Chisholm, a medical practitioner attached to the British military command in Grenada, who blamed the visit of the *Hankey* for the calamity that ensued: "[the visit of the *Hankey* led to] the commencement of a disease before, I believe, unknown in this country, and certainly unequalled in its destructive nature ...."[22] As in the case of the other sources cited in this section of my manuscript, Smith's narrative offers important first-person commentary on the ravages of yellow fever in the late eighteenth and into the nineteenth centuries.

Another source, Frank M. Snowden's *Epidemics and Society: From the Black Death to the Present* offers a comprehensive overview of epidemic diseases ranging from the Black Death or plague that ravaged several European and Asian countries from the fifteenth into the sixteenth and seventeenth centuries to the outbreak of yellow fever epidemics in the New World from the seventeenth to the nineteenth centuries. In the case of yellow fever, Snowden offers a more up-to-date medical history than the other sources identified here. Thus, for example, he notes that in areas where dengue fever was endemic, persons contracting this fever might have acquired some "crossover" immunity, informing us that "This is because dengue fever virus is a member of the same *Flavivirus* genus as the yellow fever virus". Of particular interest is his account of matters related to the Revolution in St Domingue (later Haiti), in which it appears that leaders of the Afro-Haitian forces were aware of the susceptibility of recently arrived Europeans to the yellow fever virus. Thus, he records of the revolutionary leader, Toussaint L'Ouverture, that the latter "knew full well that newly arrived Europeans perished of yellow fever every summer, while black men and women remained stubbornly healthy ...."[23] The fact that L'Ouverture was aware of the implications of the mortality profiles of the various racial groups for military strategy in the war is captured in Smith's citation of a recent study that argues "L'Ouverture had an awareness of when and where the fever would strike his European enemies. He knew that by manoeuvring the whites into the ports and lowlands during the rainy season, they would die in droves ...."

In that context, in a letter from L'Ouverture to Dessalines, one of his commanders, reads thus: "Do not forget that while waiting for the rainy season, which will rid us of our enemies, we have only destruction and fire as our weapons ...."[24] The commentary on L'Ouverture is unique in that while multiple sources on the Haitian Revolution have noted the effect of yellow fever on the French Army, few have credited knowledge of the mortality differentials between the locals and the newly arrived troops as a major part of the combat strategy of the Afro-Haitian revolutionaries. The extent of yellow fever ravages among the French forces is captured in Smith's citation of yet another source that we will comment on in this study. In citing the work of John R. McNeill, *Mosquito Empires, Ecology and War in the Greater Caribbean, 1620–1914*, Smith records him as saying: "... Napoleon despatched sixty-five thousand troops in successive waves to suppress the revolt in Saint Domingue. Of these, fifty thousand to fifty-five thousand died, with thirty-five thousand to forty-five thousand of those deaths caused by yellow fever ...."[25] We now turn to further consideration of McNeill's contribution to our summary of sources.

In McNeill's investigation of yellow fever in the Greater Caribbean, he takes some time to consider the prevailing medical therapies. He observes that "those most likely to suffer from yellow fever and malaria, newly arrived Europeans, were likely to get what medical attention they received from European doctors, usually to their misfortune. The least fortunate among fever victims avoided doctors altogether and found themselves in the care of local women, often Afro-Caribbean women, who provided basic nursing ...."[26] As we will see in the body of our manuscript, the doctors who are the focus of this study generally fit into the profile presented by McNeill.

Indeed, he asserts that the dismal record of medicine deployed to fight yellow fever and malaria has allowed these two diseases to achieve geopolitical importance in the region for over 250 years. It is not surprising that, in many cases, sufferers of yellow fever considered the medical treatment provided by military doctors a precursor to certain death. Thus, we take note of McNeill's citation of John Grant of the Black Watch Regiment, who wrote that the Royal Navy surgeons "bled us profusely [and] would have killed us, but luckily other ships were order'd and we were saved".[27] McNeill was clear that the prevailing medical views meant that doctors often tried to restore what they felt was an imbalance in the body of patients who had to be treated by such means as venesection. Moreover, some doctors considered some sufferers from yellow fever as having weak constitutions and, in some cases, being predisposed by "excited passions" and an "excess of the pleasures of Venus".[28] The prescribing of deadly medicines often countered such predispositions. Thus, as McNeill observes, "For a few decades, roughly, 1790–1830, British army doctors in the West Indies prescribed mercury for yellow fever … before concluding that bleeding alone yielded better results …."[29] As our focus shifts to considering the reports of the several military doctors in the various chapters of this study, many observations based on our sources will be found to be reflected in those reports. Before we turn our attention thereto, we might note one gem from McNeill's account that refers to the perception held by some among the Afro-Caribbean population about the susceptibility of their newly arrived European enslavers to yellow fever. This gem consists of a little ditty sung by Jamaica Blacks in taunting such arrivants. They are recorded as singing:

New[Comer] buckra
He Get Sick
He tak fever
He be die
He be die[30]

The foregoing discussion has identified some issues involved in the development of medical treatment as they relate to the yellow fever epidemics that swept the Caribbean throughout the seventeenth century and into the eighteenth century. Our attention now turns to the development of a military medical arm of the British Army and

Navy. Such an examination prepares us for a consideration of the work of British military doctors, as found in the transcribed reports that are the main subject of our investigations.

The British Military and Its Doctors

The formation of specialized medical units in the British Army and Navy dates to the restoration of Charles II in 1660. As early as 1673, each cavalry and infantry regiment was supplied with a chirurgeon (surgeon), and, as we are informed by Peterkin,[31] by 1684, each infantry regiment had a surgeon's mate as well as a surgeon. Even before the expansion of the British military into the Caribbean, British doctors had encountered various fevers, which were "divided clinically into intermittent, remittent, and continuous fevers". Thus, we would expect that some medical officers who had to deal with the administration of health care in the Caribbean theatre would have arrived in the region with some pre-set notions on the medical regime to be followed.

Roger Buckley's comprehensive study of the British Army and Navy in the West Indies traces the effect of a revolution in medicine which took place during the eighteenth century. He notes that during this time, "modern" hospital techniques began to emerge, built upon an "emphasis on observation and dissection, medical statistics, autopsy reports, pathological drawings, clinical experimentation, all of which shaped a new medical literature".[32] Simultaneous with these developments, there were new developments in the administration of military medicine. These latest developments included regular medical examinations of troops, special attention to their housing and regulations governing the operation and staffing of military hospitals. However, these developments would require some time for gestation, particularly in the case of the recruitment of medical practitioners. Over time, regulations governing the recruitment of doctors would emphasize formal medical training. Still, as we shall see in the following discussions, there was a general practice that continued throughout the eighteenth century which postponed the development of a well-trained cadre of doctors with experience in tropical medicine.

On 10 August 1738, Admiral Cavendish of the British Navy wrote to the commissioners of the Navy requesting leave to appoint a surgeon to the sloop the *Hound*. He wrote:

> Gentlemen,
>
> I am told [that] the surgeon of the *Hound* Sloop has wrote (sic) for leave to quit his employment; I take the liberty of recommending to succeed him, Mr Swan Morring, who served Doctor Swan of this town (Portsmouth) eight years, and has the character of a very able man. He is at present surgeon's mate of the *Pembroke*, [captained by] Captain Lee, and he has been on two voyages to Newfoundland with him, and has passed an examination for surgeon of a sixth rate. I ask pardon for troubling you on this account, and I am
>
> Gentlemen,
> Your most humble servant
> C. Cavendish[33]

It does not seem Cavendish's initiative paid off, for on 31 August of that same year, he wrote to the commissioners:

> The *Spry* Sloop, wanting a surgeon so long, makes me think [that] you have not many to dispose of, so [I] shall take the liberty once more, to recommend Mr Swan Morring for that sloop, in whose behalf I wrote to you the 10th Instant.[34]

In these two extracts, several issues are centrally focused. In the first case, there was a shortage of qualified medical practitioners to meet the needs of the navy and army. Secondly, the process of identifying a suitable recruit for medical service was less dependent on formal medical accreditation than on the recommendations of well-placed benefactors. Thirdly, extensive overseas experience was not required to obtain a placement in medical military service. In our further discussion, we look more closely at the second point.

On 1 November 1739, Henry Huntley, a surgeon appointed to the navy, but apparently on the verge of retirement, wrote an affidavit thus:

> The first day of November 1739, pursuant to an order from the Honourable Commissioners of His Majesty's Navy, directed to R. Hughes, Commissioner of His Majesty's Dock at Portsmouth, I Henry Huntley, late surgeon of His Majesty's ship ye *Elenor* do

Introductory Comments on the Scourge of Yellow Fever

> agree that Robert Cochran late surgeon's mate of ye *Buckingham*, shall have my medicine chest and instruments, making such reasonable deduction for ye prime cost as any surgeons in ye fleet shall think proper.
>
> Witnessed by our hands
> Henry Huntley
> Robt. Cochran[35]

In this latter document, some insights are offered into the way medical practitioners were recruited for military service. All that was required was for an individual, with or without formal training in medicine, to apprentice himself to a physician or surgeon. Once the period of apprenticeship was served (there was no formal specification of the length of service, although there may have been some common understandings on the point), the surgeon's mate, sometimes styled a hospital mate, acquired a medicine chest and doctor's equipment and armed with the requisite recommendation, reported for service. Yet another extract expands this picture. On 30 May 1738, Captain James Cornwall wrote a letter from the ship *Greenwich*, anchored at Bridgetown, Barbados, addressed to the "Honourable Principal Officers and Commissioners of His Majesty's Navy, at the Navy Office in London":

> Honourable Gentlemen,
>
> The surgeon of His Majesty's sloop *Spence*, dying in January last, I appointed Mr George Owen to succeed him. Soon after, Mr Alex Cuming, surgeon of the *Greenwich*, dying likewise, I appointed Mr Owen to succeed him in this ship; I have ordered Mr Thomas Fortescue, my surgeon's first mate at that time, into the *Spence*....[36]

The shortage of medical officers and the lack of formal procedures for accrediting medical practitioners in the military service meant that the standards of recruitment were low at the least and probably cavalier at best. The extracts above clearly identify a practice which appeared to leave any consultation with professionals out of the picture. It also meant that standards of medical treatment were likely to be seriously compromised. These issues are highlighted by Peterkin and Johnson, who note that:

> The supply of medical officers often fell far short of demand, especially in wartime. Before the formation of the standing Army, when this occurred, the Company of Barber Surgeons was usually asked to supply the surgeon required, and there were occasions on which surgeons for the Army were very low; in early times, they were often apprentices of the surgeon. Surgeons were usually promoted from the ranks of surgeons' mates.[37]

Cantlie's research on the development of an army medical department corroborates this general assessment of the status of the medical service during the eighteenth century. He observes that the pay of a surgeon, at four shillings per day (£73 per annum) was so low that few doctors would think of taking up a commission in the army, especially when a doctor in civil practice might earn four times as much.[38] Entry into the army or naval medical services was either by means of the purchase of a commission or by way of the appointments we discussed earlier. During peacetime, the opportunities for promotion were limited. However, as Cantlie observes further, the growth of the empire led to the expansion of opportunities for surgeons and physicians in the West Indies and in the Mediterranean.

For the surgeon's mate or regimental mate, however, the pay remained low, about half that of the surgeon, which, in his words, meant that "they were inevitably of poor quality, even in peacetime". Indeed, according to one source cited by Cantlie, the demand for medical recruits was so high and the supply so low that some were recruited "after the briefest training … without ever having been to a medical school or heard a single lecture".[39] Indeed, one private soldier, "after assisting the surgeon to spread plaster in the capacity of an orderly man, was appointed regimental mate".[40] While that was bad enough, we need to remember that in many cases, the mates did most of the backbreaking medical work, while the surgeon got the praise for any success. The mate might even be the scapegoat when things went wrong, as they often did.

This, then, is the background against which many medical officers who served in the Caribbean were recruited. However, late in the eighteenth and into the early nineteenth century, a number of reforms took place, which were to improve the calibre of the medical staff.

Under the appointment of John Hunter as surgeon general in the 1790s, doctors were appointed under professional control. Hunter's view was that no man "but a professional man is judge of professional merit, and even few of them ...."[41] Hospital service was also required for the appointment of regimental and naval surgeons. Hospital service brought mates under the supervision of physicians and surgeons, whose recommendation was then required for an appointment to take effect. In addition, the rank of staff surgeon was introduced in hospitals to provide another layer of promotion at higher pay. To improve the quality of medical staff, those who purchased commissions were required to be university graduates or to be at least licentiates of the College of Surgeons in London. Additionally, a candidate was required to pass an examination at the college in the presence of the surgeon general. Even with these improvements, there would still be some practitioners of the old variety for some time in the military services.

When Sir Lucas Pepys was appointed physician-general in London sometime in 1804, even more important changes took place. There was a general notion that physicians were superior to surgeons – a notion based on the superior education of the former. On his appointment, Pepys insisted that to be considered for promotion, any medical officer had to be a graduate of Oxford or Cambridge. Moreover, a candidate had to be a licentiate, member, or fellow of the College of Physicians in London. Clearly, he intended to improve the quality of the medical staff. However, in practice, Pepys's policies meant that any university graduate in Ireland or Scotland had little chance of appointment or promotion. In this context, young physician graduates without any experience in the treatment of tropical diseases were often put in charge of military hospitals in the Caribbean and other areas, superintending surgeons who, by way of postings overseas, were several years ahead in experience. Later, faced with several conflicts in the service, Pepys modified this, and officers who held MD degrees from universities other than Oxford and Cambridge were appointed. Even so, the medical board expressed its concern that from many of the Scottish medical schools, "a degree [could] be sent for by the stagecoach on paying eleven pounds".[42]

The new improvements were also reflected in structural changes. Several grades were introduced in the military service over the period 1784–1818. In 1797, the term "surgeon's mate" was abandoned in favour of "assistant surgeon". In 1801, the new grades were, in hierarchical order, surgeon general, senior surgeon, surgeon, senior assistant surgeon and assistant surgeon. Later, in 1804, these grades were again modified, and Royal Warrant substituted the following order:

- surgeon general and inspector
- assistant surgeon general and deputy inspector
- surgeon
- assistant surgeon.

By a further Royal Warrant of 1812, the grade of inspector general was placed above that of surgeon general and inspector.[43] As we will note, these structural changes represented a greater specialization in the military medical services, some rationalization of the various medical posts and some recognition of the need for formal training.

It is at this juncture of change that we are enabled to comment on our transcripts of a number of medical reports, which assist in illustrating medical practice in the Caribbean and in assessing the status of medical training and philosophy, especially with respect to the treatment of yellow fever. The earliest of these reports date back to the late eighteenth century. The reports apparently stem from a requirement for full documentation of medical histories on the part of the doctors assigned to various ships in the Royal Navy and, in some cases, a detailing of their experiences in the various colonies where the troops were placed. The reports are detailed in several files held by the National Archives in the United Kingdom, most of which have been transcribed by the author and carefully annotated as the relevant data permit. The author came across the reports in the National Archives in Kew over twenty years ago and, after several years of on-and-off-again attention to this find, has now managed to finalize the research and to prepare it for presentation to a discerning public.

British Military Doctors in the Treatment of Yellow Fever in the Caribbean

The reports that are presented in our investigation reveal a medical practice which had not moved much beyond the practice of an earlier age. In some of the cases that we shall see, the use of purges, calomel and croton oil laxatives suggests that, like their earlier counterparts, the military doctors in the Caribbean were still victims of earlier assumptions about the nature of the disease. In discussing the effects of fever, doctors were still thinking in terms of a "phlogistic"[44] theory and their treatments were thus, geared in that direction. In other cases, the references to bleeding and the use of mercury tell a similar story. Here, also, of major interest to the medical reporter is represented a commentary on the apparent relative immunity of the Black troops. We will also see the summary information on health matters for several Caribbean territories reported. What all of these have in common is that they do represent, over time, a greater emphasis on observation and statistical recording, consistent with the new medical emphases that were coming into vogue in the nineteenth century. These were promising developments in the history of medicine in the tropics. Clearly, the path of detailing minutely the diagnoses of illness, the treatment of patients and the various physical conditions under which patients were living were important advances in the knowledge of tropical medicine. The problem was that up to that point, many doctors were still their patients' worst enemy. It would be almost another century before the old ideas of treatment would disappear. The title adopted for this publication is itself based on a musing by one of the doctors surveyed, who conjectured that the cause of an outbreak of yellow fever in Barbados might well have been the presence of some Black troops whose perspiration was deemed to be particularly offensive.

The foregoing observations provide an ample base upon which we shall consider the various reports of many doctors in the British Army and Navy, as they struggled to deal with the challenge of yellow fever and, for that matter, other ailments. The transcriptions of the various reports follow, chapter by chapter. Only in a few cases is any attempt made to introduce modern spelling. Additionally, medical terms, some of which are archaic or obscure, require some annotation to make it easier for contemporary historians and medical researchers to understand their meaning. However, the author does not presume that all readers will require that kind of assistance and, thus, in many cases, some of the terms used, some in Latin or a medical jargon of older vintage, are left without comment. The first transcribed report which follows is a singular one, not contained in the same file as the body of colony reports from which the bulk of the transcriptions are lifted. This first report is that of a doctor serving in the Royal Navy in the Jamaican sphere of operations.

2. Considering a Miscellaneous Report[1]

Preview: In this first transcription of a military doctor's report on his experiences in the Caribbean theatre in the 1790s, we may note that this is not recorded in the same archival file as the other doctors' reports that will follow. Like the initial document transcribed in chapter 2, these reports were filed with the British military authorities and are now housed in the National Archives in Kew, London. Those later documents are filed under the call number WO 334/165, under the description: "Returns and reports concerning yellow fever; Report on Yellow Fever: Barbados, Antigua, Demerara, Berbice, Dominica, Grenada, Monserrat, St Kitts, St Lucia, St Vincent, Tobago, and Trinidad (1818 Dec–1840 Apr.)". It is possible that the first transcript, which is presented here separately, is listed under the call number AMD 101/83/3 and is not included in the reports of WO 334/165 because the doctor, Dr Warner, who is issuing this report, is commanded under the Jamaica area of operations, and as we will note, Jamaica is not listed in the WO 334/165 compilation. Warner's report deals primarily with yellow fever on the ship, the *Alfred,* to which he was assigned.

3rd and 4th Rates
Journal of His Majesty's Ship *Alfred*
W. J. Warner Surgeon
1 October 1797
31 March 1798
ADM 101/83/3

A narrative with remarks on the malignant fever, commonly though erroneously styled the yellow fever, which appeared on board His Majesty's Ship *Alfred* at Port Royal Jamaica in July 1796 and continued until the end of October following. This disorder having occasioned much fatality and produced a variety of opinions of the nature and treatment of it. I have endeavoured with some pains to obtain an idea of both, from my observations, aided by those of many practitioners with whom I have conferred on the subject. The following remarks are the best my judgement and ability enable me to offer.

The disorder appeared first at Jamaica in 1794, being introduced at Port Royal by the arrival of His Majesty's Ship *Pontrefid* and was occasioned to number her receiving on board a number of persons, in a sickly state, who had long been confined in prison at the Aux Cayes, a port belonging to the French in Saint Domingo. It is generally allowed to be new in the country and is considered by most practitioners a species of Typhus.

The symptoms as they appeared on board the *Alfred* at the worst period, were prostration of strength, heavy, sometimes acute pain of the forehead, a severe pain of the loins, joints, and extremities, a glazy appearance of with a bloody suffusion of the eye, nausea, or vomiting of bilious, sometimes offensive black matter, not unlike coffee grounds, often attended with evacuations by stool of the same kind, the stomach rejecting everything offered, the countenance flushed, at other times, pale and dejected with oppressive cold sweating, bleeding at the nostrils; the pulse sometimes for a short period full and quick, but more frequently languid, great thirst, the tongue white and brown at the edges, frequently covered by a white shiny matter, and as the fever advanced, became dry, brown and crusted, a fatal appearance in general, but particularly so, when attended with frequent flushing and loose stools; sometimes towards the close of the disease, a small red rash appears under the skin, and soon disappeared, having livid spots, where it has shown itself, and was always a fatal sign. In the treatment of this disease, various modes were tried, all of which I am to say proved ineffectual in very many instances. I, in speaking of them, will first mention Calomel, giving it in frequent doses to a considerable extent with a view to produce salivation, with respect to its use. I was not bold enough to give it the trial recommended.

My orders from Captain Drury were to send every person the moment of complaining on shore, and in consequence, many were sent daily to the Naval Hospital at Port Royal, where the use of Calomel[2] was made in fashion, and from its effect on those sent there, I am of the opinion it is an uncertain remedy, and in many instances is to be considered a hurtful one, as of more than two hundred persons sent from the *Alfred*, not a third part survived the third day. The same fate attended those sent from other ships. It is true that a few returned to the ship after undergoing the trial, and I am induced to think their recovery did not proceed so much from the effect of the medicine, as being favoured with a constitution capable of coping with disease, as also [to] withstand the effect of so active a medicine.

I am the more induced to favour this opinion, having observed nature do much often when assisted by our simpler methods, several of which cases I intend mentioning. And [I] am happy this is not a solitary idea, as many of the oldest and most respectable practitioners of Jamaica, Saint Domingo, Martinique, and other islands are of the same opinion relative to its effect and use. It was tried sometime at the Naval and Military Hospitals of Mole St Nicolas and abandoned from the little satisfaction the practice offered. In many cases, the symptoms were such at the time of using it, as did not afford expectation [that] the unfortunate patient could possibly live, unless assisted by other methods, half the time necessary for the absorption of the medicine to produce the desired effect, and death frequently ensued after the mouth became affected after want of retention by the stomach did not allow the medicine to remain in it and where it may [be] retained, it was frequently discovered on inspection after death in nearly the quantity taken ... in the stomach. The idea of those favouring the practice was, the disease being Typhus, they recommended the necessity of healing all the afflicted alike, whether attended with similar malignant symptoms and to use it in all stages of the disorder, and [I] have known it to be administered where apparent dissolution was evident, and further cannot help thinking the use of it frequently hastened, and sometimes produced death, as some cases occurred where a favourable turn appeared, in which the trial of it seemingly removed the prospect of recovery. Indeed, it may be asserted with much truth that those said to be cured by it generally returned to the ship exceedingly emaciated, so as to be unfit for duty for many months; in some, the faculties were impaired, others laboured under great nervous irritability or obstinate incurable dysentery where it was plain the tone of the Viscera was wholly destroyed or materially affected, in some cases the fever relapsed and was cured on board, or the patient returned to the hospital.

I am informed [that] some gentlemen on their arrival in the country were advised to take ten or twelve grains of Calomel weekly in small doses by way of preventive; the information I had from Captain Clark of the 5th West India Regiment, who dining on board about the time the fever was on the decline in the ship, informed us he was one of two persons then surviving of thirteen who had used this practice; at the time of mentioning it seemed happy in the idea of being seasoned to the climate. But lo! As all things are precarious in this life, he sickened the following day and fell a victim to the disease on the third.

I deem it unnecessary to touch on the properties of Calomel, the various effects it is apt to produce in different constitutions, as the gentlemen who may peruse these remarks are acquainted with them, and I hope will think with me that the use of it as recommended, improper in every state and stage of a disorder of the nature described. These are all my remarks on the use of Calomel and [I] come to speak on the other methods I tried or heard of.

Strong Spruce Beer has been recommended and spoken of as a specific in the disorder; [I] never tried it alone, but from information collected from gentlemen who did, [I] am induced to consider it does not deserve the character some have given it, and am of opinion it is a remedy which ought not to be solely depended on; in thirteen cases where tried onboard the *Dictator* at one time, ten died and after a trial was made of its virtue at the Hospital of Mole St Nicolas, without affording a satisfactory effect.

Emetics are condemned by many; the antimonial class with much propriety, the operation proving too violent so as to cause excessive debility. [I] have frequently administered inordinate doses of Ipecacuahana (sic)[3] on the first appearance of the complaint, sometimes when puking had commenced and am not dissatisfied with the practice, having frequently found it beneficial, prescribing the common saline mixture after it, which often removed the irritability of the stomach; where it failed, succeeded sometimes by prescribing the saline mixture in an effervescent state. Water moderately acidulated with cream of tartar, joining eight or ten drops of *Tinct Opii*,[4] taking a dose once in two or three hours often afforded much satisfaction, in quitting the stomach, which is sometimes so agitated as to reject the most simple drinks offered, and was frequently salutary where diarrhoea accompanied the vomiting. [Taking] ten grains of Salt of Tartar in two ounces of water either alone or with similar doses of *Tinct. Opii*[5] often produced pleasing effect when the stomach evacuated acrid or bilious matter and when violent griping with loose stools prevailed.

With respect to the use of bark, [I] seldom found the stomach capable of retaining it during the height of the fever, and when capable of retention, was seldom able to give it in any other form than an infusion; a few cases excepted when the stomach was not affected, in which I experienced much benefit from it. Some of these cases I have mentioned.

Bleeding is recommended by some practitioners, and one time [I] was induced to think it a reasonable practice in the early stages of the disorder, but the symptoms of inflammation where (sic) so doubtful or of short duration that I was deterred from it, fearing the system might be suddenly lowered by it; and from the mucus attending it when tried, gave up the idea, considering it but an uncertain and perhaps dangerous experiment.

A navy surgeon of my acquaintance bled in three cases, which he thought favourable to the purpose. Extreme debility followed, and death soon, and [I] have many reports similar from other gentlemen.

Before I conclude my observations, [I] have to mention Dr James's Fever Powder,[6] given at the commencement of the disorder, though with great caution, as many cases occurred where appearances did not justify trying it (such as were attended with great debility). The cases in which I found it useful where (sic) such as appeared the most inflammatory, and when the stomach was not agitated; to the use of it in such cases, I feel myself much indebted for some recoverys (sic), always using it in small doses, having sometimes found five grains too powerful in the operations, and seldom prescribed a second dose what (sic) (once) that quantity had been taken. My general plan was to direct a pill of three grains at first, repeating it four hours after, according to Calomel, to circumstances when it often produced salutary effect in promoting moderate vomiting, evacuation by stool, and generally occasioned moderate perspiration; without lowering the system considerably (a circumstance to be carefully avoided), as in many cases, where the fever with all the alarming symptoms (save debility) have disappeared, convulsions and delirium came on, and death followed in an hour or less; and in most instances, these alarming symptoms did not shew themselves untill (sic) a short time preceding death. In the common fever of the country, [I] often found it a desirable remedy, prescribing it in a similar way ... In cases where the head was principally affected, attended with palpitations, and great dejection of the spirits, [I] found Camphor[7] a valuable medicine, joining it with the common saline medicine, but these were such as where the stomach was not affected, some cases of which I shall mention.

In cases where it appeared necessary to procure stools, generally found two or three grains Calomel combined with Castile Soap[8] and Rhubarb answer the purposes in a satisfactory manner.

The opinion of Dr Allenby, the most eminent practitioner of St Pierre Martinique who has observed the fever since the first appearance in the Leeward Islands, is to evacuate the intestines the moment of attack, using at the same time the *Mist. Salin*,[9] or any other calculated to act easy on the stomach, and promote moderate perspiration, and says if these effects take place early, in most instances, the event will be fortunate. He thinks the complaint proceeds from redundancy of bile, or undigested matter, which, if not evacuated soon, becomes vitiated and produces the direful symptoms mentioned; he observes it is a fever, very different to ague which used to be peculiar in the country, and agrees with me that terming it generally the yellow fever is improper, as he scarcely was met with it since his residence in the West Indies; of the number of cases which came under my inspection [I] did not see more than two or three, where the Complection (sic) of the skin before death could justify the appellation; sometimes a jaundiced ting (sic) appeared on the patients becoming convalescent,

Considering a Miscellaneous Report

and was thought a favourable criterion. Dr Young,[10] inspector of general of Army Hospitals at Martinique, with Mr Gillespie,[11] surgeon of the Naval Hospital, are of this opinion and, I believe, most of the faculty who have seen much of the disorder. Dr Young highly disapproves of using Calomel[12] in the manner beforementioned, as also of combining it with Jalap, giving frequent doses so as to act copiously and repeatedly on the Bowells (sic), and at the same time operate to affect the mouth, agreeable to the mode favoured by Dr Chisholm,[13] which I am fearful has too often been a very unfortunate trial for the afflicted. From my own practice, [I] am convinced [that] an indiscriminate adherence to any method of treatment must in many instances fail, whereas by consulting the most leading practitioners, and adopting medicines calculated to remove the most obstinate or relieve where nature seems much depressed, will in great many instances end favourably if resorted to early.

Having experienced a pretty severe attack of fever, [I] feel myself the more enabled to speak on the subject, which I will relate concisely; the leading symptoms, a heavy pain of the forehead and eyes, considerable pain of the loins and extremities, thirst, tension with uneasiness of the abdomen (a common symptom) (which I omitted mentioning in the beginning) a depressed pulse, and sense of nausea; considering it necessary to produce stools, and knowing that my bowells (sic) were very easily moved, fearing a rough medicine would derange too much, the medicine I thought of, as most proper under these considerations was Rhubarb *puls gr* x Calomel (*fr Japon Venet fr* made into two pills), they soon operated, occasioning five or six stools of a loose and offensive smell, the day following felt myself much relieved, on the third day debility came on, which can be only described by the sufferer, accompanied by profuse perspiration, difficulty of respiration, faultering (sic) of the voice, sudden and frequent dizziness, with palpitation of the heart; for three days I laboured under these alarming symptoms which were a great deal increased by excessive sultry weather occasioned by a south-west wind prevailing and is always unhealthy at Mole St Nicolas, the natives being much affected by it. Good Madeira was the remedy. I resorted to taking a glass when most affected and was much relieved by it; my common drink was an infusion of Tamarinds with a small wine glass of brandy to a quart; on the eighth day, I began to fancy food, and regain strength in a small degree, which was never wholly restored while in the country.

The *Alfred*, on her arrival at Port Royal in the middle of July 1796, had not more than a dozen men in the sick list, convalescents in dysentery or less trifling complaints. The fever appeared on board in less than a week after, and [I] cannot help thinking it was occasioned in some measure by the people being much harassed in clearing a *Prize* on board of which were thirty persons confined to bed, others were at the same time employed to fit out the *Malabar* newly arrived from St Nicolas, where she buried most of her officers and crew of a malignant fever, supposed by Dr Weir,[14] physician-general to the Army, there to have originated at Spikes Island near Cork, where the troops were quartered previous to the embarkation for the West Indies; many were attacked on board of her or immediately on returning to the *Alfred*.

The cases I have mentioned were attended by myself and came under my inspection at the time the disorder raged with the greatest violence, being such as appeared the most favourable and many as during the first six weeks of the disorder. The daily list excused fifty, inclusive of those sent to the hospitals and [I] have to lament the mortality was so frequent that many feared complaining on being taken ill, desiring to be sent on shore, and it is not unusual for them to hide away and were not (sic) discovered untill (sic) the disorder had sometimes made such advances, as to afford little hope of recovery. Such was daily the case notwithstanding my custom of going twice round the deck daily, and Mr Hendrick Frederick Schricht, my only mate at other times, to whom the service is much indebted for his indefatigable and humane attention to the sick at all times. The first mate died at the hospital about ten days after the complaint first appeared, and the *Alfred* left England with only two people.

We were free from the fever for three weeks previous to the *Alfred* sailing from Port Royal, when it was again introduced by receiving a large draft of raw hands from His Majesty's Ship *Adventure* just arrived, with Supernumeraries from England being sickly on her arrival at the same time, another draft was received on board, part of the *Undaunted*, Frigate's ship's crew, who had suffered much on the Morant Keys, where the ship had been recently wrecked. They consisted of near two hundred and were no sooner on board than the fever broke out among them and upward of a hundred and twenty sickened in the course of a fortnight, of which numbers died on the passage to Mole St Nicolas. Thirty of the worst were sent to the hospital on arrival there, the majority of whom were returned to the ship in tolerable health. Bathing the forehead with Vinegar and Camphor afforded much relief to the pain of the forehead, as also putting the legs in warm water as high as the knees. The natives are accustomed to rub the body with lime juice or vinegar in such complaints, and I am informed great benefits often arise from the practice.

After cases of the common fever of the country occurred in the months of November and December, all of which soon did well, giving way to an emetic, evacuations by stool, as James's Powder,[15] taking the common saline mixture a day or two, afterwards the Cortex, which sometimes disagreed, whenever *Infus; Quassia*[16] or some other stomachic tonic was prescribed. About forty cases of Malignant Fever occurred on board the *Alfred* in 1797, all of which did well, being treated as related according to the symptoms which attended the attack, one of which is particularly worthy of remark, being attended toward the termination of the disorder, with alarming haemorrhage from the nose, fortunately, the stomach was not too irritable.

Pulv Cort[17] was prescribed hourly with good effect, gradually checking the discharge, and apparently supported the system which was in a very low state; this was the only case which did not prove fatal when attended with that symptom. In speaking of this fever, [I] have mentioned its introduction in Jamaica, but as the disorder has not been confined to that Island but been general all over the West Indies, it is perhaps sufficient to ascertain the precise source, yet I think some probable means may be assigned why it was more general at particular times and places. At Mole St Nicolas, its effects were inconsiderable untill (sic) the arrival of a body of troops in May 1796, amounting to seven thousand men in the space of two months. These numbers were diminished nearly half, and on our arrival, then the latter end of September, the number of the garrison in and out of hospitals did not exceed thirteen hundred. This was the fever which raged on board the *Malabar* and every other ship which brought troops out at that time. Dr Weir, as I beforementioned, thinks the seeds of the disease were brought from Ireland but did not break out in great force until the said arrival; several died on board of her, the *Dictator*, *Abergavenny*, and other ships during the passage.

Such disorders have often prevailed among soldiers experiencing a change of climate, after a long confinement on board transports, inadequate to the convenience or comfort of such numbers, add[ed] to which the mode of living and diet of such people should be considered as predisposing them for the reception of such disorders.

These causes may, I think, be considered the grand foundation of the disorder becoming so general on the arrival, also in the Men of War employed as troops ships, and such as from necessity were obliged to have an intercourse with them. In 1797, this fever was more general at particular places, and I think from local causes. At Port Royal, Martinique, now Fort Edward, the garrison lost great numbers, while the troops in the town were healthier and quite so in the garrison of Fort Bourbon, also at Saint Pierre. At the Saints, where the *Alfred* lay during the Hurricane months, the disorder hardly showed itself, whereas at Prince Rupert's Bay Dominica, a few leagues to Leeward, the disorder was fatal to almost all who were attacked with it; the same was the case at Mount Bruce above the town of Roseau in the same Island. The unhealthiness of Port Edward, I think, may be ascribed to the following causes: The building is contiguous to the Bay on one side, is very old, and much caverned in the foundation. Behind the Carenage runs a confined piece of water, from which arises foul offensive vapour.[18] At Prince Ruperts, the barracks are on two eminencies called the Cabrites; a deep hollow separates them; here, the rain, which is frequent and heavy, drains down and occasions a damp lodgement from whence a thick and offensive fog arises which does not dissipate untill (sic) the Sun has acquired a considerable altitude, add[ed] to which on the land side are swamps with heigths (sic) and the back much covered with wood.

Mount Bruce is an eminence with a swampy plain between it and the town of Roseau and surrounded by sloping heigths (sic) much covered with wood. Places so situated, I believe, are always considered unhealthy. The native and people who have been any time resident in these places are very subject to obstinate agues which disorder is an endemic at Port Royal, Martinique, in the wet season.

W. Warner, Surgeon
His Majesty's Ship, Alfred

3. Reports from Antigua

Preview: While the report from Dr Warner is singular in that there are no other contributing reports, the reports that follow under the filings of yellow fever reports from Antigua and other colonies in the National Archives give us several viewpoints on the yellow fever outbreak, and also on its causes and treatment. Again, we point out that a value of these transcripts lies in the fact that there are few first-person narratives available to us in the quantity and quality that we see here. The following transcribed reports from Antigua cover the period between the 1820s and the 1840s. Eleven doctors, who were assigned to what was called the Windward and Leeward Islands Command, report on what has been happening in various regiments, troops and on some ships. Some of the reports also include references to happenings in other Caribbean locations. Notwithstanding the inclusion of material from other locations such as Barbados, Trinidad and British Guiana, the reports transcribed here are listed under the heading "Antigua", indicating that the reporters are under the control of a central command in Antigua.

Extract of Half-Yearly Report of the Detachment Hospital 35th Regiment Monks Hill from 21 June to 20 December 1821. Also Remarks on the Fever Which Prevailed among the Forces (Possibly Penned by Dr Tegart of Whom More Will Be Said Later)

I don't mean to say that causes for fever do not exist in swamps, ships, holds and so on. What I wish to inculcate is, that intemperance is the most common of all causes with the above description of people and that before we proceed to investigate other supposed ones; we ought to be thoroughly convinced that excitement from the use of spirits is not the cause, as will appear in the sequel. On the 2nd of last November, I was ordered on board His Majesty's Ship *Pyramus* to take charge of the medical duties, the assistant surgeon being dead and the surgeon non-effective from sickness and on shore. On my taking charge I found one severe case of fever viz a lieutenant of the Royal Marines. There being no medical man on board when he first took ill, [he] was not treated so actively as he would have been otherwise. The fever still continued. On the first attack, he had about twenty buckets of seawater dashed on him at his own request. Two hours afterwards, he had himself bled by a loblolly boy[1] (in the same capacity as a surgery man) but not to any extent; Bowels were opened by some of the *sulph: magnes* (magnesium sulphate). This gentleman was the most temperate man in the ship, in every respect. I saw him on the following morning about 10:00 (he complained on the night of the first). The fever was then slight, but evidently of the yellow type. In the course of the day, it increased considerably. I wished to have sent him to the Detachment General Hospital here, but he appeared averse to the measure. Staff Surgeon Hartle[2] also wished him to go on shore, but he would not hear of it.

With this solitary case of fever, we left English Harbour for Barbados on the evening of the same day. In this case, I was convinced that the fever was produced from other causes and not intemperance. We were eight days on our passage, and during this period, there occurred three more cases of a similar type. These were two midshipmen and a private of marines. One of the young gentlemen was very temperate. The other quite the reverse, and the marine a determined drunk; all of them however did well. The ship anchored in Carlisle Bay on 9 November, and the same evening I landed them together with the lieutenant of marines in a convalescent state and conveyed them to the Naval Hospital by the desire of Mr Tegart,[3] inspector of hospitals, who also requested that I would send every case of fever on shore as soon as possible, should any more occur.

• • •

I continued doing duty on board of the *Pyramus* for three weeks after our arrival; and during the time, I sent from four to seven patients on shore every evening. This rapid increase of fever now became rather alarming. From a wish to find out the cause, if possible, Mr Tegart came on board and examined every part of the ship. The crew were mustered, all of whom appeared clean and healthy. The ship throughout was in the highest order. As to the arrangements respecting the men's comforts, duties and etc; nothing could be better; indeed, from the observations I had an opportunity of making during the time I was attached to the ship, it appeared to me that the captain and officers endeavoured to study the comforts of the crew more than they did of their own. On the very day Mr Tegart had visited the ship, twelve cases of fever were reported after dinner. They were all attacked very suddenly with a giddiness followed by violent pain in the head and became delirious in the course of five minutes. This staggered everyone, and a board of medical officers was ordered to assemble the day following in order to investigate the cause. Subjoined is a report of their proceedings after a minute examination into the economy of the Frigate.

It is a singular fact that not 1 man recovered who had the slightest taints of *Scrophula*[4] in the constitution. In such cases, the stomach was disorganized very rapidly, and the black vomit came on sooner than it usually does. Mercury had no effect upon the system whatever. Ten grains of Calomel given every half hour for nearly two days scarcely moved the bowels.

Barbados 23 November 1821
Proceedings of a Board of Medical Officers held in consequence of the following department orders.

Department Orders Barbados 23 November 1821
A board of medical officers consisting of Dr Menzies,[5] dept. inspector hospitals; Dr Bone,[6] physician to the forces and Mr Elliott, surgeon to the forces, will this day at 11:00 a.m. proceed on board HM Ship *Pyramus* to examine into the state of that ship and investigate the probable cause of the sickness which prevails on board. The board will also report upon what may appear to them the most likely means of checking the progress of the disease or removing the cause of it.

Signed
Edwd. Tegart
Inspector of Hospitals

In conformity to this order the board proceeded on board the *Pyramus* at 11:00 a.m. and having examined minutely into the state of the ship, finds that she is an old vessel lately completely repaired and injected with coal tar. She is a very tight vessel. The coal tar being rendered fluid by the heat of the climate oozes from the captain's cabin beams, and from every part of the ship, particularly from the hold where the heat is greater.[7] The coal tar mixing in the hold with the bilge water produces a very offensive effluvia (sic), particularly aggravated by the admixture with fresh water, escaping during the operation of pumping the water thro' canvas hose, from the iron tanks to the cistern. The ship was clean and in good order, but the atmosphere of the Orlop Deck[8] and Hold was close, oppressively hot; and the smell of the bilge water and coat tar was very perceptible. On pumping the ship, the bilge water was black and smelled of coal tar and offensively. The board finds that the *Pyramus* arrived at Barbados on 25 July last since which she has been at different times thirty-four days in English Harbour. She was lately there from the 11 to 19 October. Then left for St Kitts on 31 October where she remained seven days, returned on 1 November to Antigua, where she landed her sick and then proceeded to Barbados, where she arrived on the 9th inst.

The sickness recommenced at English Harbour and subsequently considerably increased on the departure of the vessel from St Kitts. With respect to the predisposing causes of the disease at present prevailing in the vessel, the board are inclined to attribute something to the stay in English Harbour. The continuance of the disease the board attribute to the state of the vessel as described, and to her lying with her head to the wind, and also to the season of the year, and to the description of the crew being all newcomers, and to the great alarm that exists among them, the impression on board appears to be general. That much is also to be attributed to the coal tar oozing from the vessel and mixing with the bilge water, but the board has not sufficient data to be able to determine how far that cause operates.

With respect to the most likely means of checking the disease, the board are of the opinion that ventilation by every means, the frequent introduction of salt water into the well, and pumping with a view of diluting and purifying the bilge water is essential. The board are of [the] opinion that the vessel should put to sea as soon as possible to cruise in the vicinity of the island and in the meantime should put a spring upon her cable when practicable, and that Brodie's Stoves[9] should be used. And as the surgeon of the vessel is at present non-effective, the board are of [the] opinion if it can be done, an experienced and active naval surgeon should be put on board her, as being necessary to inspire the crew with confidence and that, if possible, a sick berth should be fitted up; As the collection of fresh water in the hold arises partly from the leakage of the canvas hose employed in conveying the water from the tanks to the cistern, the board recommends that leather hose should be substituted.

Signed
Alexander Menzies, MD
Department Inspector of Hospitals[10]
Hugh Bone[11]
Physician to the Forces

James Elliott[12]
Surgeon to the Forces

Approved
Signed *Edward Tegart*
Inspector of Hospitals

These proceedings took place while the ship lay at anchor in Carlisle Bay, Barbados, at the time specified. The board seemed to lay great stress on the admixture of fresh with the saltwater in the ship's well. It supposes that freshwater escapes during the operation of pumping the water through canvas hose from the iron tanks to the cistern. But this really is not the case. From the tanks the freshwater is conveyed thro' leather hose to the cistern, consequently not a drop hardly escapes. When it does it is in starting the butts into the tanks; and then a small quantity runs through the canvas hose used for that purpose. But this only happens when the ship takes in water from the shore, which may be once in five or six months. The quantity then must be so small that the bad effects, if any, could hardly produce fever. Leather hose would be the means of saving this waste of water, but as to answering any other purpose, it does not appear to me very evident. As to [the] atmosphere of the Orlop Deck and Hold being close and oppressively hot, and the smell of the bilge water and coal tar having been very perceptible to the board, it may be asked how it could be otherwise in this climate; when every timber in the ship is injected with coal tar, and which oozes at every crack. The heat and closeness of this deck must be expected, more or less, as much depends on the weather. If wet, wind sails cannot be used; and unless the wind is pretty strong, very little air is conveyed by them. Consequently, the atmosphere must be close and hot, of course.

From what has been stated, the board could not have had any serious thoughts of the fever having been produced by any of the above causes; from its chiefly recommending the ship to cruise in the vicinity of the island of Barbados and the use of Brodie's Stoves. The board has enumerated so many different causes that it leads us to conclude that a combination of causes tend to keep up the febrile excitement. I have no doubt in my mind, but that the chief cause of this fever issues from the hold of the ship. Everyone knows that fevers of the worst description have been produced on board ships and even at sea from the effluvia of a foul hold; and which ceased only on the hold being cleared. Notwithstanding the *Pyramus* has only been about six months on this station. It is more than probable the cause of sickness is confined in her hold. How long it requires for foul air to generate I cannot say, but this I know from very good authority that shortly after the *Pyramus* left England for Barbados, a lighted candle would not burn in her hold until measures were adopted to pass fresh air into it by means of a wind sail. From this, it will appear that there was a predisposition in her hold for the generation of foul air. And it is but reasonable to suppose that the effects of this climate on the coal tar and the other etc, etc, etc, must increase that predisposition. Altho' the present state of the hold be such that a lighted candle may be taken into it without being extinguished, yet there is an invisible cause, which melancholy experience has but too plainly convinced us of, and which has been sufficient to extinguish many a valuable life of youths.

"The hardest heart might melt to hear,
even man might drop his iron fear."

I have been informed that the hold of the *Pyramus* has been stowed now for nearly twelve months. In an old vessel such as she is, together with the great degree of sickness which has prevailed for such a length of time without relaxing, [this] is almost a proof that the cause is local. By having her cleaned out, will be the only means of getting at the bottom of it.

Signed
John H. Freer
Hospital Assistant to the Forces
Antigua
December 1821

Half-Yearly Report Dated Shirley Heights 20 December 1821 by Thomas Hall,[13] Hospital Assistant to the Forces

The continued fevers of this country seem to be of a very different class from those which occur in Europe, not different in their general symptoms, but in their progress and termination; the excitement in the former very great and running rapidly if not subdued to dissolution, in the latter more gradual, as must be evident from the number of critical days marked by Hippocrates. It must be evident that in the newcomer, disease there is of frequent occurrence, not from the tone of his fibre only, but oftener from an unguarded use of spirits from the still, the propensity to which, opens his body for the reception of fever dysentery and etc., roused into action by miasmal influence or solar exposure, the symptoms varying according to the intensity of the cause or the constitution of the patient; not only has the robust habit of the soldier in many instances to contend with this poisonous potion (New Rum) but frequently with narcotics as tobacco infused producing as it were a sudden depression of nervous energy and susceptibility to febrile excitement.

One form of continued fever which proved very mortal to Europeans lately arrived is that denominated *Icterodes*.[14] This malignant endemic appeared on board of His Majesty's armed transport ship *Dasher*, in the month of September last. She arrived here on the 22nd. While at sea, six cases occurred, two of which were lost, and no sooner was the anchor dropped than two cases were reported in nearly the last stage of the disease. At this period, I was doing duty at the Detachment General Hospital, where the sick of that vessel were conveyed to for treatment, and thirteen were afterwards admitted.

Having embarked in this ship by order of the inspector of hospitals for Antigua, I was six days on board. My berth was furthest from the main cabin – that is by the side of the main hold where all her stores and etc, were discharged from. I shall here remark that the effluvia issuing from this place and extending to my berth was the most offensive I ever experienced. Never did I go upon deck and come down to it that I did not suffer more or less from headache. This circumstance I related to the principal medical officer here, apprehensive that in the autumnal months an aggravated type of fever would occur, and my anticipation was realized. Before leaving England, I carefully perused all the works written upon this form of fever (yellow), particularly the very eminent one from the pen of Dr Jackson[15] that I might, if possible, ascertain its nature, well aware I should meet it, in some part of my service in these colonies. I had formed an opinion that the disease arose from local causes. On my reaching Barbados, it was then prevalent and to my amazement more discussion arose upon its contagious power than I ever heard upon any paper in the societies of Edinburgh. Such was the discrepancy of opinion and such the discordance in the treatment, that I was, altho' having formed an opinion half inclined to scepticism, but from recent occurrence here, the doubt has vanished, and the paths are now open to me.

The assistant surgeon of the *Dasher* and I spent some hours together, he relating a history to me of what had happened on board. My very eminent and indefatigable chief had frequent conversations with him on the same point, and through no source could we trace even a suspicion of contagion.

Mr Hartle[16] was not here contented but sent him a number of official queries, which were all negative as to its contagious principles. These being answered it was proposed by Mr H that the crew should be landed and encamped in order that the vessel might be cleansed and fumigated, which proposition His Excellency Commanding, readily acceded to. These I thought in my own mind, having before experienced the stench, were the only means of arresting this formidable enemy.

But where was the cause of disease? Beneath the limber boards[17] where the miasmal effluvia was so very great that even the negroes employed for the cleaning were all more or less affected according to exposure and one who I attended along with Staff Surgeon Hartle was labouring under the same form of fever, and of so serious a nature, that had he been a sailor of the ship, he would in all probability have paid the debt of nature.

As to the officers and men admitted into hospital, I was a newcomer and an attendant on them. The orderly of the 35th Regiment, the most attentive I have met with, only eight months in the country, gave them injections,[18] removed excrements and supplied their numerous wants. Several navy officers without my approbation visited Assistant Surgeon Maclean,[19] the first mate, and clerk of the ship, still in no one instance was there a person caught with the disease except those who were exposed to the local sphere. The same happened when the sick of the *Pyramus* were admitted. No person in attendance or any other was ever heard to have received the disease.

I regret much that my sickness and removal precluded the possibility of my being an attendant on them as well as those very interesting cases of Idiopathic Gastritis,[20] which subsequently happened to the crew of the *Dasher*.

• • •

Will these facts not prove locality? Prove it they do to my own satisfaction and am I to blame, to support its non-contagious power until either stronger ones be made public; or ocular demonstration prove to the contrary. One particular symptom of the *Typhus Icterodes*,[21] and mostly a mortal one, is the black vomiting, altho' foreign to this report. I hope for indulgence in offering an opinion upon a medicine of modern date – the Croton Oil.[22]

• • •

The 35th Regiment having during this period been remarkably healthy at their headquarters; the barracks were regularly inspected by me once a week since I took [over], and any symptom of disease checked. The women and children (certainly numerous) have also been healthy. Some few cases of common continued fever occurred among the former, arising generally from costiveness. These I attended at their quarters and the symptoms were speedily removed by a persevering use of Cathartic Medicine. Rubeola was pretty general over the island, but with little mortality a few cases occurred among the children of this garrison and of a mild character. There are many of them, fit subjects for vaccination, and I am happy to say that I have this day been sent a packet of *visces* by the principal medical officer, he having received some as an honorary vaccinator of the institution. It is pleasing to add that the officers have enjoyed the best of health, no death; having taken place amongst them since that of Major Johnston.

I must now bring this report to a conclusion by expressing my regret that the short period I have been in charge of the regiment will not afford me greater field for extension.

Signed
Thomas Hall
Hospital Assistant to the Forces
In charge of 35th Regiment Hospital

Shirley Heights
20 December 1821

Extract of Annual Report for the Period from 21 December 1825 to 20 December 1826 from Antigua by William Munro,[23] Staff Surgeon

It appears to me that endemic disease is too often believed exclusively to originate in swampy grounds, but these supposed causes are always present, and undergo little change whilst endemics are of only occasional and uncertain occurrence. The effluvia arising from swamps would seem to require some undefined extrinsic agency to bring them into noxious activity. Montserrat which was some years past so very sickly has been uncommonly healthy during the past year. An indirect proof of the great obscurity which prevails over the exciting causes of fever. There is a swamp or rather a piece of alluvial land at English Harbour partly surrounding the base of the low hill on which the Navy Hospital is situated, and to windward of it, it forms a part of the shore of the harbour, where it terminates in mud and ooze on which the mangrove grows. This ground was long regarded as a source of disease, but whatever it may have been now that its noxious qualities are no longer perceptible, it is regarded with indifference.

• • •

During the wet and tempestuous weather which prevailed in the latter end of January, and in February, several cases of intermittent and remittent fever appeared at English Harbour. The subjects attacked were chiefly coloured children. Probably if white children had been similarly exposed, the symptoms would have been those of a continued type.

• • •

About the same time, the brigs of war *Ringdove*[24] and *Primrose*[25] were here refitting, the crews being lodged in the dockyard, several cases of fever are recorded to have appeared amongst them though it seems only one (remittent) was admitted into hospital. The causes are, I think, firstly attributed to intemperance and the proverbial improvidence of sailors.

Signed
Wm. Munro
Staff Surgeon

Extract of Report of Antigua, Dated 10 January 1836 by A. Cumming,[26] Surgeon 74th Regiment

Antigua, 10 January 1836. Having only joined the 74th Regiment at Grenada on 24 October, I feel quite incapable of entering into any detail of the medical occurrences of the Corps beyond the brief period which has elapsed since my arrival in the West Indies.

On 17 November, the regiment arrived in this island after a three days' passage in the *Columbia* Steamer. Yellow Fever had been epidemic for some months previous, from which the 36th Regiment had suffered severely; and two or three cases of the most concentrated form were in the hospital and in a moribund state about the time of our arrival. Fortunately, however, not a single case has occurred amongst us here.

We furnish[ed] a detachment of one officer and twenty-two men to the island of Barbuda which is situated betwixt twenty and thirty miles to the north of Antigua. There, several cases of the disease have appeared and at the time which I now write, three of four have proved fatal. The detachment of the 36th Regiment which that of the 74th relieved had been perfectly healthy. If I thought any further proof necessary of the non-contagious nature of yellow fever; what I have first stated might, I conceive, be urged with considerable effect

Signed
A. *Cumming*
Surgeon 74th
Regiment

Extract of Report of Medical Transactions and Prevailing Diseases in the 14th Regiment of Foot from 1 January 1836 to 31 March 1837, by R. Dowse,[27] Surgeon, and 14th Regiment (Headquarters – Antigua, 1 April 1837)

St Kitts is considered to be one of the most healthy islands of any of the Western Archipelago, and certainly ought to be from its state of cultivation and porous nature of its soil yet it is at times in common with the rest visited by that scourge of mankind in the tropics, "Fever", and unfortunately at the time of the 14th Regiment's arrival that malady began to appear as an epidemic of a most aggravated nature among both the European and coloured population of the island. It made sad ravages, old and young, climatized and non-climatized suffered equally its attacks, and great was the mortality which it caused; under such a situation it was not to be expected that a regiment such as the 14th just arrived from Europe and composed principally of young men should escape, and such proved to be the case, for in a very few days after the arrival of the headquarters, it made its appearance in two patients in hospital with slight surgical diseases, both of which proved fatal previous to 15 May; from that period, there was admitted in that month 18 cases, June 36, July 44, August 53, September 88, October 54, November 22, December 20, January 8, making in the course of the nine months in all 343 cases of fever treated in hospital out of a garrison the average strength of which was about 400 men.

In the month of July orders were received that one-half of the regiment was to hold itself in readiness to embark for Antigua. The detachment from Tortola was recalled and one officer, and thirty-one men detached to the island of Montserrat. This movement served to increase still more our number in barracks. The number of sick went on daily increasing, and the stage of convalescents (sic) so protracted that it was thought advisable to recommend that a house be hired close to the seaside for the accommodation of the convalescents, which was accordingly complied with, and I am happy to say it proved of considerable relief to our numerous sick list and the recovery of many almost hopeless cases of debility was the result. The only change in the diet of the convalescents from the ordinary ration was the issue of two extra days of fresh meat in the week. Those patients from hospital who were selected for the convalescent station required little or no medical treatment, and they were visited daily by the staff surgeon.

Those men occupying the bomb-proof barracks in the fort were found to suffer more from fever than those in the wood barracks on the parade, and as the crowded state of the whole prevented the possibility of thinning the men in the small rooms by putting some of them for a time in the barracks below, it was thought advisable to recommend another house to be hired as a temporary barrack, as near the seaside as possible for the reception of the men occupying the bomb-proofs. At the suggestion of the staff surgeon, the measure was adopted by the commandant and a large airy house on the seaside was after some delay procured at Sandy Point, capable of accommodating seventy men to which they removed on 24 September. The rooms in the fort [were] cleared out [and] the walls and roof [were] whitewashed with hot lime. The floors [were] thoroughly washed and [were] left open and unoccupied for a considerable time. At the same time, the whole of the regiment was by a general order supplied on the recommendation of the senior medical officer, with two additional days of fresh meat in the week. These measures could not but be considered to check the ravages of an epidemic fever immediately, the causes of which must be looked for in perhaps the constitution of the atmosphere, or in other sources equally as incomprehensible; but certainly after the bomb-proof barracks were vacated, a great diminution in our number of sick took place. Though many cases of fever were admitted from the detachment at Sandy Point, yet, in general, they were not of so very aggravated a nature as formerly.

In the latter part of November, the detachment from Basseterre rejoined headquarters. It had suffered severely from fever in the latter part of June and early part of July, having lost in the course of a fortnight twelve men. I understand the barracks the detachment then occupied was in a very confined situation in the Iowa and that as soon as it was moved to Bloff Point on the seaside where the men were put, part in a temporary barrack and part under canvas, not a single case of the fever occurred afterwards. On 12 December, the detachment of Sandy Point was recalled into headquarters and again occupied the bomb-proof barracks in Fort George without any renewal of fever, which was then gradually disappearing from the garrison and island altogether.

On 30 January 1837, agreeable to the general order received in July last, the headquarters consisting of 11 officers and 235 men embarked onboard the *Moira* Transport which had brought out from Europe a draft from the depot of 2 officers and 22 men; one officer and 7 men proceeded with headquarters to Antigua, and 1 officer and 15 men landed and joined the Left Wing at Brimstone Hill, St Kitts.

On 2 February, the headquarters arrived at English Harbour, Antigua, landed on the same day and took up temporary quarters in the dockyard, until the morning of the 4th when they marched to the Ridge and now occupy the quarters there and at Shirley Heights.

The distribution of the regiment is as follows:
Headquarters Ridge Antigua – 11 officers; 235 men
Left Wing Brimstone Hill, St Kitts – 7 officers; 164 men
Nevis – 1 officer; 30 men
Montserrat – 1 officer; 31 men
At Barbados recommended for change of climate to Europe – 3 men

• • •

In the return of diseases, the cases of fever are classed as remittent and continued, but in the remarks which I have attempted to make on the symptoms, progress and treatment of the epidemic which prevailed so long in the garrison and island of St Kitts, I have taken the liberty of treating of both under the one appellation fever, as at the onset of the disease in June, July and the early part of August, it presented itself invariably in the continued form and of a most ardent and aggravated description. In the latter part of August, the rains began to fall more abundantly and as the weather became more unsettled during the hurricane season, it gradually assumed the remittent character, so that in the greater part of September and throughout the remaining months of the year, it was solely in the remittent form of fever the disease presented itself. During the early part of the season when the continued form prevailed, it generally made its attack in the most urgent manner without any premonitory symptoms, the patients commonly being seized suddenly with violent acute pain in the head, back and limbs, redness and suffusion of the eyes with more or less contraction of the pupils and intolerance of light, flushed countenance, pungent heat and dryness of skin, hard and quick pulse, more or less irritability of the stomach and pain on pressure at the epigastrium with constipated bowels; such were the symptoms which ushered in the disease and continued for the three first days of the attack in those of a strong and robust habit of body but much mitigated in the feeble and very insidious in the enervated and dissipated subjects in many of whom delirium tremens[28] was superadded. In those which terminated favourably, the symptoms began to moderate on the fourth day when a diaphoresis[29] took place and generally subsided gradually about the fifth or sixth with those in which it proved fatal. Gastric irritation and determination to the head were the most prominent and urgent symptoms, the former being incontrollable in defiance of every means used. Delirium came on generally on the third day, in some serious, in others low and muttering, hiccough and *subsultus tendinium*[30] on the fourth when the vomiting of black coffee-coloured matter and in some profuse haemorrhage from the gums with other atoxic symptoms closed the melancholy scene in most cases on the fifth day.

As the rainy season advanced, the ardent continued, fever subsided and patients were no longer suddenly attacked nor perspiration through any stage of the disease found to be a critical symptom. In general, the attack was preceded for some hours by alternate chills and flushes of heat, lassitude and feebleness in walking with a tendency in many to diarrhoea, which symptoms went on increasing until a violent paroxysm obliged the subject to be immediately brought to hospital; among those who applied for admission to hospital on their first feeling unwell, the disease was in general more easily managed. In the aggravated cases, the patient after ailing some hours was commonly seized with a severe rigour, followed by intense heat of skin, profuse perspiration at the same time that the sensation of cold continued, excruciating pain in the head, back and limbs in some, pallidness of countenance, in others flushed, great irritation of stomach and pain on pressure at the epigastrium, pulse commonly quick, small and depressed, tongue furred and dry in the centre with the edge of a fiery red was observable in many cases. At the outset and in others, that member was clean and moist for the three first days, when it became dry, red and glazed; thirst craving and incessant; bowels in some constipated in others relaxed extreme feebleness and prostration of strength with disposition to syncope[31] and vertigo, on being placed in the erect position. In a few instances, it made its attack as suddenly and in as aggravated a form as it possible (sic) could have done in the most marshy locality, the subject being at once affected with such a depression of nervous energy and disposition to collapse as to afford on their admission little hope of reaction being produced; in some that object never was attained, the stage of collapse continuing until death took place on the fourth or fifth day, the patient in such instances complained of nothing, his body and extremities were cold and bathed in a cold clammy sweat. Pulse at the wrist and other parts scarcely to be felt, action of the heart equally feeble and irregular, tongue moist and cold, thirst incessant, irritability of stomach at first not excessive, voice low and feeble, hands, feet and posterior part of the body gradually became of a livid colour with the palms of the former slightly corrugated, in this state he generally remained for twenty-four or thirty-six hours free of all pain, perfectly sensible, and asserting he felt better. After this period elapsed the gastric irritation increased until the vomiting of black matter became incessant, great jactitation came on for a few hours, followed by low-muttering delirium, picking at the bed clothes, hiccough and involuntary evacuations which terminated his existence. In those in whom reaction was produced, the fever that followed was of a low typhoid type, tedious in its course, and the convalescence slow and protracted. The stage of extreme excitement in general lasted forty-eight hours after which a strong disposition to collapse was observable but if the gastric irritation could be conquered before the fourth day, recovery was certain if not or that it returned on or about that day, death almost invariably followed on [the] fifth or sixth day. In many, a deep icterus[32] tinge appeared about the third day and went on increasing for some days. It was considered rather a favourable incident, for in the cases which proved fatal it seldom made its appearance until the fourth or fifth and then slightly until after death when the tinge in a short time became much deeper. Many complained of painful deglutition,[33] particularly those in whom the tongue was dry, red and glazed, and a similar appearance was found on examination to have extended itself to the fauces[34] and no doubt to the mucous lining of the oesophagus, the extreme prostration of strength, gastric irritation, tenderness on pressure all over the abdomen, and tendency to diarrhoea which were present in all such cases indicated plainly that the mucous tissue throughout the whole of the alimentary canal was in a state of sub-acute (if not acute) inflammation. The congested state of the vessels of the stomach and the abrasion of its mucous membrane which was invariably found on the post-mortem examination of those who died of this fever, plainly pointing out the source and cause of that truly fatal symptom, black vomit. In some, haematemesis preceded (a few hours) the vomiting of the black coffee-coloured matter which must ever be looked upon as most alarming and almost certainly fatal. Yet I am happy to be able to say that many cases recovered where haemorrhage from the stomach took place and also the vomiting of black matter to a considerable extent. In all such happy terminations, critical alvine evacuations[35] of the colour and consistence of tar in considerable quantity considering the brisk and copious manner in which the bowels had been previously acted upon, always took place and seemed to be the way in which the wished-for event was brought about, as the patient almost immediately after one such dejection expressed himself relieved and the vomiting and irritability of stomach quickly disappeared. This fortunate result was not found to follow in those cases where the purging of black watery matter existed but only in those in which the black *gluey tar-like dejection took place. Haematuria*[36] was present in a few of the fatal cases but only in one of those recovered. In all, a strong disposition to haemorrhage from the gums was observable and in many to a considerable and alarming extent yet the dissolution of none can be fairly laid to its apparent exhausting influence. Death followed in many in whom it was present, and considerable numbers recovered where it existed to a great extent. It was noted that as soon as ptyalism[37] took place that the haemorrhage ceased and this led to the supposition that mercury used to the extent of inflaming the system might be the cause of it, as it was observed that the gums of many were much ulcerated though ptyalism never was produced in consequence of which the use of that drug was much diminished in the treatment, and not given with the view of exciting its peculiar action in the system, but merely in combination with aloes or extract of Colocynth as a purgative and emulgent of the liver. Yet a disposition of ulceration of the gums was apparent in many and the haemorrhage in several so treated. Profuse epistaxis[38] occurred in some cases, where weight in the head was more complained of than acute pain, and seemed to prove salutary.

On the decline of the epidemic several of the remittent fevers which had got over the most urgent symptoms gradually fell into fever of a typhoid character accompanied with *petechioe vibices*,[39] abscesses and sloughing bed sores, all but one so affected recovered but their cases were protracted and required [a] nourishing regimen and a liberal allowance of wine and porter to bring them through their difficult struggle. Erysipelas[40] supervened in four instances on the sixth or seventh day of the attack of fever and in one in which the head and face were the parts affected, proved fatal. In the other three the lower extremities were the parts affected, suppuration took place and after discharging pus for a considerable time, the abscesses gradually heated as the patients' constitution gained strength and vigour.

I will not presume to offer a remark on the cause of those fevers which every few years visit those islands, as the subject has long been a source of professional controversy and still remains unsatisfactorily explained. The idea that the fevers of this country are contagious has, I believe, long since ceased among most members of the medical profession, and I had an opportunity of witnessing the non-contagious influence of similar fevers many years ago in this country to my perfect satisfaction. Yet in the visitation lately experienced in St Kitts, I am obliged to observe that scarcely a patient who came into hospital with other diseases but was in a few days attacked with fever and so certain did it become that it was considered advisable not to admit any labouring under trifling affections that could be treated in barracks, the medical officers and all the servants of the establishment except one orderly were attacked with the disease. Many of the men who were brought from barracks to attend upon the immediate wants of the dying comrades returned to hospital the next day or two following with an attack of fever. It is true all were exposed equally to the exciting cause whatever it could be, but certainly those immediately in the hospital and about it suffered more in proportion than those in barracks. Every attention was paid to the cleanliness and ventilation of the wards and that of the persons of the patients by changing their bedding and linen frequently and the quick removal of every nuisance. The cots and bedding of those who died were instantly removed, the floor covered with a solution of the chlorate of lime and the articles not again brought into use until they had been washed and exposed for some time to the air.

Such are the facts as they occurred and were they in the hands of an able advocate of contagion might be made strongly available to his views of the subject, my own opinion is that nothing like contagion exists in the epidemic fever common to the West India islands but that an unhealthy state of the atmosphere may be engendered in and immediately around a hospital where such a very great number of cases of fever of the very worst description were being treated is, I think, possible notwithstanding the utmost vigilance and care being taken of the cleanliness and ventilation of the establishment.

The post-mortem appearances invariably met with in both forms of this fever were considerable congestion of the vessels of the brain and its membranes, diffusion of serum between the Tunica Arachnoidea[41] and Pia Mater[42] with effusion of similar fluid into the ventricles and base of the cranium and more or less air in the veins ramifying on the surface of the brain. Lungs congested and in those where tubercles were present more or less of inflammation in their immediate neighbourhood was found to exist. Heart in almost all instances sound but together with the large blood vessel gorged with blood only in very few was anything like inflammation of that organ detected, and such was in subjects that never could be roused from the state of collapse in which they were admitted. Peritoneal lining of the abdomen and its viscera highly vascular.

Liver in many enlarged. In others contracted, of a high yellow or deep orange colour, and so friable in its texture as to crumble into pieces with the pressure of the hand. Its vessels gorged with viscid black blood oozing out in considerable quantity on incisions being made into its substance. Gall bladder empty or merely containing a small quantity of thick dark bile. Stomach in general much inflamed, presenting on its internal surface softening and in many abrasions in parts of its mucous membrane, partly filled with black matter similar to that which was ejected before dissolution. A like inflamed appearance of the mucous membrane of the intestine was found in general to have extended itself throughout the canal. The spleen was seldom found increased in size but often with its outer covering inflamed and its substance so softened and pulpy as not to admit of its being detached without its breaking in the hand.

The kidneys in many were also inflamed which state in some was found to have extended along the victers[43] to the bladder. In fact, the whole viscera of the abdomen may be said to be found in general more or less inflamed. In two of the most protracted cases of fever, abscesses in the liver containing well-digested pus were found. In one, the liver was much enlarged weighing about fourteen pounds, extending considerably into the left Hypochrondium[44] with two distinct abscesses on its right lobe containing nearly two quarts of matter. In the other, the liver was contracted in size and contained throughout its whole substance eighteen abscesses about the size of an egg each, filled with well-digested pus.

The recovery from this fever was marked by a long and protracted stage of convalescence even in many of those who had passed mildly through the attack was debility so great particularly in the lower extremities, that several weeks often elapsed before they had strength sufficient to resume their ordinary duties. In others who had suffered severely, the deep yellow tinge of the skin only gave way with their return to full health and strength, and it is surprising how robust and corpulent many of them now are whose permanent recovery a little time ago was scarcely to be hoped for. In those where the yellowness of skin was but trifling or did not exist, icterus followed some time or other during their convalescence and, in a few instances, very much retarded recovery, producing still further debility and great emaciation. However, all recovered by the use of aperients and tonics.

In the first weeks of October, the weather for a few days became suddenly unusually wet and cold, when eight cases which were progressing favourable (sic) in their convalescence became suddenly affected with a renewal of fever attended with such gastric enteric affection, as speedily in their weakened state to prove fatal to six of them. With the exception of the above which may be fairly attributable to the sudden change of the weather, relapses were not in general numerous.

Signed
R. *Dowse*
Surgeon, 14th Regiment

Abstract of Annual Report to Accompany the Annual Return of Sick and Wounded of the Troops in the Windward and Leeward Islands Command for the Period from 1 April 1838 to 31 March 1839 by T. Draper,[45] Inspector General of Hospitals

Barbados

In the early part of November, the 52nd Regiment arrived here from Gibraltar and occupied the barracks lately vacated by the 36th Regiment, who sailed for Halifax. Fever of the Remittent form had for some weeks been prevalent in Bridgetown and its environs amongst the civil population, but the military had been quite exempt from it. Shortly after the 52nd landed, however, a few cases made its appearance amongst the men, but it was not such as to cause any serious alarm and soon disappeared. Six cases only terminating in death. Amongst the officers, however, things were very different. They occupied the barracks vacated by the officers of the 36th Regiment who had enjoyed uninterrupted health; tho' it is fair to state that Major Cross, 36th Regiment, was attacked with remittent fever the day after he embarked in the *Hercules* 74 and died before she sailed from Carlisle Bay and was buried on shore. Fourteen officers only of the 52nd Regiment arrived with the Corps, and the commanding officer was quartered in a house allotted for him at some distance from the barracks; and the medical officer was quartered near the hospital. Thus, it will appear that twelve officers only were quartered in the barracks, ten of whom suffered from this fever and three terminated fatally; and all had narrow escapes, for the fever was of a very aggravated form. There are some circumstances also that deserve notice. The paymaster with his wife and daughter about nineteen and son about twelve years of age occupied the quarters vacated by Major Cross. He and his wife died; the daughter and son narrowly escaping with life. The Regimental Orderly Room was also in this barrack and next to it the quartermaster's store of clothing and etc. Now it is strange, but no less true, that every individual who had any duty in that Orderly Room were (sic) attacked with fever, even the commanding officer who attended there every day suffered from a severe attack, although he was quartered in a separate house some distance from the barracks. The orderly room clerk, the paymaster sergeant and two mess waiters died, and the paymaster sergeant of the 69th Regt. who went there to assist also fell a victim. In fact, out of twenty-four individuals who were connected with this part of the building (the lower or ground floor), only two females and four young children escaped. In the upper floor, fever was equally prevalent but less fatal. Under these distressing conditions, I recommended the entire evacuation of the building and that the officers should for a short time be allowed to go into lodgings with a view of having a thorough examination of the rooms and under the floors and to have them painted and coloured, which they much needed. The general consented at once to my recommendations and from that period no case of fever has occurred although the barracks are again occupied, and many fresh officers have since arrived from England. Now, the cause of this unusual and severe epidemic, it is difficult to account for unless, indeed, it be attributed to atmospheric influence; and I am more inclined to give some credit to this from the circumstance that the disease was confined to the officers' barracks and the commanding officer's quarters, the latter being nearly in line with those barracks. All this time, the men were very healthy, and their barracks are situated about one hundred yards distant and in a different direction. I am, however, to observe that there was nothing under the flooring or elsewhere to which the cause of this fever could be attributed. Of Staff Surgeon Franklin[46] and Assistant Surgeon Spence 52nd Regt.,[47] I cannot speak too highly. Their attention was unremitting and their kindness the source of much comfort to those who recovered and most soothing to those who fell victims to that awful and unmanageable disease. The garrison has since been healthy.

British Guiana
The 69th Regiment was removed from this colony to Barbados during the first quarter of the year and replaced the 70th Regiment from headquarters. This meeting of the two corps did not fail to produce increased intemperance and to fill the hospital; yet, during the three first quarters of the year, the troops throughout the colony were generally healthy. In the last quarter (from 1 January to 31 March),

however, this noble colony was again visited with a most destructive epidemic, in the shape of bilious remittent fever of a most malignant type. The disease commenced in early part of February, but March was by far the most fatal month; in the beginning of which the Left Wing embarked for Barbados taking with it all the sick and weakly men of the Corps capable of being removed. It may, therefore, be stated that out of thirty-six men who died of fever and its sequelae, they were mostly from one wing of the regiment amounting to about two hundred men. Every remedy was tried without much benefit, for medicine seemed to have no effect. Gastric irritation was incessant and could not be overcome. The detachment of the 1st West India Regiment then quartered there was healthy during this lamentable epidemic, which caused such a loss of life to the European soldier. The civilians also suffered but little. Berbice also continued healthy.

Trinidad

During the month of May, remittent fever made its appearance amongst the 89th Regiment in rather a serious form; 105 cases were admitted, 15 of which terminated fatally viz 10 at St James and 5 at St Joseph. It fell particularly amongst the newly arrived drafts, chiefly young Irishmen. This fever also prevailed in the town of Port of Spain amongst the inhabitants with greater severity than the troops. Towards the end of the quarter, the character of the fever assumed a much milder type and had nearly disappeared the beginning of the second quarter. However, about the beginning of July, it set in at St Joseph and was of the most malignant character. Out of a detachment of sixty-eight men, ten died there, when it was removed to St James (being then removed by black troops) when nine more died making a total of nineteen deaths out of that small detachment. The Africans did not suffer.[48] The epidemic appeared to be little under the control of medical treatment and proved equally fatal, however treated. St Joseph had always been considered a very healthy station. The surgeon [of] the 89th Regiment stated that the "water in the well adjoining the barracks, which was always considered excellent quality, became offensive to the smell and water was then procured from the village considerably lower than the barrack. In a short time, it was found necessary to bring it from the river as the whole of the wells became in some degree putrid". Can this fairly be attributed to any other than atmospheric influence? The post of St Joseph was very healthy during the third quarter, but it was garrisoned by the black troops upon whom the climate had no effect but assistant staff surgeon, Dr Duncan,[49] died of the same description of fever that had proved so fatal to the 89th the preceding quarter; but sickness seemed to follow that Corps for fever made its appearance at St James' and no less than nineteen cases terminated fatally besides three officers. The season was very wet and in consequence the underwood that surrounded the barracks was not cut down as usual; and this was the cause in the opinion of the principal medical officer (PMO) of the epidemic; for when the rains ceased and the men were enabled to clear the ground, the fever disappeared. However, the change of weather might also have been one cause. Every treatment was tried but medicine had but little effect. Black vomit appeared in all the fatal cases. It is strange but true that the population of Port of Spain (not three miles from St James) was healthier during this period than they had been for the last ten years. The 89th Regiment was relieved during the last quarter of the year by the 74th Regiment and now Garrison Antigua and St Kitts and have much improved in health since their change; and the 74th which went from St Lucia and Dominica has not suffered. With respect to Trinidad, it will be seen that it has been much more fatal this year than even Demerara, in proportion to its strength, and it is not unlikely that may prove the case every year, unless Negroes are employed when necessary to keep the brushwood under, for it is too extensive to be kept properly cut down by the military.

Tobago
This garrison has been uniformly healthy during the year.

Grenada
During the first quarter, the troops composing this garrison enjoyed excellent health, but in the second quarter, fever made its appearance and did not disappear until the later end of November, and not even then amongst the inhabitants. This fever appeared as an epidemic of great malignity and the symptoms were those of true yellow fever.

Reports from Antigua

In no case when black vomit appeared did the patient recover. It commenced among the artillery in a fort near the town and soon appeared in the 70th Regt. on Richmond Hill, an elevation of several hundred feet above the level of the sea. The crews of the shipping also suffered and particularly her Majesty's steamer, *Columbia*. The garrison was augmented in the third quarter by 40 men of the 1st West India Regiment, which was composed of 202 white and 112 black troops. Of the former, 122 have been under treatment and 18 died, whilst from the latter only 13 were treated and no fatal termination,[50] thus, giving another very remarkable instance of the little susceptibility of disease in the African compared to the European. During the last quarter of the year, the garrison was healthy. The civil population both whites and coloured (the former amongst the most respectable) suffered in at least an equal degree with the military.

St Vincent

This island was very healthy, indeed the first three-quarters of the year, but in the month of March, remittent fever in a very severe form made its appearance although it did not prove very fatal. The surgeon of the regiment suffered by it and the Adjutant of the 70th Regiment died from it. Forty-four cases (all whites) were admitted into hospital and three ended in death; also, the sergeant major died, but he died in quarters in the fort (being a very good man, he was allowed to remain there, to be attended by his wife).

St Lucia

There is nothing particular to remark upon at this island. It has been amongst the first in health this year although a number of young African recruits have joined.

Dominica

The troops in this island suffered much from remittent fever which made its appearance in the early part of May commencing in the artillery whose barracks are close and to leeward of the town of Roseau. The strength of the detachment was only fifteen, of which number twelve were attacked and eight died. About 28 May, this fever appeared amongst the 74th Regiment on Morne Bruce and continued to rage until the end of September, when it ceased altogether; not suddenly, however, for fewer and milder cases were admitted during September than any of the four preceding months. The form of this fever was very insidious commencing generally with slight arterial action, clean moist tongue and skin, but little above the natural heat. As the disease progressed, the powers of life gradually declined without any organ appearing to be particularly affected, and the patient was calm throughout the whole period. Haemorrhage from the gums and throat was common but, though alarming, not always a fatal symptom. There were no rigours, exacerbations or remissions. From these circumstances, I should be inclined to think the fever was of a continued form terminating in typhus. The garrison to period before mentioned viz 30 September was 240 strong composed of about equal numbers of white and black; of the former 102 were admitted and 35 died whilst of the latter only 11 were admitted and none died. This subject is certainly worthy of serious consideration. Three officers also died during this period. The third and fourth quarters the troops were healthy, and nothing occurred worthy of remark except that the 74th Detachment was relieved by the 14th Regt. in January.

At Antigua and St Kitts, the troops were healthy during the year. The 14th Regiment was removed from those islands in January and the 89th Regiment from Trinidad and Tobago, and now occupy St Lucia and Dominica, no occurrence requiring observation. The sickness and mortality has fallen, however, more on the young than on the old soldiers as will be seen on reference to the accompanying casualty return; for out of 344 deaths, 254 have occurred from 20 to 30; whilst from 31 to 36 only 63 died and from that to 45 only 27 took place; one cause of this however maybe fairly attributed to the greater number of the former than the latter ages in the regiment. However, the proportion of mortality is greater even in the young than the more advanced in life, and more fatal cases have occurred in those recently arrived and during the first 18 months in proportion than amongst the longer residents.

Signed
T. Draper
Inspector General of Hospitals
Barbados 30 July 1839

Extract of Annual Report on Diseases Treated in the Regimental Hospital 89th Regiment from 1 April 1838 to 31 March 1839 Dated Ridge, Antigua by Surgeon J. Duncanson,[51] 1st West India Regiment

There is one circumstance, however, I may advert to, peculiar to Antigua, which is that much less rain falls there than in any of the other islands. Its climate consequently is drier. It enjoys also a nearly uniform and equable temperature throughout the year. The soil is generally very shallow with a rocky substratum. The land has no great elevation above the level of the sea, the highest point not above eight hundred feet perhaps. The island is not therefore subject to those hidden alterations of temperature which are experienced in St Lucia and other islands abounding in steep lofty and inaccessible mountains, densely covered to the summits with forest trees. The only water used in Antigua is rainwater which is collected in tanks and cisterns, there being no springs or river. Antigua is formed as might be expected from its geological and physical features to be one of the healthiest islands in the West Indies. The average annual ratio of mortality for twenty years being under three times less than that of Jamaica, Tobago or St Lucia. Prior to 1836 when an epidemic fever manifested itself, the island had been for upwards of twenty years entirely free from such a visitation and had been consequently remarkably healthy, and happily it is now and has been for some time past in the same satisfactory state. For the only cases of fever, I have met with since my arrival here were all the intermittent type and were cases of relapse, the disease having been originally contracted in Trinidad or Tobago.

The average strength of the regiment throughout the year has been 271. The admissions into hospital have amounted to 748. Of these 166 were cases of intermittent fever, 209 remittent fever, and 69 continued fevers. The deaths in hospital during the period were 58; of these 47 were fatal cases of remittent fever. Besides it appears by the accompanying annual return that four officers of the regiment died. One of these was Surgeon Orr[52] who died 21 January last. The same epidemic, it is stated, also proved fatal to nine women and nine children. But this number of fatal cases among the women I have twice found is far from being correct. For I have a list of no fewer than 16 soldiers' wives who died during the year. Since its arrival in the West Indies in December 1835, I have ascertained that the 89th Regiment has lost twenty-eight women and forty children. I find on referring to the historical register that from 1 April to 30 June 1838, the regiment being at the time with the exception of one company stationed in Trinidad, a great and unprecedented sickness took place accompanied with fearful mortality as it is expressed. The wet season it would appear set in prematurely. The rains were attended with storms of thunder and lightning. The atmosphere is described to have been sultry with occasionally complete calms and from this the increase of the sick list it is stated commenced.

Fever of the remittent type or rather bearing more the appearance of bilious continued as it is termed then became prevalent among the men. A detachment of ninety-eight men which had arrived from England in March preceding are said to have been by far the greatest sufferers and many fell victims to the disease. The general symptoms were heavy pains in the head and loins, flushed face, quick suppressed pulse at times quite tremulous, eyes suffused, a white, loaded tongue, skin hot with a harsh and parched feel, great nausea, and irritability of stomach, occasional vomiting of green matter, pains of the limbs with urgent thirst, great restlessness with an incessant desire to drink water. On the fourth or fifth day, the tongue, teeth and lips were covered with sores. The patients then became comatose and were seized with black vomit and generally expired on the sixth or seventh day in a state of insensibility. The body in these cases invariably became yellow two or three days previous to dissolution. Some of the cases assumed a milder and more insidious form having on admission no symptom calling for particular attention. The patients in these cases usually complained of slight headache, pulse about eighty, skin scarcely above the natural temperature and moist tongue always loaded but on the third day the character of the disease underwent a change for the worse. About the middle of July, the epidemic assumed a still more malignant and destructive character.

But of a detachment of eighty-six men stationed at St Joseph, nineteen have died. St Joseph had always been reckoned for many years a remarkably healthy station until May last when fever attacked a few of the men lately arrived from England. The inhabitants of the neighbouring [area] suffered also from the same fever but not in an equal degree with the military. Some ascribed this epidemic to malaria arising from a marshy piece of ground about half a mile from the front of the barracks caused by the river having changed its channel and the early and partial fall of rain. The water in the wells became offensive and putrid. *(The correctness of this statement with regard to the water becoming offensive and putrid is very doubtful, for on making enquiry I have been told by an officer who was stationed at St Joseph the whole time of the sickness as well as by other officers that the water in the wells during the period referred to did not become either offensive or putrid but possessed its usual purity unchanged: Audi alteram partem, signed J. D.).* It was therefore found necessary to bring water from the river for the troops. After a comparatively healthy interval of a few weeks the epidemic again manifested itself about the end of October and after a very heavy fall of rain, and with extremely fatal results. It set in with the usual symptoms, on the third day, the body became yellow; black vomit supervened with coma and generally on the fourth or fifth dissolution took place. The subjects of five of the fatal cases which occurred from April to June were young recruits recently from England, and the same number of fatal cases were those of old soldiers, all of whom were men of drunken and dissolute habits. The post-mortem examination exhibited a turgid state of the vessels of the brain with effusion of serum in the base of the brain and ventricles. The liver enlarged and gorged with blood; gall bladder collapsed and nearly empty; stomach and intestines distended with flatus and black matter resembling the sediment of coffee. Mucous membrane of stomach described to be inflamed and softened; spleen generally large and of soft consistency.

Signed
J. Duncanson
Surgeon 1st West India Regiment
(in medical charge of 89th Regiment since 28 March 1839)

4. Reports from Barbados

Preview: The Barbados Reports begin with a particularly detailed filing from Dr John Arthur on the situation in Barbados during 1821. Dr Arthur had been appointed as surgeon to the 60th Regiment of Foot on 5 September 1811. He was subsequently promoted to physician on 3 August 1815 and had a further promotion as deputy inspector of hospitals (D.I.H.) on 27 May 1825. His report offers fascinating insights into the surrounding social and environmental conditions recorded during the yellow fever epidemic he witnessed. For historians researching the prevailing medical philosophies of early nineteenth-century practitioners in the New World, Dr Arthur's report discusses the questions of contagion, miasmata, and other philosophies in the diagnosis and treatment of yellow fever. He also introduces notions of racial difference in the immunity profiles of various social groups. It is an excellent backdrop to the several other doctors' reports submitted under the Barbados filing, which follow sequentially up to the 1840s in our study. Incidentally, it is Dr Arthur's surmising on a causal link between the housing of Africans ("Congo") in the Bridgetown environment and an outbreak of yellow fever, which is a partial source for the title of this manuscript.

Report Submitted by John Arthur, Physician P.M.O., Barbados, 17 March 1821

In my remarks on the diseases of the first quarter of the last half year, which I forwarded with the return for that period, I had the satisfaction of noticing the healthy state of the garrison and the small number of deaths that occurred during it. But in the return for the last quarter, the list of deaths will be found considerably lengthened.

Yet considering the circumstance that the malignant epidemic with black vomiting, which has been prevailing and spreading through this island very destructively now for more than eight months, had actually got into this garrison in three or four instances, manifesting its usual malignity of character by the rapidity of its progress (till fortunately arrested in its course by prompt measures that were adopted in each instance for that purpose with the happiest good effect). [With] the large proportional mortality amongst those affected by it within a short space of time, we have reasons to consider ourselves singularly fortunate. For on analysing the deaths the regular strength of the garrison will be found to have suffered in but a very slight degree from it. What I may call the irregulars rather attached to than actually belonging to the army (and thus not under the same control and restraint that the others were subjected to), such storekeeper's department now forming a branch of the commissariat. The Barrack Department, the various occupations of the persons employed in which necessarily requires them to be widely scattered about, etc.; with the women and children constituting the greater part of the bulk of the sufferers.

The 21st Fusiliers, the only complete white regiment in the garrison, 619 strong, up to the date of the return, lost but four persons by it, and these were all detached men from the corps viz; The two John Fallon and John Andrews were with the barracks Department, the one occupied a small house at one side of the barrack yard gate, the other worked in a saddler's shop at the opposite side of the same gate all the week, but on Sundays when he mounted guard, the one was admitted into hospital the day after the other. The third was John Windle, a surgery man. The regimental hospital in which there was then a man, John Watts, labouring severely under the same disease which he seemed to have contracted in some of his private irregular rambles to town; when admitted into hospital, he came from punishment drills which he was under for having absented himself during the night times from his guard at Government House and acknowledged that he was in the habit of privately visiting a girl in or near the town. He recovered, and I clearly ascertained from him that very shortly before Windle was attacked with the disease himself, he had repeatedly administered to him medicines and injections and had dressed his blisters. He though in direct opposition to orders, black servants having been specially appointed for the express purpose of attending to such cases which were carefully kept separate from the others and though he had been but a very short time released from quarantine in which I had myself put him along with other white orderlies, having caught them similarly employed about John Fallon, the man that first died of it. The unfortunate man at length fell a victim to his temerity in thus rashly persisting in disobedience of orders intended for his own security. The surgery man of the Naval Hospital, also one of the 21st Regiment, suffered a severe attack of the disease from the very same cause but recovered.

The fourth fatal case in this regiment was Taylor Wilson, living at Colonel Popham's, the deputy barrack and quartermaster general, in whose family the disease was prevailing severely when this man was taken ill with it. These four detached cases were the only deaths from fever in the regiment for the quarter up to the date of the return, during the entire of which the malignant fever with black vomit was prevailing as an epidemic so fatally in the neighbourhood. Such were the good effects of the arrangements and precautionary measures hereafter to be mentioned that were adopted for its preventions, which were carried into effect and strictly enforced by the officers of the regiment who have, in consequence, experienced the benefit of them and who deserves much credit for their care of and attention towards the men.

Since then, there have been two alarms in the regiment. On 23, 24 and 25 December, some severe suspicious-looking cases of fever were admitted in hospital from one company, the 6th, one of whom, Thompson, admitted on the 23rd, died with black vomit on the 25th; another, Robert Reid, from the next berth to that of the last one admitted the same day, died with the same symptom on the 28th. Another, Lewis Burk, also contiguous as to his place in barracks, was admitted on the 25th but, after this symptom had made its appearance had a remarkable, unexpected recovery. All from the one company and the same part of the barrack being from contiguous berths; other severe, strongly suspicious cases that recovered were intermixed with these being in the neighbourhood of them and of one another. It was, therefore, manifest that the malignant fever had got into this company and was spreading through it. After the appearance of black vomit in the first mentioned instance of Corporal Thompson of the 25th, which removed all doubt on the subject, it was determined to encamp them in the same manner as had been done two months before with the Artillery Sappers and Miners under similar circumstances with complete success. This company was accordingly encamped on 26 December immediately in the rear of their barrack, a little to windward but in the close vicinity of it all. Communication being, at the same time, prevented. The best and most favourable result was the consequence, an immense and complete cessation of the fever in that company, not a single case from it having occurred in the encampment, nor indeed an admission for any disease for fully two or three weeks when a solitary case of bowel complaint being a recurrence of an old chronic affection, presented itself and was admitted into hospital. But shortly afterwards a fresh alarm was raised in the 9th Company, the next adjoining one to the former in the same barrack room. Corporal Roome, having been admitted from it on the 2nd and who, died with black vomit on 6 January. He had been preceded by a man from the next berth to him in the same company (Marcus Burns, who had been admitted on 29 December with severe fever, which after a little time was attended with black stool but who recovered). He was soon followed by his particular friend Sergeant Patterson, who also slept in a corner neighbouring berth by himself and who soon shared the same fate. The assistant, in some written remarks, states, "Roome was in the closest intimacy with Sergeant Patterson and whatever writing he may have had to do was always seen as the sergeant's table". The sergeant was one of the oldest and most respectable non-commissioned officers in the regiment, had got some property and was shortly about to return to England when he was taken ill of this disease on 4 January, of which he died after much black vomit on the 7th. John Brown, the comrade of Roome, was admitted into hospital the same day as the preceding man, ill from fever which proved a severe, suspicious one, but he recovered.

Alexander Fleming of the 8th Company lately reduced from a sergeant attached to Sergeant Patterson, therefore remaining in the 9th Company where he slept in the next berth to him. In some remarks of the assistant, he was stated "to have been in the habit of cleaning Sergeant Patterson's accoutrements and was constantly about his person". His case was last in the garrison, attended with black vomit. He was admitted on 6 January and died on the 10th. This company as the preceding one when it was clearly ascertained by the occurrence of black vomit in Roome's case that the malignant fever was in and spreading through it from berth to berth was on 6 January encamped in the same as the former one and with nearly the same success. But two cases of fever were admitted from it afterwards. Thomas Hogan on 9 January and Frederick Lake on 11 January, both from the same tents (but three or four men at farthest were placed in each), and both in barrack had slept in the next berth to Roome's. They, though severe cases, recovered.

These were all fatal cases in the 21st Regiment attended with black vomit, and such was the progress that disease was making in each instance till measures adopted for arresting it, which proved successful. The remarkable circumstance of the contiguity of berths of those affected was first observed by the officers themselves and mentioned by the assistant. No doubt, as usual at all times, several cases of the common ardent from the ordinary causes also occurred. But taking into consideration all the attending and consequential circumstances of each, no two diseases can be more distinct or different. Indeed, the difference in each case was generally discernible by an experienced eye at an early stage of the complaint and confirmed afterwards by the after appearances and events which generally removed all doubts on the subjects. I find the number of these common ordinary cases as elapsed in the accompanying half-yearly returns under the head of common continued fever to correspond pretty nearly with the number of the same cases for the same period of the year before. That in this one is in the former immediately after Christmas from the great inebriety practised and various excesses and irregularities committed in celebration of the holydays. Several such cases occurred but which were recognized as such at first and kept as carefully as we could, separated from them, they of the malignant kind. They came from all the companies indiscriminately in very nearly equal numbers or an average for the first fortnight after Christmas day, about two per company. As even of this fever, an odd case will every now and then prove fatal but unattended with that strongly distinguishing characteristic black vomit, so general in the numerous fatal cases of the other.

I think it but right and proper to ascribe to this head two if not all of three other deaths from fever that occurred in this regiment, in none of which did black vomit appear and in two of them, at least this disease was not communicated to any other person. The particular of these three cases were as follows:

First: William Dougherty of the 9th Company admitted on the eighteenth and died on 21 December, though in this case, there was no black vomit, nor any appearance of it found in the stomach or intestines on dissection after death. I am yet led to entertain suspicions of its having been a case of the malignant epidemic from the shortness of its course having terminated so speedily in death and the disease having shown itself decisively so soon afterwards in the neighbouring berths. For a reply to my request to the adjutant for information respecting the situation of his berth, he was kind enough to inform me "that Dougherty slept near Roome and Sergeant Patterson".

Second: Edward Cluning of the 7th Company admitted on the 23rd and died on 28 December. No black vomit thrown before death, nor any found in the stomach afterwards, but as he passed dark-coloured matter by stool (a suspicious though much more doubtful and equivocal symptom than black vomit – very dark bilious stool, being not infrequent in different diseases of warm climates). His comrades that were in the same berth with him were immediately encamped for the greater security of the company. The disease, however extended no farther; no other case having appeared in that company.

Third: John Miller of the 10th Company was admitted on the 25th and died on 31 December without black vomiting or purging. His case appeared so little like the malignant epidemic that [no] steps were deemed necessary to be taken to prevent its spreading, nor was any other person taken ill afterward in his or the adjoining berths.

An interval of more than two months having now elapsed since the appearance of the last case in garrison, and as it seems to have been declining for some time in the town and country, though, I am sorry to say cases of it are still occurring there every now and then. I hope we may calculate with some certainty on the termination of it for the present among the troops. It is now highly gratifying to contemplate this fine regiment about to embark for Demerara and Berbice after nearly two years' service in this island and being the two first since their arrival from England, with such very trifling detriment or loss as they have experienced even after having encountered this usually dreadful formidable disease. Their total loss from fever during the entire prevalence of the epidemic up to this date has been altogether but twelve men. They have not lost an officer by it, nor a woman or a child – not an officer of this regiment has died in this island since their first arrival, though in the very same quarters and barracks in which the 2nd or Queen's Regiment suffered so severely in 1816 when this island was last visited by the same epidemic.

These remarks, of course, apply to this regiment only during their residence in this island. Two companies that were detached from hence in September last to Tobago and which returned in January were far from being so fortunate. In a short space of time, they lost four out of five of their officers, including their medical officer, and more than thirty men. The remains of the two companies of the 4th regiment that had served there before then, then came up here, reduced to one-third of their original strength and with but one surviving officer out of five. They also lost a medical officer, Mr Ward,[1] that had been sent there from this debarkation. They were immediately marched to Gun Hill, a distant elevated post in the interior of the island, where they continued healthy. The companies of the 21st on their return were encamped, and communication with the rest of the regiment for some considerable time prevented. They also continued healthy. The melancholy fates of the two detachments afford not bad specimens of the destructive effects of this malignant disease. On its having broken out and prevailing there among civilians generally as well as the military the latter end of 1818 and beginning of 1819, I witnessed the ravages which it made amongst both pretty equally. I reported then on the subject and the abstract of the sick returns of the troops in the island for the thirteen years preceding, [from]which, annexed to that report, may be seen the very healthy state of the military during that entire period. The principal garrison, which was then suffering and which has since experienced such great losses, had been one of the healthiest and with as little mortality as any other in the West Indies during the entire of that long interval though quartered in a miserable condemned old wooden barrack on the same site with the present ones. Indeed, in it the disease first broke out and raged for some time till the men were removed into the present new stone barrack and from which removal it received the first check. The seeds of it, however, appear to have been somehow retained in that island and from which it has been since renewed and proved to be destructive to the succeeding new detachments there – the next most numerous bodies of white persons in the garrison here. The Ordnance Department, consisting of the artillery, the Sappers and Miners, the Engineers and the civil branch, suffered more severely though still comparatively speaking in but a slight degree. The artillery containing 138 men, 28 women and 27 children, lost but 8 men, 5 women and 4 children, all of whom except for one man attacked in hospital were outliers in huts, not quarters, or on detached charges or duties. For when the disease seemed to be spreading to the artillery from the Sappers and Miners quartered in the same barrack with them (the upper room of which a fine, spacious and usually very healthy one was occupied, one-half by the artillery and the other half by the Sappers and Miners who were more early and more severely affected by the disease) one man, Drummer Bernard Reily of the artillery, being admitted from that barrack on 25 October ill with very severe suspicious-looking fever of which he finally recovered. All the artillery from it were encamped the following day, the 26th, by themselves round the Cenotaph at one side of the parade and not a fatal or severe marked case occurred afterwards in that camp.

The man attacked with the disease in hospital was Gunner James Vamplew. He had been a patient there from 6 October with venereal warts, was seized with fever on the 25th or 26th, and died with black vomit on the 28th. These had been treated just before in the same common ward with him and the other patients, a decided case of the disease. John Kinnaird, Sappers and Miners, was admitted on the 20th and who died on 24 October. He was taken ill so suddenly and severely whilst exposed to the sun as an orderly to his commanding officer on his way to town that it was considered and marked as a case of *Coup de Soleil*. I pronounced it in the first instance to have been a case of the malignant fever but not being believed. I was determined to satisfy myself as far as possible by dissection after death, as he had not thrown up any black vomit. Mr Donnelly,[2] assistant surgeon, was present to perform the dissection, but as I thought I perceived in him a degree of dislike and unwillingness to expose himself to the hazard from it, I begged of him to give me the knife. When I went through it myself in his presence, and on taking out the stomach, found it loaded with the matter of black vomit, which I afterwards exhibited to the inspector Mr Green[3] and the surgeon Mr Bradley,[4] and which of course brought conviction to their mind Mrs Berry of the Sappers and Miners to be afterwards particularly mentioned when tracing the commencement of the disease in that corps, was his washerwoman. No such occurrence happened afterwards in any of the hospitals, with those ill with malignant fever being carefully separated from the other patients.

An orderly of this hospital, Gunner Archibald McMullin, was also attacked with fever about this time, being admitted as a patient on 28 October. It may be that this was also from the same source. Still, he likewise, for some days before being taken ill, attended the spring cart that conveyed the malignant cases from this to the Naval Hospital appointed for the reception of all such cases by which also, perhaps, he might have been exposed to the cause of the disease. His case was not a severe one and he recovered. This kind of danger was also obviated afterwards by the regulation that black servants alone should attend on and be employed about those ill of this complaint which when observed was attended with eminent success when infringed with imminent danger.

I have already related the instances of two surgery men, the one at the Naval the other at the 21st Hospital. A third happened in the steward of this hospital. Sergeant Lovath, whom I have repeatedly found in the observation ward about patients ill with fever – indeed, I must say frequently of necessity from the extreme stupidity and inattention of the persons first employed. In consequence, both himself and family suffered from it. The Sappers and Miners earlier affected (and who, from what I have to state hereafter seemed to have received it from the people of the Storekeeper's Department) suffered in proportion to their small number far more considerably. Out of forty-six men, thirteen women and twenty-six children, they lost nine men, one woman and four children.

In this party also were experienced the beneficial effects of removal and separation from the infected by means of encampment, to which, of course they were confined in the same manner as the others. By 26 October, the entire family of Mr Berry of this corps, the father, mother and five children and nearly every person that had any communications with them were affected with the complaint. One, Mary Berry, had already died with black vomit on the 25th. John Kinnaird quartered in the barracks, whom Mrs Berry washed as before mentioned, died on the 24th when the matter of black vomit was found abundantly contained in his stomach. The sergeant major of the party, Jameson, who kept one child constantly and received two others into his quarters on the admission of their parents into hospital and in whose house, I first saw these children when taken ill, was himself admitted on the 25th, proved a very severe case and had a very narrow escape. His recovery was unexpected by me as I saw very dark matter thrown up by him. Mr Graham, draughtsman in the Engineer Department, had another of the children, and his wife was taken ill on the 20th a weak elderly woman. The fever, in her case was rather a low lingering one. She died on 2 November. Mr Graham himself was attacked on 26 October, but he recovered. They had no children. These were all quartered in different situations. Some others at this time were admitted from the out quarters and huts, which proved fatal with the same most usual appearance in these cases – black vomit.

From the barrack of the Sappers and Miners on 23 October, William Bowden was admitted with fever – he recovered. On the 25th, from the same place were admitted in the same state, three, of whom one only, Owen Connor, recovered. The other two died. Henry Rickie on the 28th with black vomit and Robert Armstrong on the 31st. Appearances now were very alarming. [A large number of admissions from this small group presented a very serious picture, along with] the large proportional number of deaths with that malignant symptom, black vomit, hitherto unknown for some years in this island. The disease appeared about to rage with all the usual violence and fatal consequences which it had manifested at former periods in this garrison, as well as more recently in those of other islands. The alarm was consequently very great when, at the suggestion and recommendation of Mr Green, the party from barrack was encamped on 26 October at one side of the parade between the engineer's house occupied by Captain Smith and the morning and evening guns. From this to 31 October, when I embarked for Tobago, things looked more favourably (sic). Not one admission occurred from camp of a fatal or severe case. But on my return about 8 November, I found that three fatal cases had been admitted from the camp. William Russell and James Bell on 31 October, and both I understood, died with black vomit on 3 November, and Mr Veitch,[5] who had been admitted on the 1st, died on 4 November. The particulars of these cases I could not be personally acquainted with, having been absent. They may have been affected before going into camp. I understand that William Veitch declared that he had slept when in barrack next to one of the men that had been affected with it, or I should not be surprised from a knowledge of their great irregularity and how much they were addicted to drinking, so had they contrived to stray away from the encampment which was by no means difficult, particularly after this during the long period that they remained in the camp.

But one more fatal case occurred. Mr Johnson, a cook, admitted on 18 November and died on the 20th with black vomit appeared, and as a cook, he was absent a day from the encampment for the purpose of cooking in the kitchen. But then he may have gone wherever he pleased. He only slept in the encampment at nights. The families of both artillery and Sappers and Miners were encamped in two parties – one on a part of the parade grounds towards one side and the other on low ground a little outside and below the garrison near where a lime kiln has been lately erected. I do not find or know of a single case of any kind admitted from or placed under canvass (sic), with the exception of a very trifling one, Esther Tupe, admitted on 15 November. The wide difference between this and what happened to others not so situated was very striking and remarkable, as all the deaths must, of course, have happened among the latter. This also serves to account for the deaths not having been more numerous among the women and children in general of this department. Of the officers and their families of the ordnance department, the only persons affected were the following: Assistant Surgeon Donnelly, much exposed by his professional duties but particularly in his attendance on a woman, Mrs Boyde, whom he delivered while labouring under this disease and who died on 30 October of haemorrhage of the uterus that followed. He was taken ill on 3 November and died on the 8th with black vomit. The woman that attended her in her accouchement, Mrs Borde, was also attacked with the disease, admitted into hospital on 29 October, recovered. Mr Donnelly was soon followed by his particular friend, Captain Roberts, Commanding engineer, in whose house he had always lived till the breaking out of the sickness when, for the purpose of being more convenient to his hospital duty, he moved up to one of Mr Bradley's rooms in the hospital. Captain Roberts was assiduous in his attentions to him during his illness and was with him in his last moments. He was taken ill on 13 November and died on the 17th. Mr Bradley, surgeon, Royal Artillery, in whose bedroom Mr Donnelly had died, was also taken ill about the same time had a very severe attack but recovered. I before mentioned the cases of Mr and Mrs Graham as connected with the sickness in the family of the Berry's (sic).

In the next quarter close to his forming, I may say part of the same building was Lieutenant Andrews, Royal Artillery, and his wife Mrs Andrews was ill with fever, the particulars of whose case I am unacquainted with, but the servant that was in the house at the same time, James Lindsay, was admitted into hospital on 28 October and died 2 November with black vomit. I do not know of any other officer or of any of their families of this department (who, of course, are not being exposed in a similar way) having been even affected with the disease. Of all persons connected with the military, far the most unfortunate in point of suffering from this severe malady were seven families of decent working people engaged in various employments in the storekeeper's department, consisting of seventeen persons, men, women and children, of whom they lost nine. Two of the families were entirely carried off by it, viz, Mr Catchlove with his wife and child and Mr and Mrs Ford. The disease appeared malignant early among these people than any I have yet mentioned, and I have already stated that it seems to have been communicated from them to the Sappers and Miners, those amongst whom the progress of it was last treated of, the particulars of which will be presently explained.

I do not include with these the Assistant Storekeeper General Mr Haversatt and his wife as though he paid every due attention to them during their sickness [he] cautiously avoided coming in contact with them in compliance with a recommendation he had received for his own security. They, in consequence, were not exposed to or affected by it, while the others attended one another without any such precaution and were accordingly attacked in succession. The situation of the dwellings was supposed by some to be the cause of the sickness amongst them. Houses were, therefore, hired for their accommodation on Collymore Rock Road. A situation reputed as one of the healthiest in the island, but being near the town and as, the only object was change of situation and not separation of the healthy from the infected, which, to my own knowledge and against my wish and directions was neglected, [no] benefit resulted from the change. They suffered as much in their new as in their former residency, to which their survivors have since returned and are now enjoying good health. The quarters occupied by the four families first attacked with this disease were situated as follows: the main road from the garrison through the bay to the town passes off obliquely at an acute angle from one corner of the garrison (which being on higher ground at first with a gentle descent) to the more low-level course of the bay road. At a little distance from this corner, a short by-road of about fifty or sixty yards in length runs off from the side of the garrison directly at right angles with a steeper descent to meet the former ones and in the flat triangular spaces below, included between these two roads before meeting. The rocky cliffs of the garrison ground behind and to windward is the engineer's yard. In this yard, at the angle of junction of the two roads, is the quarter then occupied by the Berry family and at the opposite side of the main road directly facing the short one are two wooden houses so near each other that it is easy to step from the door of one into that of the other – each divided into two rooms by a centre partition so as to leave one good one for each of the four families abovementioned. These people, not being distinguishable from civilians in general by any particular dress could not be stopped by the sentries and therefore had constantly a free and unrestrained communication with the bay and town where the disease had been prevailing for some time before. Mr and Mrs Turner, occupying one of the centre rooms were the first affected. He was taken ill on 1 October, and she about the 3rd. he recovered, but she died on the 11th in her quarter. Hers though a fatal was not a strongly marked case. She stated that she had been in town the day before being taken ill and that she had been in the habit of going there repeatedly. The inhabitants of the other centre room were next seized with the fever, the husband, Alexander M'Carlo, on 17 October and the wife on the 19th. They were taken up to the Naval Hospital, and both recovered. In the next room, an end one in the same house, the family of the late Catchlows lived, which was soon entirely carried off by it. Mr Catchlow was attacked on 20 October and removed to the Naval Hospital on the 25th, where he died on the 27th. His wife complained on the 30th, remained in her quarter and died there on 3 November. Their only child, Henry Catchlow, taken ill on 2 November, was removed to the Naval Hospital on the 4th, where [the child] also died on the 7th. The only remaining individuals of this party not yet affected were of the family of the Truemans occupying the other end room. They attended the Catchlows and took care of the child till its removal to hospital. They appeared to be the next destined subjects for the disease. Still, as it was ascribed by some entirely to situations, it was expected to save them by a change of residence to a healthier one, which was carried into effect about this time, but to no purpose. For in the new quarter, Mrs Trueman was very soon (on 4 November) attacked with the same disease. She recovered, but her husband, taken ill on the 8th, died there on the 12th with black vomit, and more lately, as will appear presently, other families that removed here at the same time from other quarters also shared the same fate. Thus, it ran through the four families, not exempting from attack a single individual belonging to them. During its entire course, there had not been the least interruption of a free and friendly intercourse amongst them. They visited, attended and gave every assistance to each other throughout the entire [time], which was necessary from their not having had servants.

From what I have already stated respecting the relative situation of Corporal Berry's quarter and the houses occupied by these people, their proximity may be understood, they being opposite to one another on the same road, only the breadth of the road distance between them, and that a close friendly intercourse also subsisted between the inhabitants themselves is certain from the acknowledgement of Mrs Berry that she had dressed out the body of Mrs Turner, the first of these women that died, adding the remark that "a fine corpse it was". Thus, the origin of it in this family that suffered so severely, having lost four children in consequence of it, is sufficiently and satisfactorily accounted for and its introduction from thence into the corps it belonged to and by which the garrison, in general, was so much endangered through the media of those different persons who from having had connection or personal communication with them when sick as before stated were themselves affected with the disease though living in different situations.

The Sergeant Major Jameson, in whose house I saw some of the sick children and who was himself very soon after severely attacked, lived in a very comfortable quarter close to the top of that short by-road before described, leading into the garrison. Mr Graham, Draughtsman, who had another of the children and lost his wife by it, lived in a quarter up in the garrison itself. And Kinnaird, that died of black vomit for whom Mrs Berry washed, was the first person in the barrack affected with it and, after which it soon began to spread through that barrack.

Thus, is clearly made out the source and progress in this instance of this malignant disease in the garrison hitherto healthy and which continued so to those not exposed to it by some communication with the sick.

The 21st Regiment in the same garrison, I may say from the facts I have already fully mentioned, continued very healthy and unaffected by it for two months afterwards. The three other families of the Storekeeper's Department lived at first in the dockyard but what remained of them were removed in the beginning of November, the same time with the others also to the hired houses on Collymore Rock Road. Previous to this change, Mr Ford had been taken ill on 29 October, removed to the hospital on the 31st, accompanied by his wife, who insisted on attending him, where he died on 5 November with black vomit. The wife had been taken ill on 1 November and died on the 4th. I have already stated that the Truemans were early affected in their new quarters, and a week had hardly elapsed after the death of her husband when, to my surprise and annoyance, I saw Mrs Trueman mixed with the other people. The total disregard and neglect of precautionary or preventive measures among these people was, therefore, very evident. In consequence, it was no way surprising that while the disease continued to prevail about in different directions, it should have reappeared amongst them even after a residence of more than five weeks in their new, usually reputed, very healthy quarters.

On 10 December, Mr Hussy and Mr Clarke were both attacked with fever. The one remained in his quarter, where he was attended by a private practitioner and died on the 14th. The other was removed to hospital the following day, where he also died the same time as the former. Both had black vomit. The child of Hussy was soon afterwards affected but recovered. Mrs Clarke, though she attended her husband throughout, entirely escaped. Thus, all these families have suffered, none, whether in the new or the old quarters, experience an exemption from this fatal epidemic.

The white persons of the quarter and barrack department consisting principally of artificers discharged from the old corps that have served in this command (several of which are now reduced) and mostly employed as non-commissioned officers in this department in their several avocations and to superintend and direct the coloured and black people in the employ of the department. They are thus mostly old residents in the country and a much more unconnected set than any. I have yet mentioned each having a separate residence (all out of the garrison) many of them distinct charges and generally employed separately in their respective businesses, but a most dissipated set. For from their high rates of pay and the nature of their situations, they have both the means and opportunity of indulging in drink, which they do to great excess, squandering away all their money on it and by which they shorten considerably [the] periods of their natural existence. Their cases are always severe ones. Of necessity, the same restrictions could not be imposed on them as on the military in general. They had liberty to pass and repass the sentries and thus enjoyed a free communication with the bay and town. Consequently, one of the very first cases from the military connected with the garrison admitted into the hospital with this malignant disease, which I am treating, was from amongst them and others from the same party occurred afterwards. Corporal Bradshaw admitted 12 October died on the 15th with black vomit. He had most usually lived with a woman in the bay. Sergeant Banks, who had come out with the 21st Regiment from England but now employed in this department, was taken ill about 6 November while living in and in charge of Colonel Popham's house at Collymore Rock Road during the absence of the family at St Lucia. He remained there 'till the black vomit had made its appearance when he was removed into a small neighbouring house, and his sickness reported. He died there on 13 November. I shall have to mention this case again as the source of the disease to Colonel Popham's family, though his wife, who attended him, escaped. They were but lately married and had no children.

Sergeant White from the dockyard admitted into hospital on 23 November, died on the 25th furiously delirious. Mrs Vaux, from the same place, was admitted on 28 November with a severe case attended with dark-coloured vomit but notwithstanding which she recovered. She was followed by her husband on 8 December, a less severe case, and who also recovered. From a neighbouring quarter in the same dockyard was admitted on 16 December, William Raisbrook, and who died after much black vomit on the 19th. His wife had left him and was living with another man. Neither he nor the preceding man had children. Corporal Rodusky and Farrar, also from the dockyard, were next admitted on 20 December. The first one died on the 24th after having passed much black matter by stool. The other recovered. The houses of these people, though a separate distinct one for each, are all in a cluster near each other. The two latter men were single, but the last one of all, Corporal Farrar, had a mustee[6] woman known by the name of Beccy Mand living with him, whom when I went to see Mrs Vaux and had to order her up to the Naval Hospital; I found sitting behind her on the bed supporting her in her arms. I soon afterwards heard of this woman having died after a very short illness. When Corporal Farrar, the man with whom she lived, was brought to hospital, the bed on which he lay in the cart that brought him being merely a palliasse case filled with shavings was observed to be stained with dark coloured marks which he declared himself were from the black vomit of his wife as he termed her, who had lately died, and which required several washings before they could be completely removed. The shavings were burnt. The palliasse case is yet in store here. Such was the connection between these cases which I thus accidentally became acquainted with.[7]

Lieutenant Palmer lately of the 63rd Regiment, [in] charge of the Africans employed as military labourers, resided in the dockyard in a good, large house, but one closet of which was separate from part of the house occupied by Mr Forde before mentioned by only a very slight wooden partition. On 17 November, one of his children was attacked with fever and soon afterwards, two others in quick succession. The only remaining one, the fourth, was sent to the country and escaped. Mrs Palmer was next taken ill, and lastly, himself worn out and exhausted by the fatigue and anxiety in attending on and watching over his wife and children (for two days before his illness, he had not taken off his clothes or gone to bed regularly) was seized with it after much black vomit and died on 1 December. The others of the family recovered. One of the children lay for nearly two weeks in a very doubtful, almost hopeless state. Its stools were black, and it was only supported for several days by brandy and water till, at length, on the 14th day, a favourable change took place. Mrs Palmer having been confined in her bowels just before her attack with the fever, I directed some plain Calomel[8] pills for her with the double purpose of opening her bowels and by affecting the system slightly to counteract the liability and even the effects of the disease itself should it come on. But on being attacked, she took the pills faster than I directed so that the mouth became much sorer than I could have wished, which, however, I think, rather tended to mitigate the disease and promote her recovery.

I have already stated the circumstance of Sergeant Banks being taken ill with the fever of which he died while living at and in charge of Lieutenant Colonel Popham's house at Collymore Rock Road, which was formerly the residence of the Barrack and Quarter Master General. It is a very fine large house and has always had the character of being one of the healthiest in the neighbourhood of the town or garrison. I have known it resorted to on this account by Colonel Dolphin, well acquainted with the island when commandant and in a bad state of health with the hope of being benefited by a change to a situation so remarkably healthy. Sergeant Banks occupied a bedroom of one of the young ladies and remained there unknown to be sick till after black vomit had actually shown itself. The family in a few days, returned to the house. The inspector, Mr Green, informed me that the young daughter, the first of the family taken ill, had slept on a temporary bed made on two easy chairs that had been in the room occupied by Sergeant Banks and on which he observed himself some dark suspicious-looking stains. Sergeant Banks had been taken ill on the 6th and died on 10 November.

An African named Thomas Bull, employed in the house and who had most likely attended Sergeant Banks and assisted in his removal, was next taken ill with fever, for which he was admitted into hospital on the 12th and died on the 14th. Another African, Lord Blarney, also employed among the domestics in the house, was admitted on the 24th and died on the 26th after having thrown up much decided black vomit as reported to me at the time by Mr Caverhill and whose notes on the subject I have given to the inspector. The young ladies of the family were in a few days affected. This affected Norma

Popham, a fine, grown-up young girl about sixteen years old. After that so frequent symptom, black vomit [she] was carried off by it on 3 December. They also lost a white female servant, and Taylor Wilson of the 21st Regiment, living as coachman there, was admitted into hospital ill with fever on the 11 December and died on the 14th. Such was havoc it made in this family, though in a situation remarkable for its salubrity, so little respect does this disease pay to the situations of either places or persons.

Mr Caverhill,[8] hospital assistant, whom I mentioned in a former report as having resisted and entirely escaped the disease when it prevailed epidemically in Dominica in the year 1817, has not been, I am sorry to say, fortunate this time. He was attached to the barrack department and had charge of the military labour hospital which always did him great credit. He was acted on by the cause, being deeply depressed in spirit and affected with great anxiety and uneasiness of mind that evidently weighed heavy on him from an unpleasant circumstance that had then recently occurred. On 3 December, he slept in Colonel Popham's house and had, I am informed, voluntarily assisted in putting the body of Miss. Monica Popham into the coffin. He was also otherwise exposed in attendance on a private patient as well as others then labouring under the disease. He was taken ill on the night of 7 December and died on the 9th, having thrown up much black vomit and been but about forty-eight hours ill.

The small detachment of the staff corps forming part of this department, but the men being quartered in the garrison in the same barrack with the 21st Fusiliery entirely escaped [unlike] the Sergeant Ludford with his family living out of the garrison in a detached house near the large lime kiln before mentioned as marshy. The situation of an encampment of one party of the families that were put under canvass in its neighbourhood and while these thus exactly similarly situated as to ground and situation and though more exposed to the weather but not exposed to the cause of this disease by any communication with the infected were enjoying good health. The disease ran through this family, though sheltered in a good, comfortable dwelling and carried off both the father and mother. Sergeant Ludford was admitted on 15 November and died on the 17th with black vomit. Mrs Ludford was taken ill on the 19th. She could not be persuaded to leave her house or submit to be removed to hospital. She died also with black vomit on 25 November. Four children had been previously affected with slighter attacks of fever for which they were treated in Mr Caverhill's hospital and recovered. After the death of their parents, the children were taken up to the Naval Hospital, where they were taken care of and kept out of the way for some time. Luckily, it seems from some circumstances there had been no communication whatever between this family and the rest of the corps, which was in the barracks in the garrison, nor with the people encamped in the neighbourhood, which was positively forbidden. Therefore, no ill consequences ensued amongst them.

But two white women of the 1st West India Regiment, Mrs Minden and Mrs Best, whom the surgeon doctor McCreery[10] informed had been clearly ascertained to have gone into the house to see Mrs Ludford while sick and the first mentioned one in my presence acknowledge[d] to have taken the infant child of Mrs Ludford from the house and to have suckled it the day of its mother's death, were themselves soon afterwards attacked with fever and admitted into hospital. Previous to this not a single case any ways resembling this fever had occurred in this regiment. Mrs Ludford had died on 25 November, and these women were admitted into hospital on the 29th. Mrs Minden's was a severe case. She passed first much black and afterwards bloody matter by stool. They both recovered of the fever, but Mrs Minden ultimately died on 24 December of a recurrence of chronic dysentery that she had before laboured under and which there supervened on the fever.

On dissection after death, the large intestines were found extensively ulcerated after this one decided. Two suspicious cases occurred among the few white non-commissioned officers of this corps; the paymaster sergeant Frawly admitted on 25 November, but as delirium early appeared and principally prevailed afterwards and from his known habits of intemperance it was marked and considered as a case of delirium tremors (sic). I saw him daily and even [from] the general appearances throughout the course of the case rather thought it a very suspicious one. Drum Major Matthews, a very singular case, was admitted on 6 December. I was present and examined him when he first entered the hospital. He complained only of general debility and pains in his bones; his pulse was perfectly tranquil and regular skin natural, and no other appearance of fever present that I could perceive, and he continued so till about four days afterwards when delirium and decided black vomit (which I saw myself) came on, he was then removed to the Naval Hospital where he finally recovered. Sergeant Armourer Brandt was admitted on 17 December with fever, died on the 22nd. No black vomit appeared, but his skin was very yellow before death. Not a commissioned officer of this regiment was affected.

In a former report on this disease, as it prevailed at Tobago the latter end of 1818 and beginning of 1819, I mentioned that the blacks, though far less subject to it than the whites, were not altogether exempt from it, of which I then gave a few instances.[11] In this one, I have already stated the cases of two young Africans, Thomas Bull and Lord Blarney, who came from Colonel Popham's house, the last of whom threw up black vomit abundantly before his death. Sometime before this, there was shown to Mr Green and myself by Mr Caverhill some matter of black vomit that he had just found in the stomach of a young African who had died after an illness of but two or three days and on going into the dead house to see the body found the eyes of it quite yellow. About that time, I observed also in his hospital other cases of fever of a very loss character among the same description of persons that seemed to suffer from the bleedings which he then practised with confidence and success but which now rather required wine and stimulants to rouse and support them and by the use of which they were evidently benefited.

I have thus gone over in detail the deaths caused by this malignant epidemic amongst the military in and about the garrison from its commencement till its termination. I have, therefore, had to include those that occurred since 20 December, the date of the accompanying return, with the double purpose of giving a corrected view of the entire from beginning to end and for completing my remarks up to the time of being relieved as principal medical officer by Dr Menzies,[12] deputy inspector of hospitals. I have dwelt the more, particularly on the deaths, the cases terminating thus having been the most strongly marked one in which we had also the advantage of dissection afterwards to aid us in our decision on them, therefore the most unequivocal in their nature and as being in themselves strongly positive certain facts of undeniable occurrence altogether best fitted for drawing inferences from or founding conclusions on.

By a contrary course too generally pursued from an overwhelming desire of generalizing and a consequent neglect of proper discrimination all cases of fever occurring in this climate from the slightest febrile attacks merely following a debauch and subsiding of itself by rest and temperance for a day or two to those of the most malignant epidemic as well as the marsh fevers endemic in some places, are all confounded together as one in kind, originating from one cause and only differing in degree from each other, whereby the most false doctrines both as to theory and practice have been deduced from them thus all lumped together and been supported with much keenness [as to] some degree of plausibility. Such has been the principal source of all the doubts and difficulties on the subject and from which I have known some fatal errors in practice.

Before entering on the rise and progress of the late epidemic generally in the island as far as it fell under my own observation or came within my knowledge, I wish to premise that since my return to this island from England in May 1817, though during the remainder of that year, the entire of 1818 and till the close of 1819 while in this island, I had the charge of and attendance on the sick in General Hospital and have always during the entire time been in the daily habit of visiting outpatients. I can positively declare I have not seen one single instance of black vomit in any of the various cases of fever that came under my care or inspection here during the entire period till the commencement of the late epidemic, so very frequently attended with that symptom which prevailed here last half year.

On this point, as a matter of fact, I am happy to have the concurring testimony of the other medical officers in charge of hospitals however differing from mine in opinion. I annex the answers by each to the questions proposed by me to them individually on the subject. The only exception real or apparent that has fallen within my notice was in [the] year 1817 in the case of Mr Pitman, a commissary, when I attended jointly with Dr Bow,[13] who states that he threw up black vomit but which I was not present at and not having been laid by for my inspection, I did not see. But more lately, in the same year, I was present at the examination of a body after death where port wine that was found in the stomach which, to my knowledge, the subject having when alive been my patient had swallowed just before death, and which was then distinguishable by the smell was mistaken by him for black vomit and which would have been very apt to have deceived any person not aware of the circumstance. To Surgeon McDermott[14] of the 4th Regiment, lately arrived from Grenada, I proposed verbally the same question and received a decided answer to the same purport, that though during nearly two years which they served there since their arrival from England, they experienced some losses by deaths from fever, yet in not a single instance had he seen black vomit there. This simple fact of the entire absence of it in the one case while it so generally prevails in the other, thus well attested by these different persons of itself marking decided distinction and a wide difference between the fevers ordinarily to be met with and this occasional visitant as a malignant destructive epidemic I conceive sufficient to remove all doubt on the question of their identity or diversity. Indeed, their general character, consequent and attending circumstances are altogether so little alike that I am at a loss to perceive the slightest affinity between them.

While other places with which this one constantly maintained a free unrestrained intercourse were suffering under the wide-spreading calamity, it was not to be expected that this could have long escaped it. When it had commenced to rage at Demerara, apprehensions were entertained of its reaching this island from the very frequent communication generally passing between them. Regulations were therefore instituted by the Governor Lord Combermere for the examination of vessels coming from thence and to prevent the landing of any persons or things from them till after such examination should have taken place in order, if possible, to guard against the introduction of the disease this way. But soon afterwards, when in consequence of a captain of a mail boat having concealed the death of a passenger, Mrs Spread, an actress who died of the disease on board his vessel while on the passage to this place till it was discovered when the other passengers [who] had landed were separated and scattered through the island. It was wished to inflict some penalty on him. The discovery was made that there was no law or authority whatever for it in force here. The regulations, of course, were no longer observed or even thought of, and even afterwards, the communication was totally uncontrolled and unrestricted. It is well known that some of the vessels that called here on their way home were, at the time infected and continued to suffer even after having left this island. I have also heard of persons lying ill of the fever in town just after their arrival from thence. It would, therefore, be only surprising could this place have escaped under such circumstances and would have afforded no bad plea against the idea of contagion. However, the reverse as was making to have been expected has unluckily happened.

The first cases that this time came under my own observation were in the latter end of July, the last in two discharged soldiers from the 66th Regiment. On 29 July, when returning home, I was called into a small house on the roadside to see the first, Mr Freeman, a baker. He told me that he had been ill with fever for two or three days. He was then to my concern and alarm for the garrison throwing up black vomit and died the same night. I had asked him if he saw or knew of any other person affected the same way. He said one of his comrades who worked at the same business and place with him [was] also ill. I made him out the next day and found him in the same state, also throwing up black vomit and, which was followed by the same event, death, a few hours afterwards, though in neither case would state of the pulse which in both was tolerably full and regular, nor indeed any other of the symptoms or appearances but black vomit have indicated the extreme danger that they were then in. The last man was sitting up out of bed, and his skin was very yellow when I saw him. I lost no time in making Mr Green acquainted with the circumstances, and which were also purposely made known generally throughout the garrison as a caution and in order to put all persons on their guard. Mr Green also visited and saw the last man himself. The bodies were interred as expeditiously as well could be by Black Pioneers, and other precautions recommended so that no ill consequences ensued.

I learned that they had both worked and lived together at a Mr Maurey's, a French baker, at the end of the bay within a few doors of the bridge leading into the town till seized with sickness when they withdrew to the small wooden dwellings of the black or coloured woman that they had before co-habited with. Passing Mr Maurey's house the following week on my way to town, I enquired how the rest of the family were and was told that a white servant woman or housekeeper was lying ill with fever above stairs, who they asked me to look at. She was then labouring under irritability of stomach, which I understood afterwards to have been moderated or stopped by the expressed juice of wormwood[15] given in teaspoonful doses, but after a very short interval, black vomit supervened with an excessive haemorrhage from the uterus. She died on 14 August. On coming down I found a black man belonging to Mr Maurey lying stretched across the bottom of the stairs, also ill with fever which had just commenced and proved a severe long continued one, though he eventually recovered. Mrs Maurey complained to me a few days afterwards (when again passing the house and asking how they did) of slight febrile symptoms, not so severe, however, as to confine her to bed, though she was evidently alarmed, and her eyes were yellow. She appeared of a delicate habit, perhaps it might have been but a slight bilious attack. She and her husband were both Creoles and had no children. I went into the bakehouse, and the persons working there, being to the best of my recollection one white and two black or coloured men, told me that they had all lately experienced more or less severe attacks of fever so as to have obliged each of them to have absented himself from his work for some time. I asked Mr Maurey if he knew of any other persons in his neighbourhood having been lately affected or dying of the disease. He immediately pointed to the house directly opposite at the other side of the way belonging to a respectable merchant, a Mr Allen, from which two young men comrades had just before died. The one in the country at an estate belonging to Mr Allen, I understand, between town and Speights, on going down to which the young man sickened and after a few days died. The other soon shared the same fate in town and followed his comrade, which account I had confirmed from others afterwards. A short time afterwards, Mr Jenkins, a purveyor's clerk of whom I used to make enquiries as living at but a little distance from Mr Maurey's, informed me that a black servant girl of his next door neighbour, a Mr Luke, who had been in the habit of visiting and sitting with the other women at Mr Maurey's when sick, was herself taken ill and also died of black vomit. It then spread to others of Mr Luke's family, of whom altogether two died and two recovered. Mr Jenkins himself suffered a smart febrile attack. In a house almost directly opposite to his, the family of a Mr Caves was nearly annihilated by the fever, for out of five persons, there remained but one survivor, and that one after an almost unexpected recovery from a very severe attack. The fever continued to make [such] ravages in the bay that I never passed through it without meeting the bier conveyance away of the dead.

The bay, as it is termed, is merely the road of about a mile and a half in length between the town and garrison adjacent to the seashore and lined on each side nearly the entire way by a continuation of houses, most of them poor, small wooden ones. Above Beckles Spring (which forms a good stream of clear, pure water constantly running across the road into the sea) and towards the garrison, there is one small part that has generally a damp, unfavourable appearance. In consequence of, the water from the ground above having percolated through the porous coral rock and spread over the low-level ground below before it finds its way to the sea. But I have not usually perceived any bad smell from it nor heard of the houses there being particularly unhealthy, nor was it near this that the disease commenced or mostly prevailed. It had also spread through the town in different directions, causing much mortality and even reached Speightstown (between which and this one, large boats are daily passing), where I am informed, it likewise made havoc, and different cases of it that proved fatal occurred here and there in the country. The last that I heard of and which were but very lately too, were of a Mr Bascombe who died in the bay. His niece died the same day in town. Both, I am told, with black vomit. And his brother, residing in the country, who it seems visited him when sick and was seen at his funeral, was shortly afterwards attacked, but I suppose recovered. I have not heard of his death.

The garrison had continued, for a considerable time after the appearance and prevalence of the disease, all about being healthy and perfectly free from it. The men, having been forbidden and prevented from going to either the town or bay, not being permitted to pass the sentries placed around. The first man admitted into any of the military hospitals was William Green from Kings House nigh the town, who had been a servant to Captain Campbell, aide-de-camp to Sir Frederick Robinson, commanding the forces at present. He had been one of a party of recruits for the patriotic army in South America wrecked in a vessel off the back of the island, several of whom deserted and remained behind here after the others had got off. He had been hired by Captain Campbell as a groom but dismissed for misconduct by him. When leaving this [island] for Tobago, having obtained an artillery man to look after his house during his absence, this man, after having been away some time, returned on the night of 25 September begging and praying the one then in charge who had succeeded him to admit him into a small house he occupied near the stables as being very sick and entirely destitute of any shelter or support who moved by his distressed situation, admitted him, spread his great coat for him on the floor and when he found him in the middle of the night so very ill, gave up his own bed to him.

These circumstances, becoming known the following day among the other servants reached the family of Sir Frederick Robinson then here and excited considerable alarm amongst them. The man was, therefore hurried off to hospital that evening, and the medical officer that received him, not suspecting the complaint, placed him in a ward with other patients. His admission was unknown to me till his death was also reported the following morning when I likewise learned that he had thrown up much black vomit, part of which was on the wall beside his bed. After the removal of the body, the doors and jalousies being closed, the ward and all in it were thoroughly fumigated by means of fumigating lamps and burning port fires in it, which happened to have been at hand. The (sulphurous acid fumes from which may be supposed to be of use) while another ward was equipping with fresh, clean beds, drapes, utensils, etc., for the reception of these patients into which they were immediately removed after being cleaned and purified and having left everything behind them in the other ward for the purification of which also every pains were taken before the admission of any fresh patients into it. The man, having been so short a time in the ward, only for one night, it is most likely that there had been no personal contact between him and any of the others, so that, it happened, no harm was done nor any other patient affected in consequence.

I directly afterwards went to Kings House and found the bedding and things used by this man spread out to dry and learned that no other person had used them after him. I had them collected by a black pioneer and put in the house that he had been admitted into, the window of which being secured, I locked the door, keeping possession of the key myself and having obtained the inspector's sanction, had the man that had admitted him removed to the Naval Hospital, where he remained under observation in a place by himself for twenty-one days. He, I am glad to say, entirely escaped, not having suffered the slightest attack.

The house was soon after thoroughly fumigated in the presence of Mr Green and myself through a hole cut in the door by means of a machine constructed according to his directions. The wooden bedstead that he had lain on was also burnt in our presence and the remainder of the things which were capable of being washed were removed in a cart to the Naval Hospital for that purpose. The house, after having been well-ventilated for some time through the jalousies of the windows that were left constantly open, was well-cleaned and whitewashed, and I then surrendered the key. No case whatever occurred afterwards among the family, their servants or the people living in any of the outbuildings within the precincts of Kings House.

The next cases connected with the military were at Rickett's Battery at the very opposite remote end of the town from that towards the garrison in the family of Gunner Carson, who had been left there alone with his family in charge of the place. His son, who was his only child, died in the morning and his wife on the night of 4 October. It was reported to me on the 5th by the surgeon of artillery, who was only made acquainted with it himself the day before when the child had already died, and the mother was dying with black vomit. They having been attended by a private town practitioner, called in by them, when Mr Green and myself, in company with the surgeon, went the same day to visit the place, we found sailors drinking there, and from the bottles, liquors and apparatus around it was clear that he had kept a kind of canteen or grog shop for the resort of such persons. It was even mentioned to us that one of the patriots before alluded to had been seen lying sick in his place but the week before and that he was then warned of the danger that might result there from. This was told to us by the Brigade Major Crittenden captain of artillery who had been informed so by some of his own people, but the man, in the most solemn positive manner, denied it. He was taken up to the Artillery Hospital and placed under observation in a room by himself, where I saw him after a day or two suffering under a smart attack of fever, but which speedily terminated in a free copious perspiration, and he quickly recovered. It was of such short duration that whether it might have been a slight form of the same fever as the wife and child had died [of] or had been only induced by personal fatigue joined with mental uneasiness. I will not pretend to say; I merely state the fact as it actually happened. The place he had occupied at the fort was fumigated, cleared out, cleaned, white-washed in the same manner as I have described to have been done to the place at Kings House, after which another Gunner was sent there to succeed him, and no fresh case has appeared there since.

Thus, widely had this disease extended itself in different directions, though as yet the garrison at St Ann's remained healthy and quite free from it. But as the danger became so extensive and threatening and by possibility might reach us notwithstanding the preventive measures adopted, which from what I have already stated will be seen to have been carried into effect but incompletely and partially, it became necessary to take some steps for the reception of it in order that while every care and comfort was provided for and secured to the sick, yet by counteracting in every possible way its great tendency to spread from them to others, it might be arrested in its further course and progress and the evils to be dreaded from it if not altogether, prevented at least thus considerably reduced by being confined within very narrow limits. The late Naval Hospital was cleared of all. Still, one maniacal and two leprous patients who, however, were kept apart in detached places by themselves, and it was allotted exclusively for cases of the malignant fever being kept closed off as it were in a state of quarantine.

Black orderlies were procured from the 1st West India Regiment to attend on such cases but turned out so totally useless from extreme stupidity that it was found necessary to hire for this purpose black-coloured women natives of the island, who proved very useful and intelligent and who having been in the island when the disease before at different times prevailed in it, were little likely now to catch it.[16] Fumigating lamps and materials were supplied plentifully and were kept constantly in use in the wards while there were any sick in there. In each of the other hospitals, the most detached room was appropriated as an observation ward for the reception of all slight, ordinary or doubtful fever cases, which were also attended by black servants, all others having been strictly forbidden to enter it and where fumigation with nitrous or oxymuriatic[17] acid gas by means of fumigating lamps was constantly practised. In twenty-four hours, the character of such malignant cases as might have been before doubtful generally became sufficiently developed to enable us to decide on their nature and to determine on their removal to the naval hospital in which discriminations and decisions I usually assisted in my daily visits to all the hospitals. In a very few cases, the fatal symptoms came so rapidly that we had not time for their removal, and on some occasions when the sick in this ward were becoming a little numerous, amounting to perhaps four, five or six persons and that a decided malignant case had appeared amongst them, the entire were removed to the Naval Hospital, but the slighter cases avowedly as such were carefully separated and put in distinct wards from the others and the observation ward being thus cleared out was well cleaned and made ready for the reception of fresh cases. The bedding, clothing, and so on that had been used by these people while in hospital, as well as those belonging to themselves, always accompanied them when removed and were afterwards burnt or well purified, washed and aired as circumstances required. The bedding of those that died were always burnt, all articles belonging to persons attached with fever were required to be sent along with them to hospital where they were well-washed, cleaned and aired by black pioneers before they were again restored to them. In the Naval Hospital, a store was fitted up, made close and provided with a fumigating apparatus made according to Mr Green's orders, where these things were first received and well fumigated before they were given to the black women, constantly employed for the purpose of washing them and afterwards were exposed to the air for some considerable time before they were restored to their owners on being discharged from hospital and who were also after this report for two or three weeks at an intermediate place called a convalescent hospital on full, fresh rations before being allowed to join their companies to do duty in the garrison. The surgeons and medical officer in charge of parties or departments were required to be particularly attentive in their inspections so as to have separated immediately on being taken ill and sent to hospital all persons affected with the slightest appearance of fever.

I have already stated the beneficial effects from encampment in arresting the progress of the disease and putting an entire stop to it. After it had been clearly ascertained to have got into the barracks of the 21st Fusiliers of the artillery and of the Sappers and Miners and of having by the same means saved several families altogether from it though while under canvass. They experienced some severe wet weather to secure them the better, from which the tents were generally made double by putting one inside the other and to raise them a little from the ground. A flooring was made in each tent by some rough, un-planed boards being laid loosely over two or three joists. The timber was obtained from the barrack department. There was no trouble in preparing it nor any expense incurred as it continued unaltered and fit for the original purpose of building.

The tents were also rather served by the airing they got [which] were but for three or four persons at farthest placed in each. They had been supplied with palliasses and pillowcases stuffed with thrash (sic) to lie on and blankets to cover them. They expressed themselves as being very well-contented and very comfortable. The encampments took place not at one and same but at different times and with the same decided good effects each time as before fully detailed. The final result of all these measures will be manifested by contrasting the very trifling losses experienced by those bodies of persons amongst whom they have been carried into effect fully and completely with what others suffered who had not the full benefit of them. From partial or total non-observance of them, and with the ravages uniformly committed by this dreadful disease whenever and wherever it has made its appearance (unless opposed by some such similar steps) which has happened in other islands and places very lately and in this one in the year 1816, when last visited by this malignant epidemic and at which time the white troops were exactly similarly situated as those last year. They having been both quartered in the very same barracks. It is now to be hoped that as the practicability and utility of preventive and precautionary measures have been incontestably proved that, theoretical speculations will give way to practical truths more particularly where the interests of humanity are so deeply concerned and that the lives of men may not be made the sport of or sacrificed by any self-confidence in private opinions or obstinacy of prejudice in opposition to positive incontrovertible and well-established facts. The benefit and efficacy of these measures can be no longer presented as problematical or as a mere subject matter of opinion or doubt. They have been thus tried and proved in practice. They have been put to the trial, and the proof has been decisive. They have been subjected to the test of experiment and the result has been conclusive and not in the instances only I have now related. For I have seen myself before the same decided beneficial effects from similar measures adopted and a similar course pursued in Gibraltar in 1810, on the same principle of separating. Keeping carefully separated and the preventing as far as in our power the coming in contact of the healthy with the infected, or with any thus capable of communicating the infection, which they practised afloat by means of hulks hired for the purpose of removing the healthy into them from the infected ships and ashore by means of encampment on the neutral ground to which the infected with the things belonging to them, most likely to communicate the infection were kept away and confined from all communication with the rest. The result afloat was that while those that remained in the infected vessels in communication with the sick suffered most severely and with considerable loss, the others that were removed entirely escaped and ashore, the inhabitant[s] and troops were, I may say, completely saved from the danger that then threatened them similar to what they had before experience[d] in 1804. Having been a principal and performer there then, I can fully attest all the circumstances as stated by Mr Pym in his book on the subject. Indeed, on the facts that there fell under my observation were my opinions first founded without my previous thoughts on the subject till then and which have been since fully confirmed by all my subsequent experience.

It is to be fairly presumed that the same effects will always be produced by the same measures under similar circumstances if only carried into full and complete effect. To obtain which will, however, require the utmost vigilance, care and attention as many efforts will be too often made by the thoughtless or interested to elude them. If attempted in only a partial, careless or indifferent manner from a want of confidence in the principle, it may be as well neglected altogether. An instance in proof of this occurred at Dominica in 1817. The disease, having committed some ravages among the troops on Morne Bruce, was completely arrested by the removal of the healthy part of them to Point Michel, where they remained perfectly free from it for two or three weeks, but immediately after the arrival there of some men direct from the hospital at the Morne with their baggage (which had been in store while there), the disease was again renewed amongst them and ran its course in its usually destructive manner. I might also adduce other similar instances but, which I trust is unnecessary. While it is not a little gratifying to me to have been at all instrumental towards producing the happy, good effects that resulted from the measures adopted, as I have fully detailed, had the contrary happened and, could I have had to charge myself with any of the numerous deaths that might have ensued from a neglect of them, my mind and conscience would have been very ill at rest indeed. A sentinel on his post before an enemy, if found wanting in vigilance, would be liable to suffer the punishment of death should a health officer in which light I consider all public medical men be considered less culpable who aware of such danger threatening would fail to use every possible means to avert so dreadful a public calamity was the possibility of doing so only barely probable but how much more so when it has already been actually ascertained and decidedly proved by past experience.

The few objections started in opposition to the use of preventive and precautionary means are so very futile and trivial compared with the dreadful fatal ill consequences resulting from a neglect of them and hardly to deserve any notice. It is too puerile and weak to be offered by any experienced person in their senses that the necessary alarms to warn persons against positive imminent dangers of this magnitude should not be raised from the fear of truly frightening them out of their lives. Equally groundless, at least in this part of the world, is the apprehension of the sick being deserted by and not receiving every due care and attention from their friends or attendants. Quite the contrary have I always found it the case even when the persons themselves were very sensible of the danger incurred by it where those concerned were their near relatives. Among friends, it is considered indispensable to pay visits and show civilities during the time of sickness by which practice the sick are too often improperly harassed and their friends uselessly exposed to danger. It is also the time usually chosen by the coloured and black people to ingratiate themselves with the whites by the kindness and diligent attentions paid to them then and by which they generally succeed those bestowed then being seldom forgotten afterwards so that I have generally had reason to complain of the presence of too many persons in the sick chambers. At all events, there can hardly ever be any scarcity of persons to be obtained for hire to attend the sick from the number of black, coloured, and even white persons who having passed through the disease need not be afraid of it that are constantly in want of employment and glad to be any ways employed. There was no difficulty found in procuring nurses for attending or/ and taking care of the sick in the malignant fever hospital here last year. The applicants for the situation of sick nurses in the hospital were very numerous. Though I was always concerned and had nothing whatever to do with the appointment of them, I have been repeatedly solicited and teased for my interest on the supposition that I might have had sense in obtaining it for them.

Reports from Barbados

As to commerce, could the interests of it at any time or rate be put in competition with or allowed to interfere with those of humanity[?] Could human lives be thought so cheaply of as to be put in the balance against or as it were to be trucked or bartered for pecuniary gains to be obtained in the way of traffic? Yet, in this case the losses that could possibly arise from any health regulations that might be instituted would be so very trifling indeed as to deserve very little weight or consideration. The little internal commerce carried on between the islands and colonies themselves alone could be affected, and that only occasionally and temporary with perhaps a single island or colony at a time during the prevalence of a contagious complaint in it, which usually soon runs its course and is of but short duration. The communication with the mother country, as well as with British North America, would not be likely even to suffer any interruption at least on account of this complaint. From the one are constantly arriving manufactured goods and articles of provisions and from the other, lumber, flour, cattle, etc. There is, therefore, no likelihood of ever experiencing any want of these necessary articles from any restrictions that might be imposed for the warding off of this pestilential complaint. The horrible scourge of this part of the world, which I am convinced by judicious regulations, might be completely eradicated and, if ever again renewed be early arrested and prevented from extending itself to any great distance. It is well known from the history of this island alone that there have been lapses of long periods for several years together during which it has been perfectly free from it and remained healthy.

As to the cause of the commencement and progress of the late epidemic in this island from all the foregoing facts as premises, I conceive, but one conclusion can follow showing it to have depended on the highly contagious nature of the disease and the total want and disregard of all health regulations in the island generally. It continued through all the months between June and February following, only affected by the measures that were opposed to it amongst the military. During the period, several varieties of weather occurred particularly. As to drought or moisture, it was yet progressive in its course till very lately. It seems to have died away from the want of fresh subjects susceptible of and being exposed to its influence. There has been no correspondence or similarity between the state of the weather last half year and that for the same period of the year 1816 when it before prevailed. That one was reported to have been remarkably wet and to the excess of which the disease was then ascribed, while the last has, on the contrary, been rather a dry one and the crops in consequence but very indifferent. Had it as an epidemic depended on any particular constitution of the atmosphere or state of the weather or season, it must have been more general, more simultaneous and left under our control. On such a principle, is it possible to account for the numerous exemptions among the military, mostly possible as being newcomers, breathing the same atmosphere as others and particularly exposed to the influence of the weather by night as well as day from the nature of their duties[?] Not an officer of the 21st died, much less was even affected though quartered in the very same barrack in which those of the Queen's Regiment had suffered so severely, and it is to be recollected that the trade wind constantly blowing is very uniform in its direction varying only a little to the northward or southward of east. Those of the 1st West India Regiment were equally fortunate, and of the Ordnance Department, only though few suffered or were affected who were well known, as I before stated, to have been fully exposed to the contagion of it by communication with the sick and the same remark also applies to the men of the garrison generally. Those only having been attacked with it of whom from all I have related it will be seen that there was either positive or strongly presumptive proof as to their having been exposed in a similar manner. If it depended on anything in the atmosphere breathed at the same time equally by all would it be so tardy in its progress as to have been nearly three months in the bay and town before it made its appearance in a single case in the garrison and on such a supposition would not the very steps taken to retard and arrest it and which proved so successful have rather tended to promote and forward it in its operation and have been the means of rendering it more general and destructive by removing the men from the shelter of five large comfortable barracks of mason work and exposing them the more freely to all the influence of the weather by placing them under thin canvass only, and could any miasmata or exhalation from the earth be supposed to have contributed to it would they not have been inhaled the more freely by them lying and sleeping with their noses so close to the very source of them?

Marsh fevers are, however, very different and totally unknown here except when now and then an odd case may arrive from some other island but which are generally much benefited by the change and soon disappear. The situations chosen for the encampment had no advantage over those of the barracks. In one or two instances, it was decidedly the reverse and the two companies of the 21st Regiment, when encamped so close to the rear of their own barrack and to the windward of it that in this respect there could have been no difference whatever.

From the detail of facts given, it may be seen how little it has been confined to any particular situation, not having respected even the healthiest. Colonel Popham's family suffered, as I have stated in Collymore House, remarkable for its salubrity. The families of the storekeeper's department, after a residence of five weeks in the quarters chosen for them as healthy on Collymore Rock Road were not less fortunate in this respect than in those previously occupied by them reckoned unhealthy. Therefore, deserted by them for a time, but in which the survivors are now enjoying good health. The surgery man in the Naval Hospital (always reputed as healthfully situated) as well as the one in the General Hospital, in which places they were constantly employed and continually remained, were both attacked with this disease and of which the last one died as before mentioned when the causes of their attack were also at the same time I trust clearly and satisfactorily made out, while on the other hand, it is a remarkable fact that the 21st Regiment which escaped so well mounted a small night guard during the entire prevalence of the sickness in the dockyard considered the very worst and most unhealthy situation about the garrison. I have been in the habit of examining the men whose cases proved serious as to the guards they had mounted shortly before being taken ill. I only recollect one instance of such at all connected with this guard. Lewis Burk of the 6th Company, having gone on this guard in the evening, was taken ill with fever, relieved of it early the next morning and taken into hospital. Whether the situation of his berth in barrack with respect to the other men that had been affected with the fever, or of this dockyard was the most likely cause of his illness will appear from the circumstances then and now stated.

The general character and marked features of the disease as it appeared here exactly correspond with those manifested by it as the different times and places that I have before witnessed it. However, individual cases of it may vary in many particulars. A marked malignity speedily destructive of human life independent of any increase or diminution of action in the system locally or generally is prevalent in and characteristic of the disease. In my report on the disease at Tobago I mentioned two cases in which no febrile action whatever was perceptible. The same has occurred here, this time in the case of the Drum Major of the 1st West India Regiment with whom black vomit and delirium came on about the 4th day, though his pulse had been perfectly tranquil and regular, skin natural and no appearance whatever of increased irritated or even oppressed action as is noticed in Dr McCreery's report and which I also have before stated in this one.

The cases of Thomas Berry and a few others were similar, and in many was the danger extreme, death approaching fast when the more purely febrile symptoms were moderate or even apparently favourable so that the appearances of them served but little frequently to indicate the danger being not at all in proportion to it. The remarks that I have made on the particular symptoms of the disease as it prevailed at Tobago, as well as on the distinction between this and the different other fevers, it is unnecessary for me now to repeat being applicable and corresponding equally to what I have seen of it here only that more recoveries after black vomit had come on had occurred here than I ever before witnessed. I have seen three myself and have heard of a few others. Those that I have seen myself had not been bled. Of the others, I cannot speak so positively. I only state the fact. As worthy of attention hereafter without attempting at present to draw any inference from it as to any connection between recovery after this usually so very fatal a symptom and the circumstance of their not having been bled.

The appearances on dissection I have also divest[ed] on a little in that report, and what I have stated in it in have only found confirmed by what I have seen since. The first and last fatal cases were dissected carefully myself. The first one, Kinnaird in the Artillery Hospital, in presence of Assistant Surgeon Donnelly and the last one, Fleming in the Naval Hospital, Mr Palmer,[18] assistant staff surgeon, being present but unable to perform it himself in consequence of cuts on his finger. I must acknowledge that from all I have seen I am not a little sceptical on dissection reports in general and am convinced that they should be received with no small degree of doubt and caution. Natural appearances or those brought on only by accidental circumstances are frequently considered and marked down as morbid and essential ones. Indeed, it requires considerable experience and practice to be able always to distinguish properly between them, and all appearances are very generally greatly magnified, exaggerated and not infrequently distorted and perverted to suit the imagination and meet preconceived notions. I have seen two persons at a dissection differ widely as to the colour of a part. In the moments of dying, we observed a change of colour in the skin from the blood settling and lodging, particularly in posterior and most dependent parts of the body; may there not and does there not, in fact, a similar change from the same course operating at the same time take place in some of the interior parts then concealed from our view and which is seldom or never taken into account afterwards? How much must the appearances in the head as to quantity of blood and apparently increased vascularity depend on the position of it as to being more or less prudent at the time of dying and during the operation of opening it so frequently done with great violence from the want of valves in the veins and sinuses allowing the blood so easily to recede in them? I have known adhesions that are constant and natural made as morbid ones, and when the appearance of the brain appeared to me hardly changed from natural, I have seen it noted down as highly vascular and inflamed. Principally, I believe because the person noting it conceived it ought to be so to meet his view of the case. In the thorax, the appearance of the lungs is apt to be varied and affected by the longer or shorter duration of the sickness, the quantity of blood in the system generally as well as by other incidental circumstances. In the abdomen, I have been in the habit of paying particular attention to the state of the stomach and have, in all cases of whatever complaint the patient may have died, found the posterior side towards the lesser arch and the cardiac orifice of a more or less red vascular appearance and have known it when so in a slighter degree after this than other very different complaints noted down as indicating high inflammation. Perhaps the very prevalent use of ardent spirits may contribute to this appearance, so generally here, accidental scratches from the nails of the operator are overlooked at the moment of happening. I have reason to think to be sometimes mistaken for abrasions, erosions and, etc. From the delicacy of the mucous membrane and its being so easily detached, I abstain even from applying a rough sponge to it and merely rinse it out in water. The effects of the gastric juice on it should be also considered and, which I am inclined to think sometimes tends towards the apparently increased vascularity of the black part by leaving the blood vessels there more bare of the coats covering them and thus bringing them more into view. I have certainly never seen any disorganization of the coats of the stomach by gangrene in this complaint, though I have known slight superficial discolorations marked such. In some cases where, at first view, the small intestines generally looked very healthy on unravelling, tracing them along and drawing out the most dependent lying hid in the pelvis on the very lowest parts of these, I have found vascular or bloody flaking patches. After this, as well as other complaints, on dissection of the last subject, Fleming, who was examined very soon after death on cutting through the steguments preparatory to sawing the cranium, there spewed about twenty-four ounces of blood from the blood vessels of the head which was collected in a small basin. I observed [it] coagulated afterwards and separated regularly into crassamentum[19] and serum. The crassamentum was rather lax in its texture and amounted in weight to a pound, and the serum filled an eight-ounce measure and coagulated firmly on the application of heat.

    On washing the crassamentum till, part of the fibrina appeared clear of the red particles and, in the form of white membranous substances (which was a very tedious process), was reduced to the weight of but a few ounces and the washings on the application of heat formed a coagulated serum on the surface. It must have, therefore in coagulating, retained a considerable portion of the serous or albuminous part. About twelve ounces of pure-looking black vomit was found in his stomach, which I had also laid by for further examination. The experiments on which [were] necessar[il]y crude from the hurry that they were performed in and the entire want of apparatus and tests but what the medicines in the surgery afforded, though therefore of little importance in themselves, yet may possibly lead to others more important hereafter. The black matter had not unpleasant smell. I have asked patients throwing up black vomit what taste they perceived from it, and they generally state that what was thrown up at first was bitter, as if mixed with bile, but after some time, when vomiting without much effort or straining, they made no complaint of any bad taste in it. That collected from Fleming on being filtered through blotting paper, there came through readily at first about eight ounces of a clear, bright transparent fluid of the colour of rather pale Madeira wine. What then remained on the filter was so thick and viscid, passing through very slowly, and having already acquired a highly offensive smell, I poured off the thinner part and allowed the remainder to dry on the paper. In a small portion of the clear filtered liquor on being subjected to the heat a coagulum formed. Another small portion on the addition of spirit of wine immediately became turbid, being clouded throughout with innumerable small whitish flocculi which gradually subsided to the bottom, forming a white sediment and having the liquor above transparent and of a clear straw colour in which state it at present continues. The addition of all the mineral acids diluted with water under the liquid more or less turbid and caused a sediment to form, which appear to me now to have since rather diminished and the colour of the liquids to have become a little changed those with the sulphuric and muriatic acid to have become darker and so on. In that with dilute nitric acid, the sediment has nearly disappeared, and the liquor is a clear, bright pale-yellow transparent colour. The solution of metallic salts, as sugar of lead, corrosive sublimate and lunar caustic, on being added to separate small portions, threw down copious precipitates which yet remain.

The addition of the solutions of the subcarbonates of the alkalis only heightened the colour, rendering it more dark without diminishing the transparency of the fluid. I now find that since a slight brownish sediment has formed, the black part that dried on the paper adhered to it so tenaciously that I could not separate it. I, therefore, merely cut the paper with it into slips, which I put into small vials filled with all the foregoing tests. In one with ether and another with simple water retaining the upper end of the slip between the cork and the neck of the bottle, the remaining part suspended in the fluid, none of which appeared to have dissolved or to have had any action whatever on it with the exception of a strong solution of the subcarbonates of the alkalis particularly of a soda which was immediately darkened by it and I now find a darkish sediment towards the bottom and suspended through the fluid which is of a clear, dark brown colour and the paper has still a good deal of the black matter adhering to it. In the bottle with plain water, there appears to have been also a little detached from the paper, which has fallen to the bottom. The water is still clear but has acquired a slight yellowish tinge. The paper, when I was employed about it, had a most highly offensive smell, so much so that Mr Palmer, who was beside me, was obliged to withdraw, saying that it made him sick. I continued over it for at least two or three hours and about four days afterwards was attacked with fever myself, which I am inclined entirely to ascribe to having dwelt so long over the putrid matter on the paper, not knowing any other adequate cause for it. It assumed rather a low typhoid character and confined me to bed nearly a fortnight. I intended also to have made some examination of the bile found in the gall bladder but was disappointed, having lost it by accident. However, it had a perfectly natural appearance.

On the treatment, I can have little to add to what I have already given on the subject in my report on the disease at Tobago. Each of the medical officers in charge of sick practised according to his own mode, and it is hard to say which was most successful or, rather, which was least successful. An appearance of success can be always maintained and which I am sorry to say is too frequently done by blending cases of ordinary fever with those of the malignant kind. Some of the early cases that were treated by bleeding and so on, just having sunk and died soon after. A prejudice prevailed with many against the use of the Lancet[20] altogether in this fever, though the patients continued to die without as well as with it. The practice was again renewed in the 17th Regiment, and on going over the deaths with the surgeons, I found that exactly one-half that terminated this had been bled, and the other half had not. I would not entirely reject bleeding used with discretion and moderation which I conceive thus managed may be useful in many cases as preparatory or auxiliary to other means. But I am decidedly averse to large or indiscriminate bleedings.

The case of Mr Caverhill made a very strong impression on my mind and decided me in a great measure on this point. He was a strong, robust young man of apparently a plethoric habit. I had been with him in his surgery for a considerable time the day before his illness when he had no appearance nor made any complaint of being ill. On the following day, I saw him. He was under the operation of purgative medicine that he had already taken and was in a free perspiration, bleeding being proposed. I recommended to wait for a short time to see the effect from the operation of the medicine and the perspiration that he was in but consented to its being performed afterwards in moderation, should he not experience relief. When visiting him in the evening, I was surprised to find that two large finger glasses (holding, I should think, at least three pints) had been filled with blood from him. He had felt some relief of the pain and uneasiness in his head while bleeding and, therefore, urged them to go on with it to that extent. Early the next morning, I received a note saying that his pulse was not to be felt. He was roused a little for a time by the use of strong stimulants, but black vomit came on that evening, and he died that night having been barely forty-eight hours ill.

Calomel was very generally used by some, combined with acrid purgatives and others with antimonies, both which combinations though I considered very injudicious, yet I have seen some recoveries after the use of them, particularly where the mouth was affected. It was given by others singly or joined, with small opiates[21] or aided by mercurial frictions, the more speedily to affect the system, and I believe for the most recoveries have been after the use of this medicine in one shape or other. I have seen it freely used and that successfully too, in one case, by or at least with the consent of a person in the habit of railing violently against it when the two cases of it that had been just before treated by him had both died and they were all officers. It was at the commencement of the disease in the garrison.

I have now, in conclusion, only to hope that as the disease has always proved so extremely unmanageable and so excessively fatal that, the value of preventive and precautionary measures may be duly appreciated and not easily forgotten.

Signed
John Arthur[22] Physician P.M.O.

Half-Yearly Remarks on Diseases from July to December 1821 by Edward Tegart,[23] Inspector of Hospitals

Yellow Fever, that important and justly dreaded disease, is next and last to be noticed amongst the febrile affections. The name is not correct because the yellowness is as often absent as present in the complaint, and it never appears at the commencement – It is an effect, not a cause – Yellow suffusion is present in many other disorders besides this one. Therefore, this ought not to be called yellow fever, but perhaps less harm may result from this denomination than from others that have been given to it. It has been called [1] pestilential, [2] malignant and putrid. What fatal errors might result were the treatment of this disease to be influenced by these titles! Who would use the Lancet or employ strong purgatives in diseases of this type? It is to be lamented that no appropriate name has yet been given, expressive of its action on the human constitution, because great mischief may accrue from improper significations being given to diseases from arbitrary or assuming writers. There ought to be a standard name for the endemic fever of the West Indies. The Synocha of Cullen[24] would perhaps convey a clearer idea of this disease to the English practitioner than any other I am acquainted with. I believe the two diseases to be essentially the same; the difference in symptoms and post-mortem appearances are occasioned by the climate, not by the heat of it, for if that were the case, they would be much more aggravated and the disease consequently more fatal in other countries than in this. We must, therefore, suppose it to be a peculiar state of climate and atmosphere that causes the Synocha in England and the endemic of the West Indies.

But the name is not the only point upon which writers and practitioners differ; the cause and the nature of the disease have been long disputed and often with much heat and acrimony. It is, however, fortunate that although the contagionists and non-contagionists may differ in opinion on those heads, the modern practice is nearly the same. Both parties agree that the fever is an inflammatory one and treat it as such. None, I believe, at present entertain the opinion of its primary action being of the low nervous and putrid type.

• • •

Barbados – During the first four months of the period embraced in this report, the garrison enjoyed an uncommon share of good-health. As sickness appeared so late as the middle of October, we had well-grounded hopes of escaping what is considered the sickly season in this island, namely the last three months of the year. But in the middle of October, a number of the 4th Regiment were sent to hospital labouring under fever of the remittent type. In a few days, some of the cases assumed a more concentrated [form] and in two instances the matter of black vomit was formed on examination. Many of the sick, however, had very alarming symptoms such as irritability of stomach, determination to the head, and yellow suffusion. It was difficult to account for the cause of this fever; the barracks are supposed to be the best and most airy and cool of any in the command, and the weather at this period was not so hot nor so dry as it had been when the men were so healthy. It was, however, observed that more cases were taken ill in the lower part of the barrack than the upper.

This division (one-half) of the regiment was put into tents, and in a very short time, fewer sick were sent to hospital than the other half, and the cases became milder. It is a remarkable circumstance that not one sick man sent from camp died during the six weeks they were under canvas, and when they were relieved by the other half, these latter only lost one man in the same space of time. This result has been so favourable that all the stations in the command have been ordered to be provided with camp equipage that the white troops may be encamped every autumn or whenever any serious illness may appear amongst them.

The first decided cases of *Icterodes* attended with black vomit appeared about the middle of November in the Artillery Hospital. Many others followed of the same description.

The barracks of the artillery stand high and are well-ventilated, but the habits of the men are not favourable to health. They have the means and the inclination of indulging in the use of strong spirits; they are worse subjects for attacks of fever than any others in this garrison. The disease commenced with them and was generated by them and proved fatal to several when no others in the garrison were affected with it, nor were any of the people in Bridgetown.

The artillerymen were encamped on 7 December when their health evidently improved; few fresh cases appeared amongst them until the Christmas holidays when several severe and fatal cases occurred from the renewal of the existing cause – hard drinking. So few cases of fever occurred towards the end of December and the beginning of January that on the 8th, I reported the garrison in a healthy state. The camp was broken up, and the restrictions under which the troops have been placed were removed, and the extra allowance of fresh meat was discontinued.

• • •

Tobago – Considerable anxiety prevailed at the commencement of this half year for the troops in Tobago, as several cases of yellow fever occurred, and some loss was sustained. Half the white troops were removed to Grenada to avoid the disease, but they have been recalled, as it has entirely disappeared, and the island is reported by Mr Panting[25] to enjoy better health than it has for the last three years. The inhabitants, particularly about Courland, have suffered most severely by fever attended with all the concentrated symptoms of yellow fever except black vomit. Many of the oldest and most respectable gentlemen in the country have fallen victim to the disease. We have to lament the loss of a very deserving medical officer, Mr Arthur,[26] by this fever. No other officer has suffered by it. It is to be hoped that the draining of marshes will improve the health of Tobago, which has been bad for years.

Signed
Edward Tegart
Inspector of Troops
Barbados, January 1822

Extract of the Half-Yearly Report from Barbados, Dated December 1821 by Geo: MacDermott,[27] Surgeon 4th Regiment

Febris Remittens[28] – This fever generally commenced its attack in the evening or at night but was not confined to those particular periods, often making its first appearance in the morning or at noon. It usually set in with a rigour, accompanied by nausea, vertigo and prostration of strength, after these symptoms had continued for a period of from ten to thirty- or forty-minute[s] reaction took place. The patient became hot and restless complained of pain across the sericiputl,[29] loins and knees (the latter pain apparently confined to the patella) and a severe spasmodic affection of the calves of the legs. After some time, sweat burst forth, which, in general, reduced the heat of skin, leaving the pains and spasms nearly as before. But if the proper remedies were applied during the paroxysm, the pains diminished or quit altogether, producing a pretty clear remission, seldom of long duration. A fresh accession soon came on, but not exactly of the same description. The increase of temperature was gradual and seldom preceded by chills. The tongue, which was heretofore clean or perhaps had [a] streak or two of white froth down the middle, now became loaded with a thick coat of white or yellowish slime accompanied by a bitter or mawkish taste ... The eyes lost somewhat of their lustre. The frequency rather than the strength or fullness of the pulse was conspicuous. Thirst increased, and the night or period of the paroxysm was passed in a restless manner. Sleep, if it came on, generally failed to afford its wonted refreshment to the patient. Sweating, if generally diffused and of long continuance, brought relief and, in cases, promising a favourable termination as second remission became pretty distinct. But whether the issue ultimately proved favourable or the reverse, each succeeding remission lasted a shorter time and was less clearly defined, until the fever quit the patient altogether. In the cases which terminated favourably, you were able to make an accurate prognosis on the third day but seldom sooner. The symptoms which argued favourably were the tongue becoming clean at the edges, the eyes resuming their natural appearance, the pain across the loins (which was usually the last to quit its seat) subsiding, the skin becoming soft and cool, a cessation of restlessness, and a good night's rest.

The patient the following morning complained perhaps of great weakness, amounting often to inability to move to the night chair or sit for any length of time in an erect position without becoming faint. At the same time, he felt quite easy and expressed a wish for some wine and nourishment. Recovery from this state was quick, the patient, on the second or third day after, being able to walk about as a convalescent. If the termination was likely to prove fatal, a third remission seldom took place. The heat of skin often subsided, and the patient only complained of weakness or uneasiness as if from labour and uneasiness across his loins when he moved. In this state, on a cursory view, we might be inclined to say, "this man will do well". But on closer examination we will see many things to alarm us. The tongue still retains its slimy coat. The pulse though soft perhaps and neither full nor strong, still maintains its frequency; the skin may be cool and soft but seems impermeable to perspiration, or that secretion appears to be no longer carried on. The look becomes unintelligent. And the patient, even when conversing with you, often appears in a reverie, or in other words, to have his mind occupied by some subject different from the one under discussion. This no doubt proceeds more from confusion of ideas than from having them fixed on any particular subject. For though a question or observation may be sufficient, to fix his attention and thereby elicit a clear and correct answer, he appears incapable of arranging his thought in proper order. The next stage as far as regards the mind is incoherent speaking or muttering, which continues until the mental functions are terminated by the Hand of Death. In some cases, however, the patient remains sensible until a short time before his final exit.

In the meantime, the deterioration of the corporeal symptoms keeps pace with those of the mind. The tongue becomes brown and moist or brown and dry and furred. Sometimes, it remains loaded with a coat of viscid white slime – the frequency of the pulse increases. The bowels are inactive or else pour out a thin fluid sometimes brown, sometimes black. The eyes become dull and glassy, and the features collapsed. The stomach during this period probably remains easy and retentive. From this circumstance, we might be inclined to expect that by the administration and retention of proper remedies, a change for the better would take place, but this [is] a fallacious source of hope. The stomach will retain what is swallowed even to a very considerable amount, but it would seem as if the pyloric orifice were closed. The transmission of the contents of the stomach into the intestines [is] thereby prevented, for after the lapse of hours, the accumulated contents will be suddenly and forcibly ejected. After this, the stomach becomes irritable and seldom retains anything for a longer space than half an hour. What is thrown up becomes gradually darker than what has been swallowed until, in some cases, it ends in black vomit. After this takes place, I believe we may bid adieu to hope, but I have known the stomach, even after this occurrence, again to become easy and retentive and continue so for several hours until death closed the scene.

This fever in the aggravated form now described, is the true endemic or *Typus Icterodes*.[30] Yet in its commencement it presents no prominent characteristic that enables us accurately to foresee whether in its course it would prove to be only a mild remittent or the malignant and concentrated yellow fever.

The prognosis, therefore, during the first twenty-four hours should never be decisive, as the event often proves the most attentive and accurate observer to have been in error. The bilious suffusion which has procured this the name of yellow fever appears to me a circumstance of no great consequence. In some cases of the most violent and concentrated nature, I have known death to supervene before the skin had become yellow. On the contrary, in those of a comparative mild description, a deep discoloration has taken place days before the solution of the fever.

The preceding is an outline of the most usual form this fever assumed in the 4th Regiment this season, but many deviations were observable. Sometimes, the attack commenced suddenly with a violent pain in the head accompanied by delirium. In other instances, it began with griping and purging but these usually wasted when the fever had completely developed itself. In some, the temperature of the body ran high, accompanied by considerable arterial action. In other cases, the fever commenced and continued its fatal progress without almost in any degree hurrying the circulation, increasing the heat of skin or giving rise to any serious pain. In such cases, coma is the symptom which chiefly points out the danger. In general, during the first fortnight after this began to rage amongst the men, the heat of skin was seldom above par, and the vascular system seemed deprived of its natural degree of energy. Dissections often showed the veins of the head turgid with black blood and the longitudinal veins full even to repletion with it. The membranes in the course of this sinus perforated with numerous holes, giving exit to the flow of the blood from it when the top of the cranium was removed. The liver and lungs also often exhibited marks of congestion, seldom of acute inflammation. The stomach, in some instances where black vomit had not taken place, was full of the black fluid.

The cause of this disease, I believe, is the general nature of the climate more than local situation or other peculiarity of circumstances.

Signed
Geo. MacDermott
Surgeon 4th Regiment

Table 4.1: Return of the Storekeeper General's Department, Showing the Dates of Their Arrival at Barbados, Sicknesses, Deaths, Recoveries

Name	Age	Rank	Date of Arrival	When Taken Ill	Died	Recov.	Sickness	Residence
Walter Ford	23	Conductor	January 1819	30 October 1820	5 November 1820	-	Fever	Dock yard
Mrs Ford	28	-	-	1 November 1820	4 November 1820	-	Fever	Dock yard
E. Harmer	23	Conductor	18 January 1820	1 November 1820	-	yes	Fever	Bay at Mr Maurey's
-	"	-	-	31 October 1821	-	yes	Fever	Bay at Mr Maurey's
H. Clarke	25	Cooper	-	10 December 1820	14 December 1820	-	None	Dockyard and Collymore Rock
Mrs Clarke	23	-	-	-	-	-	None	""and return to Europe
Louisa Clarke	2	-	-	-	-	-	Fever	""and return to Europe
Francis Catchlore	43	Carpenter	-	23 October 1820	27 October 1820	-	Fever	Cottages in Crabtown
Mrs Catchlore	43	-	-	28 October 1820	2 November 1820	-	Fever	Cottages in Crabtown
Henry Catchlore	6	-	-	28 October 1820	7 November 1820	-	Fever	Cottages in Crabtown
A. McAsh	27	Carpenter	-	18 October 1820	-	yes	Fever	Cottages in Crabtown
-	"	-	-	27 October 1821	-	yes	Fever	Cottages in Crabtown
Mrs McAsh	27	-	-	19 October 1820	-	yes	Fever	Cottages in Crabtown
Mr Turner	42	Packer	-	2 October 1820	-	yes	Fever	Cottages in Crabtown
-	"	-	-	23 August 1821	-	yes	Fever	Cottages in Crabtown
Mrs Turner	34	-	-	3 October 1820	11 October 1820	-	Fever	Cottages in Crabtown
Mr Herssey	27	Packer	-	10 December 1820	14 December 1820	-	Fever	Dockyard and Collymore Rock

Name	Age	Rank	Date of Arrival	When Taken Ill	Died	Recov.	Sickness	Residence
F. Herssey	7	-	-	10 December 1820	-	yes	Fever	Dockyard and Collymore Rock
Mrs Herssey	30	-	-	-	-	-	Fever	Dockyard and Collymore Rock
Chs. Frereman	32	Packer	-	8 November 1820	12 November 1820	-	Fever	Cottages in Crabtown and Collymore Rock
Mrs Frereman	24	-	-	5 November 1820	-	yes	fever	""and return to Europe
G.F. Haversatt	38	Asst. Storekeeper General	6 February 1820	-	-	-	None	Bay at Mr Maurey's
Mrs Haversatt	29	-	6 February 1820	11 September 1821	19–20 September	-	Fever	Bay at Mr Maurey's

Signed: G.F. Haversatt, Assistant Storekeeper General

Reports from Barbados

Table 4.2: Return of Convalescents of Fever Treated in the Naval Hospital, Barbados, from 20 October to 18 December 1821

4th Regiment							
Names	Years in Barbados	Quartered	Admitted	Event	Duration	Fever	Remarks
Serjeant I. Warde	2	barrack	30-Oct 1821	discharged	27 days	Febris Continua	To duty
Serjeant Bonham	2 years 5 months	barrack	30-Oct	"	27	Febris Convalescence	Transferred to 4th Regiment Hospital
Daniel Float	2 years 5 months	barrack	30-Oct	discharged	35	Febris Convalescence	To duty
Peter Musgrave	2 years 5 months	barrack	30-Oct	discharged	24	Febris Convalescence	To duty
Daniel Blunt	9 months	barrack	30-Oct	discharged	13	Febris Convalescence	Retained till 11 December, then discharged to duty. He was sent to Gunhill, where he shot himself thro' the leg, and he died
George Hasker	2 years 5 months	barrack	30-Oct	Remanded	41	Febris Convalescence	To duty
George Webb	2 years 5 months	barrack	31-Oct	discharged	20	Febris Convalescence	To duty
John Cardell	2 years 5 months	barrack	31-Oct	discharged	15	Febris Convalescence	To duty
John Randell	2 years 5 months	barrack	31-Oct	discharged	31	Febris Convalescence	To Duty
John Ford	2 years 5 months	barrack	30-Oct	discharged	32	Febris Convalescence	Transferred to 4th Hospital
John Moloy	2 years 5 months	barrack	1-Nov	discharged	34	Febris Convalescence	To duty
Edward Smith	9 months	barrack	2-Nov	discharged	31	Febris Convalescence	To duty
Joseph Butter	5 months	barrack	1-Nov	discharged	17	Febris Convalescence	Transferred convalescent to 4th Hospital
Joseph Turner	7 years	barrack	2-Nov	discharged	28	Febris Convalescence	To duty
James Church	2 years 5 months	barrack	3-Nov	discharged	15	Febris Convalescence	To duty
Henry Wyvell	9 months	barrack	3-Nov	discharged	26	Febris Convalescence	Transferred to 4th Hospital
Luke Gibney	2 years 5 months	barrack	3-Nov	discharged	28	Febris Convalescence	To duty
Michael Swaine	2 years 5 months	barrack	4-Nov	discharged	29	Febris Convalescence	To duty

4th Regiment							
Names	Years in Barbados	Quartered	Admitted	Event	Duration	Fever	Remarks
Baptist Buckly	2 years 5 months	barrack	4-Nov	discharged	16	Febris Convalescence	To duty
Thomas Dixon	2 years 5 months	barrack	5-Nov	discharged	28	Febris Convalescence	To duty
Joseph Hunter	2 years 5 months	barrack	5-Nov	discharged	26	Febris Convalescence	To duty
William Spencer	2 years 5 months	barrack	5-Nov	discharged	26	Febris Convalescence	To duty
William Morris	3 months	barrack	5-Nov	discharged	28	Febris Convalescence	To duty
Serjeant R. Smith	2 years 5 months	barrack	5-Nov	discharged	26	Febris Convalescence	To duty
Serjeant H. Hopley	2 years 5 months	barrack	5-Nov	discharged	21	Febris Convalescence	To duty
Thos. Morrison	3 months	barrack	10-Nov	discharged	21	Febris Convalescence	To duty
Mrs Snelly	9 months	camp	10-Nov	discharged	21	Febris Convalescence	To duty
James Smith	2 years 5 months	camp	10-Nov	discharged	23	Febris Convalescence	Transferred convalescent to 4th Hospital
Thomas Roe	2 years 5 months	barrack	10-Nov	discharged	23	Febris Convalescence	Retained as Orderly
Samuel Serix	9 months	barrack	11-Nov	discharged	24	Febris Convalescence	To duty
Benjamin Holingshead	2 years 5 months	camp	11-Nov	discharged	24	Febris Convalescence	To duty
Mrs Darby	2 years 5 months	barrack	11-Nov	discharged	23	Febris Convalescence	To duty
Serjeant Geo Deakin	2 years 5 months	barrack	11-Nov	discharged	24	Febris Convalescence	Transferred convalescent to 4th Hospital
James Hayes	9 months	barrack	19-Nov	discharged	14	Febris Convalescence	To duty
John Wood	2 years 5 months	barrack	19-Nov	discharged	18	Febris Convalescence	To duty
Emmanuel Martin	2 years 5 months	camp	19-Nov	discharged	13	Febris Convalescence	To duty
Robert Gomer	2 years 5 months	Hut	19-Nov	discharged	13	Febris Convalescence	Transferred convalescent to 4th Hospital
John Arnold	2 years 5 months	camp	19-Nov	discharged	14	Febris Convalescence	Retained as Orderly

Some of the precautionary and preventive measures of 1820 and 1821 I shall state briefly in this report:

M.D.O. 17 October 1820 – All the men and women under treatment in the Naval Hospital to be removed to the General Hospital, with the following exceptions: such people as are put in observation, the lepers and the sick officers until suitable quarters can be provided for them. The servants to be left there for the present to consist of the wardmaster, the surgery man, the old black nurse, the cook, the black orderly and the white orderly in attendance on the officers. The remainder to accompany the sick when removed and to be employed as heretofore. Doctor Bone[31] will be pleased to take charge of the patients moved to General Hospital. Mr Home[32] and Mr Davidson[33] will do duty with him, the one in the male ward, the other in the female ward.

Signed
R. Green
I.A.H.

On 27 October 1820, the copy of a letter from Mr Green to the surgeons of regiments dated 17 October 1820 was inserted in the M.D.O. Books. The following are extracts from it.

The Naval Hospital to be reserved for suspicious cases of fever and for those who are decided cases of *Typhus Icterodes*. It is not intended, however, to admit all febrile cases on the first appearance unless those of a suspicious or malignant character, but they are to be admitted into the Regimental Hospital in the first instance and to be carefully separated from the other sick in a distinct room if possible, and placed there in observation until the disease is clearly developed, always with a fumigating lamp burning near the bed; and to windward of it. Whenever it shall unfortunately prove to be *Typhus Icterodes*, the covered cart is to be applied for and the individual sent to the Naval Hospital without loss of time. In the performance of any of these duties, none but black orderlies or pioneers should, if possible, be employed. When the case is decidedly one of yellow fever, the bedding and clothing which the patient has used since his illness should be burnt immediately in the presence of the medical officer, including the canvas bottom belonging to the iron bedstead on which he has slept.

In writing the foregoing precautionary measures, the inspector is induced by a thorough conviction that young Europeans, if much exposed to the influence of the miasma arising from the bodies of individuals labouring under this disease, are generally attacked and that the results also frequently fatal.[34] It is not necessary here to enter into any discussions respecting the quantum of the contagious properties of yellow fever. It is sufficient to know that when it appears in families, several are generally attacked and that in Military Hospitals, a large proportion of the white orderlies in immediate attendance on that description of patients also suffer. Fortunately, however, it has been found that Africans are not equally liable to the disease. When attacked that, it seldom has the malignant character on proportional fatal termination as among Europeans.

Signed
R. Green to the Surgeons of
R.D. 21st, 1st W.I. I.A.H. and
Hospital Assistant Caverhill
17 October 1820

"The usual returns and reports sent to Dr Arthur as P.M.O. are to be sent during his absence to Doctor Bone, Physician to the Forces, who will be pleased to sign them in the usual manner."

Doctor Arthur went to Tobago to assist in establishing military quarantine in that island. He was only absent about eight days. In establishing the Quarantine Hospital, there were several minor regulations not inserted in the Department Orderly Book but which were acted on. The Hospital Porter was prohibited from admitting any person into the Hospital enclosure, except the medical officers who resided there – Dr Arthur, Dr Bone, Mr Doughty[35] and Mr Palmer,[36] and their families or persons having business with them. And this order was posted on a board and hung outside the gate. Two sentries of the 1st W.I. Regiment were placed at the doors of the wards to prevent communication with the patients. The general orders relative to patients affected with yellow fever were two, I shall insert them. They were given by Major General Sir. F.P. Robinson.

Headquarters, Tobago, General Orders, 31 October 1820

No. 7

In the event of any officer being seized with the yellow fever, he is to be attended by black servants only, and any white servant he may have is to be immediately removed from about his person or room.

Headquarters, Tobago, General Orders, 28 November 1820

No. 3

Everything belonging to those men who have died of yellow fever, with the exception of linen shirts and trousers, is to be invariably burnt under the inspection of an officer of the medical staff upon the recommendation of the inspector of hospitals. The observation ward of the Artillery Hospital was a small room in the east end of the range of offices. The observation ward of the 21st Regiment was one of the wards of the ground floor of the military hospital. And my observation ward was one of the upstairs wards also in the Military Hospital. From my observation ward, I did not transfer any case of fever to the Naval Hospital and I did not lose any. From the Ordnance and the 21st Regiment, many were transferred and many of those transferred died. When I was acting as P.M.O.[37] My judgement in sending patients to the Naval Hospital was guided by the appearance of the tongue and eye, as indicating the state of the stomach, and by the general severity of the symptoms and place of residence of the patient. In fact, by the appearance of the gastric symptoms. It could not be expected, therefore, that Mr Doughty could have success in treating patients thus selected for him; some people, however, were sent to the hospital on suspicion of having caught the disease, and these did well in the Naval Hospital as there were no white servants in the hospital except Murphy the porter and his family; Serjeant McDonald the wardmaster and his family; and a drunken soldier of the 21st Regiment named Simon, a surgery man. The immunity or liability of white servants to gastric disease could not be proved. The surgery man had a slight attack of gastric disease with no symptom of black vomiting or of yellowness. He was a case that was adduced as having caught yellow fever by contagion. I saw him twice or thrice daily as I did all Mr Doughty's patients – therefore, I know well.

First, that the surgery man had not a disease that any contagionist would have called it, except as occurring in a quarantine establishment.

Second, that he was a muddling drunken person and had been several times sent to the guardhouse for being drunk; and third, that he lived in the small low room adjoining the surgery and kitchen, a place with two suffocators and one door to the eastward, and one grated window to the westward, a quarter which on account of its lowness and want of ventilation I prohibit any white servant from inhabiting. He recovered and has since died at Demerara.

Serjeant McDonald, his wife and son, a boy about thirteen years of age, all escaped yellow fever, although McDonald was caught one day in the ward at the bedside of a yellow fever patient making his will. Serjeant Murphy, on the 9 October, was looking for a room to accommodate Lord Combermere's gardener and wife sent to the Naval Hospital to perform quarantine. The poor old man had a paralytic affection of the left leg. The room he was examining was one of those over the stables. The stair to it was bad, and in descending, he fell from the top of the station and, broke his left thigh and dislocated his left arm at the shoulder and hurt his side. The accident happened at 7:00 am. Mr Doughty and Palmer reduced the dislocation and put splinters upon the thigh. I saw the poor old man at noon that day, and the next morning at 10:00, I called on him on my way to a medical board in the military hospital and found him yellow. Vomiting everything he swallowed and, in fact, dying with the common symptoms of yellow fever, his leg and abdomen much swollen. On my return from the board, I called with Mr Doughty again at his quarter. The poor old man was dead, and his body quite yellow. This melancholy case is in proof of a position which I had maintained in my report on Trinidad in 1818. I beg to extract the passage.

> In England, inoculation with putrid matter from a putrid body produces occasionally a local inflammation, and it does so in the West Indies as in the cases of Mr Lenon and Mr A'lounor, but it does not either in England or the West Indies communicate the disease of which the patient died, although were the inoculated

person to die of inflammation from the inoculation and were he full of rich blood, the season hot, the air dry, stagnant, bad, and yellow fever prevailing, perhaps his stomach and liver might become affected, and he might die yellow and with black vomit, and a similar result is not impossible under similar circumstances from a fractured limb; for the reigning epidemic reigns alone, but neither the one event nor the other would prove the existence of a specific contagion of yellow fever.

Mr Green left Barbados for England on 13 May 1821, and Mr Tegart assumed the direction of the medical department in this command on 16 June 1821. The medical department orders this year connected with the prevention of sickness in the garrison were not numerous.

Barbados, 16 June 1821, M.D.O.

As the inspector of hospitals will now assume the general duties of the command, the deputy inspector will resume the superintendence of the hospitals in Barbados. Dr Bone will have charge of the General Hospital. The general orders issued on the recommendation of the inspector of hospitals were first to remove all the military from the low, unhealthy ground westward of the parade and from all the bad hired huts, the following are the orders on that subject.

Brigade Order, 16 August 1821

In order to insure, as much as possible, the present healthy state of the troops during what is considered the sickly season, the following arrangements are forthwith to take place.

1. The lower part of the north barrack is to be vacated by such men as at present occupy it. The southern half is to be appropriated to such married families of the 4th Regiment as cannot be comfortably accommodated in huts contiguous to the barrack.
2. The northern part is to be appropriate to such white non-commissioned officers and privates with their families without any exception belonging to the quarter and barrack department as are at present living in the dockyard and vicinity, meaning thereby, the low, swampy ground in that neighbourhood. The Ordnance Corps will accommodate in a similar manner their married people so that the ground in question shall not be occupied by any white non-commissioned officer or soldier and families, more than is absolutely necessary for the duties of the

service for the next three months. To encamp part of the 4th Regiment and also the artillery and Royal Sappers and Miners. The following are the orders.

Headquarters, Barbados, General Orders

31 October 1821

Four companies of the 4th K.O. Regiment to be encamped as soon as possible on such ground at St Ann's as shall be pointed out by the inspector of hospitals. The commandant will be pleased to make the necessary arrangements with a view of carrying this order into effect with the least possible delay.

1. To arrange with Captain Newcombe of the *Pyramus* for allowing a medical board to examine the state of the vessel and to investigate the causes of the sickness, and to report upon the most likely means of checking the disease or removing the cause of it. This board was held on 23 November; the proceedings were next day given to the Inspector. The following is a copy of the proceedings.

Barbados, 23 November 1821

Proceedings of a Board of Medical Officers held in consequence of the following department order.

Department order 23 November 1821

A board of medical officers consisting of Dr Menzies,[38] deputy inspector of hospitals, Dr Bone,[39] Physician to the Forces and Staff Surgeon Elliott,[40] will this day at 11:00 proceed on board His Majesty's Ship *Pyramus* to examine into the state of that ship and investigate the probable cause of the sickness which prevails on board. The board will also report upon what may appear to them the most likely means of checking the progress of the disease or removing the cause of it.

Signed
E. Tegart[41] Esquire
Inspector of Hospitals

In conformity to this order, the board proceeded on board the *Pyramus* at 11:00 a.m. and, having examined minutely into the state of the ship, find that she is an old vessel lately completely repaired and inserted with coal tar. She is a very tight vessel, and the coal tar rendered fluid by the heat of the climate oozes from the beam of the captain's cabin and from every part of the ship, particularly from the hold where the heat is greater and mixing in the hold with the bilge water produces a very offensive effluvium particularly aggravated by admixture with fresh water escaping during the operation of pumping the water through a canvas hose, from the iron tanks to the cistern. The ship was clean and in good order, but the atmosphere of the Orlop Deck and Hold was close and oppressively hot, and the smell of the bilge water and coal tar very perceptible. On pumping the ship, the bilge water was black and smelled of coal tar offensively. The board finds that the *Pyramus* arrived at Barbados on 25 July last and since that period has been at different times thirty-four days in English Harbour. She was there from the 11 to 19 October, then left for St Kitts, where she remained seven days. She sailed on 27 October and, on 1 November, arrived at Antigua, where she landed her sick and then proceeded to Barbados, where she arrived on 9 November. The sickness commenced in English Harbour and subsequently considerably increased on the departure of the vessel from St Kitts. With regard to the predisposing causes of the disease at present prevailing in the vessel, the board are inclined to attribute [it] to the state of the vessel as described and to her lying head to wind and also to the season of the year and to the description of the crew all newcomers and to the great alarm that exists among them; the impression on board seems to be general, that there is much also to be attributed to the coal tar oozing from the vessel, and mixing with the bilge water; but the board have not sufficient data to be able to determine how far that cause operates.

With respect to the most likely means of checking the disease, the board are of the opinion that ventilation by every means and, the frequent introduction of salt water into the well, and frequent pumping with the view of diluting and purifying the bilge water is essential. The board are of the opinion that the vessel should be put to sea as soon as possible to cruise in the vicinity of the island and, in the meantime, should put a spring upon the cable when practicable, that Brodies Stoves[42] should be used on board, and as the surgeon of the vessel is non-effective the board are of the opinion that if it can be done an experienced and active naval surgeon should be put on board her, it being necessary to inspire the crew with confidence and that if possible, a sick berth should be fetted up.

As the collection of fresh water in the hold arises partly from the leakage of the canvass hose employed in starting the water from the casks into the tanks, the board recommend that a leather hose should be substituted.

Signed

Alexander Menzies M.D., Deputy Inspector of Hospitals

Hugh Bone, M.D., Physician to the Forces

E. Tegart Esquire, Director of Army Hospitals

Elliott, Surgeon to the Forces

The vessel went to sea from Barbados on 9 December 1821 and was put into English Harbour on 3 January 1822. and is now cleaning out her hold (she lost during that trip 10 men, two women and three officers). The quantity of filth found there accounts fully for the sickness on board. It appears that the frame of the vessel was taken at Copenhagen but that she was put together in England. According to the accounts received from English Harbour, she has lost since her arrival in this command.

1. To remove the patients from the Ordnance to the Military Hospital. The following general order was issued on 16 January 1822. "A board of Survey to assemble at St Ann's tomorrow morning at ten o'clock to inspect and report on the state of the building usually occupied by the sick of the Ordnance Department; and as much mortality has occurred in it lately, the board will also give their opinion as to the probable causes of the insalubrity thereof and suggest such measures for remedying what may appear noxious or require alteration as they conceive necessary. Doctor Menzies being unable to attend on account of his health, I was sent in his place. The board found the cellars under the offices dry but not ventilated; the building and offices in bad repair, the hospital badly ventilated in consequence of a dead wall to windward, the partition between the surgeons'

quarters and the ward the leeward rooms where three persons had been taken ill, and had died, to be ill-ventilated and unfit to be occupied as quarters. A drain running from the leeward to the windward of the hospital yard, depositing its filth on the parade windward of the hospital and producing foul air, which was blown back again upon the hospital; the kitchen and bath house to be in a ruinous state. The privy on the side of the road and to windward of it and of the range of officers' huts on the brink of the parade, and that the contents of it were carried away through part of the garrison to the sea by manual labour. The board also found the locality bad, as being too leeward of the privy and exposed to south-west winds, which usually are unhealthy in Barbados, and especially in that situation as having passed over low land which has been abandoned by medical advice. The recommendations of the board were in detail to do away with the causes of disease, which have been stated, so far as could be done by repairs and improvements in the buildings, offices and drains. But premised by an observation that should it be judged expedient to reoccupy the buildings as a hospital, the board recommends which may probably lead to the total abandonment of this building as a hospital. This hospital always appeared to me to be unhealthy, and on that idea, I advised Mr Bradley to leave it in 1820. The proceedings of this board are most important – important not only in consequence of the proceedings themselves but of the mode which the commander of the forces employed for information on the subject. The report of an individual is of value in proportion to the talents of the individual and his freedom from prejudices. But the report of five perfectly competent, disinterested individuals carries greater weight and brings stronger conviction."
2. The fifth measure I shall notice was the assembling of a Medical Board upon the barracks occupied by the officers of the 4th Regiment.

Barbados, 14 May 1822

The board was ordered by Sir Henry Warde to report upon the causes of the sickness among the officers of the fourth and upon the state of the barracks they occupied and whether removing them to other houses or quarters was advisable. The board reported to the following purport. The sickness among the officers of the 4th arose from the same causes as the sickness which lately prevailed among the men, and according to the usual march of the epidemic in Barbados, they are suffering the last. The board recommended that the officers should be removed from the barracks they then occupied and accommodated in other buildings or barracks, and that the barracks should be repaired, whitewashed, painted and furnished with glass windows.

Signed
Dr Menzies, Deputy Inspector
Dr Bone, Physician to the Forces
A. Lainsworth,[43] Staff Surgeon

The barrack was formerly judged to be unhealth[il]y situated and probably was so when the low ground to windward was not drained; yet during this season, the causes were moral, not physical, on account of which it appeared to me advisable to recommend the removal of the officers. I find that in a hospital, if several men die in a ward, the ward is apt to get a bad name, and for that reason, I frequently change the ward where the worst cases of gastric disease are treated. None of the officers were taken ill subsequent to their removal. Having given this account of the preventive measures under the contagion system of 1820 and of those in 1821, when that system had died a natural death, it remains for me in this report to state some results that have been obtained in this hospital and to conclude with some observations on the seat and causes of the epidemic, and my method of treating it.

My assistants were Dr Bain[44] and Mr Campbell.[45] The prescriptions and reports were by myself; the registers were kept by my assistant; Dr Bain kept the medical register of the males and Mr Campbell of the females. Both registers are kept neatly, very fully and give a true account of the symptoms and of the practice. The fatal cases were all opened by the assistants and myself, with the exception of three or four who, in consequence of particular requests from friends or relations, were not. The reports of the dissection are all except one written by myself, and during the examination in the dead house, the orderly of the ward where the patient died attended in the dead house. These examinations were done with great labour and care. The reports of them are entered in the register after the case, and the future investigator of the epidemic of Barbados will find in the registers of the Naval Hospital of 1821 evidence not of great talent, but labour which his constitution must be strong, and his zeal great if he can much exceed. My assistants were excellent.

The hospital servants were acquainted with my system. Those of them who prove[d] inattentive or drunken were instantly dismissed. The officers were in a good state, and the general system of economy which I observed has already been detailed to the board in any former reports; some requisite additions and alterations were added. Everyone knew the duty of his situation, and everyone performed it. The first important result which I have proved in the Naval Hospital is that the yellow fever, as it is called, cannot by any possibility be communicated from one person to another. At Santander (In Santander in 1813, about seven hundred persons were exposed to the influence of yellow fever and all with impunity. This statement in my public report written at that time ...) in 1813, none of my assistants or orderlies or nurses employed with the cases of yellow fever treated in the Casa Blanca or the Quarantine Hospital were attacked with it. In 1820, none of my orderlies or servants were attacked with yellow fever, but it might be argued that I have not the charge of the Quarantine Hospital. I have now, however, the heartfelt satisfaction of stating that from 20 June 1821 to 20 February 1822, which includes the whole period of the sickly season, not one medical officer,[46] white servant or person employed in any capacity in the Naval Hospital establishment, have been attacked with yellow fever or purple fever or any disease whatever. I consider this fact to be of first importance.

The committee of the House of Commons appointed to investigate the contagion of plague put the following questions to the learned Dr Latham, president of the Royal College of Physicians London,[47] to which he gives the following answers.

Q. *What mode would you consider it best to pursue in order to ascertain it (the plague) was not contagious?*
A. Purposely subjecting individuals to its influence, a course it would be unjustifiable to adopt for the sake of experiment merely.

Q. *A Frenchman was taken on board the* Thesens Man of War; *he had open buboes, he recovered, none of the crew got plague. Would you consider that as leading to a conviction that the plague was not contagious?*

A. If it was ascertained that a considerable number of the crew came absolutely into contact with the person of the individual, I should so consider.

Q. *Some persons did communicate?*

A. I stipulate for a considerable number.

The trial which Dr Latham allows to be decisive of the question of personal contagion of a disease has been made here, not purposely for the sake of experiment merely, but purposely for the sake of saving the lives of the sick by giving them proper attendance.

The following white servants have been employed in the Naval Hospital from 20 June 1821 to 20 February 1822, none of whom were taken ill.

Table 4.3: White Employees at Naval Hospital Who Escaped Sickness, 20 June 1821–20 February 1822

Regt./ Names		Employment	Remained 21 June or since entered	Discharged	Remaining
21st Sergt. Kyle		Steward	21 June		Remaining
Mrs Kyle		Matron	" "		"
Miss Kyle		Seamstress	" "		"
4th Edw. Yearlds		Asst. Ward Man	21 June	6 July	
" Wm Burke		"	7 July	11 Dec.	
" John Ross		"	25 November	15 Jan.	
" Wm. Wellman		"	13 December		Remaining
R.A. Jas. McDonald		Porter	21 June	18 January	
4th John Chairman		"		19 January	"
civilians	James Tinsley	Surgery Man	21 June	2 July	
	Thos. McDonald	Asst. "	21 June	7 July	
4th Sam. Harvey		"	14 July	1 August	
" John Cooper		"	2 August		Remaining

Reports from Barbados

Regt./ Names	Employment	Remained 21 June or since entered	Discharged	Remaining
" Jas. Wadsworth	Barber	21 June		Died
" Sam. Harvey	Orderly	" "	5 July	
" Edw. Harber	"	" "		Remaining
" Nicholas. Pascol	"	" "	23 November	
" Wm. Skinner	"	" "	1 August	
" Richard Marks	"	29 July	15 August	
" Sam. Harvey	"	2 August	4 September	
" Bryan Toley	"	7 September	23 November	
" Matt. Firth	"	6 November		Remaining
" Benjn. Bedill	"	11 November	8 December	
" Sam Smith	"	" "		Remaining
" Wm. Card	"	" "		Died
" Wm. Dolton	"	20 "		"
" Jno. Arnold	"	24 "		"
R. Marine Ed. Brittain	Steward to Lieut. Tothill	10 November		"
4th Sam Seex	"	24 "		"
" Wm. Burke	Asst. Ward Man	16 January		"
" John Watson	Mattress maker	21 June		"

N.B. Civilian Jagues de Grafe, repairer of bedsteads, was occasionally employed during the above period.
Total 32
Certified to be correct
Taken from Documents in the Purveyor's Office
Signed W. Pierce
Acting Dept. Purveyor

N.B.: Sergeant Kyle's family also consisted of five children, as noted in the original document.

The patients were not prevented from having intercourse with each other.

Turner, the first gastric case, was admitted on 23 August 1821. From that period to the 20 February 1822, eighty-one persons not affected with gastric disease but with other diseases or with no disease* (*children with mothers who were sick or mothers to nurse their sick children) have been admitted into the hospital. And not one of these has caught yellow fever or any kind of fever or gastric disease. The last fatal case in the Naval Hospital occurred on the 7 February 1822. The coloured persons employed in the Naval Hospital had similar remarkable immunity from sickness. Only one of them has been sick during the period embraced in this statement, and she, a person who has a Barbados leg, is subject to hysteria and had a fever and ague attack on 20 January 1822. She had pain of her back, and I put a blister on the pained part, which kept her in hospital for eight days.

Return of coloured people employed in the Naval Hospital from 20 June 1821 to 20 February 1822, certified to be correctly taken from documents in the Purveyor's Office.

Signed
N. Pierce
Acting Deputy Purveyor

During the epidemic season, the Engineer Department were repairing the Naval Hospital. They repaired it one pavilion at a time, and when that was finished, the patients were moved into it from another pavilion. The workmen, generally coloured people about thirty in number, repaired the vacated one.

None of these workmen have been affected with yellow fever or any disease since they began to work in the Naval Hospital. The total number of those exposed to the influence of the disease in this hospital is not less than 160, of whom 35 were white servants* (*officers and visitors not included) (Santander 700 + N.H [Naval Hospital] 160 = Total 860). No fumigation was employed, no oil skin gloves or jackets were used, no bedding or clothes were burnt, no quarantine prevention of communication with friends and relations was enforced or even proposed.

Table 4.4: Fatality Rate in Coloured Personnel Employed at Naval Hospital

	Names	Employment	Remained 21 June or since Entered	Discharged	Remaining
	James	Cook	21 June	_____	Remaining
	Polly	Washerwoman	"	_____	Died
	Flora	"	"	_____	Died
	Diana	"	4 November	18 December	_____
	Kitty	"	21 June	30 June	_____
	Ann Pollard	"	14 November	_____	Remaining
	Kitty	"	11 "	_____	Died
	Nelly	"	23 "	12 December	_____
	Bellah	Nurse	21 "	15 August	_____
	Ruthy White	"	"	_____	Remaining
	Mary Nobelton	"	"	_____	Died
	Betsey Long	"	18 November	_____	Died
Civilians	Eve Blackman	"	21 "	_____	Died
	Fanny	"	28 "	_____	Died
	Austin	Pioneer	21 June	_____	Remaining
	Bolt	Do	Do	_____	Died
	Cook	Do	Do	_____	Died
	Burke	Do	Do	_____	Died
	McPherson	Do	Do	_____	Died
	Tom Tough	Do	Do	_____	Died
	Dick	Carter	Do		Died
Military Labourers	Hancock	Asst. Cook	Do	_____	Died
	William	Pioneer			
Total 22					

I now take leave of the question of contagion in yellow fever. The spirit of inductive reasoning and wholesome scepticism on that subject have lately been roused in England. And so, few in the West Indies believe the doctrine that they may be very safely permitted to enjoy their own opinion; they cannot do much harm. The intelligence of the age forbids burning for witchcraft and will soon forbid imprisonment and dereliction for being affected or suspected of being affected with yellow fever.

The gastric disease, commonly called yellow fever, is a combination of two diseases. The first is a disease of the villous coat of the intestinal canal, principally of the stomach or small intestines. The second is a disease of the liver and portal system. The combination of these two diseases forms the yellow fever of authors. When these two states are combined with a tendency to gangrene of the seat of the disease and the system generally, the compound gangrenous disease is the concentrated yellow fever of Jackson,[48] the disease that prevailed in 1820 and in 1821 in this island. The stomach on dissection shows its villous tunic in various states: first pulpy and of a deep dusky red colour; second slightly of a dusky red colour in the cul-de-sac of the cardiac portion, and pale towards the pylorics. Third, pale every part of its villous tunic. In all these states, however, it is like paste and very easily can be separated from the muscular coat. The headquarters of the disease appears to be in that part of the cardiac cul-de-sac that lies between the spleen and pancreas. The peritoneal coat of the intestine does not appear to be much diseased in the structure. The appearances of the villous tunic of the duodenum and of the cul-de-sac of the stomach and of the ileum [occur] at its entrance into the colon. Sometimes the caecum is gangrenous and has an opening in it near the appendix vermiform. The ulcers I have observed in subjects who have taken large doses of Calomel, the liver during the compound gangrenous disease called the concentrate yellow fever becomes friable and quite rotten. It is generally very nearly the colour of the skin. Still, when the liver is not affected with any gangrenous tendency and is obstructed in its duct only, the bile is absorbed or thrown back into the general circulation, and the patient becomes of a bright yellow colour. If the gall ducts are obstructed and the system tending to gangrene, the yellow colour is generally dark and dirty, sometimes very pale and scarcely perceptible. The intensity of the colour given by the bile is according to the quantity of red globules in the blood of the subject.

A tumid cachectic[49] having pale bile and then watery blood does not become very yellow, but a florid young person dies livid or very yellow.

During the two last epidemics in this island, the tendency to gangrene was less than I have observed during the epidemic of 1818 in Trinidad and 1820 in Tobago. The wounds of the Lancet did not heal in Tobago, nor did blistered surfaces, but in this island, they generally did readily. The epidemic disease that occurred in the garrison of St Ann's this season and last was, in the majority of cases, diseases of the villous tunic of the intestine with little tendency to gangrene of that part and no obstruction of the liver and no yellowness of the eye or skin. This disease does not differ from the *febris continua communis* of authors. It is so easily cured that if the patient is allowed the inhalation of pure air and is well-nursed, the result is favourable and will even be favourable under very preposterous or absurd treatment. There also occurred, especially this season, many cases of simple jaundice; the bile did not find a passage into the intestine. The patient was not well but had a clean or whitish tongue and could walk about. This disease was not dangerous unless when (sic) the villous tunic of the intestine became also diseased. But there were many cases (sic) where the tendency to gangrene of the villous tunic of the intestine and of the parenchyma of the liver were evident, and these were the cases that required the treatment of a master of the healing art. These are cases, many of which can be saved by judicious treatment, but many of which will perish in spite of any mode of treatment hitherto tried. The matters vomited during the different states and stages of the disease are different. I shall describe them for this information is not to be got in books. They are as follows – viz:

    1st – contents of the stomach at the invasion of the disease

    2nd – the fluids drank (sic) mixed with green or yellow bile

    3rd – the fluids drank (sic) without any admixture or change

    4th – a fluid like indigo or China ink brought up with severe straining. I suppose it to be bile, for it coagulates with spirits of wine

    5th – a brown fluid resembling urine in appearance

6th – brownish blood, not flaky, proceeding from the faeces and germs and perhaps partly in some cases from the pulpy cardiac opening of the stomach

7th – brown flaky blood mixed with mucous matter proceeding from the germs faeces and stomach, usually the precursor of the real black vomit

8th – *the real black vomit* which also is blood altered by its passage thro' the vessels of the villous tunic. It is, in general, ejected by gulps and in large quantities; but sometimes it is only found in the stomach after death. This matter is nearly of the same specific gravity with the fluid in which it is ejected. It is not soluble in water but floats in it in rough-edged, edged, irregular shapes of various sizes. Its colour is brownish black; spirits of wine or acids do not coagulate it. They simply mix with and suspend it. I proved by numerous experiments nearly four years ago that it was not bile. This year, I mixed bile with the black vomit lying in the duodenum and also with portions of black vomit found the stomach and found that the addition of bile greatly altered the appearance of the black vomit and that the bile mixed in the black vomit could be coagulated with acids proving clearly that black vomit and bile are totally different in appearance and chemical properties.

Every person is liable to an attack of gastric disease for every person has an intestinal tube and a liver and portal system. But all are not equally liable. Spare persons of sound viscera who are active and prudent are least liable. Those who have constitutions broken by courses of medicine, irregular habits or hardships in the walk of life and those who are unaccustomed to the climate full of rich blood. And all who are unhappy in mind can with difficulty escape in the epidemic season. The tracing of the operation of the cause applied to the body and affecting first the part to which it is applied and finally the whole system, particularly the villous tunic of the intestine, parenchyma of the portal system, vessels fluids and nervous system, is a difficult task.

I shall take as an example a very common cause of disease in the West Indies, one that no person will dispute to be a cause of disease – the application of wet and cold to the body. A.B., going to dine in the country, gets wet by a heavy shower of rain. He arrives first as the party is sitting down to dinner and happens to be placed with his back exposed to a current of air. His clothes begin to dry upon him, he feels a chill upon his surface and takes a glass of wine to warm his stomach. The chill of the surface continues, however, and coldness and pain of the spine begin to be felt. He comes home early but feels headache and soreness all over him and nausea at his stomach and becomes hot and restless. The next morning, his tongue is foul and, if in the middle of the epidemic season is perhaps covered with a crust and has scarlet or purple edges, and his eyes are suffused, and his nerves unsteady. The gastric disease is, in fact, completely formed. Now, the first effect of the wet and cold applied to the extreme vessels of the skin was to constrict them and cause the general sensation of cold. These effects must be the act of the nervous system or of the whole system sympathizing with the extreme vessels, for these effects follow the application of cold and wet under the circumstances described. As the extreme vessels in this state cease to absorb or exhale, it follows that the fluids of the system must soon be changed, and they are so. The manner of the operation of the cause, however, is not easily understood, nor is it certain that difference of exciting causes produces difference of the seat or phenomena of the disease.

Do all immediate exciting causes of disease produce during the epidemic season in Barbados disease of the gastric kind?

The case of Porter Murphy seems to prove that it does, and the universal sameness of the seat of the disease seems also to prove that any injury to any part of the body or any quality of the soul will induce the gastric disease varied in character according to the subject and season. For the abdominal viscera is the weak part of the West Indians. Mephitic[50] air is a very common cause of disease among soldiers. As for example, in Seafort, Port of Spain, Trinidad, in 1818, produced disease of the same textures as did fatigue on the hill of Fort George. The phenomena varied according to the subject and residence, not the immediate exciting cause. In England especially in spring, Pulmonic[51] disease is the most common. When a person catches cold (as it is termed), the injury is doubtless first done to the trachea[52] or lungs, yet the villous coat of the stomach very soon becomes affected, and then the disease is what authors have called fever. When the disease is affecting the villous tunic of the intestines but without any gangrenous tendency and without obstruction of the gall ducts, four oz of Rochelle Salts[53] with or without two grains of Emetic Tartar,[54] taken in divided doses during the first twenty-four hours, using also agreeable diluents and warm bathing generally cures it. The convalescence may be trusted to the usual hospital discipline and diet and to a small dose of salts in the morning and a tepid bath in the evening. When the gall ducts are obstructed and the villous coat affected but with no apparent tendency to putridity, the prescriptions are to be the same as in the first state but continued perhaps for two or three days or until bile appears in the stools. As soon as the bile flows, my prognosis is favourable, and convalescence is managed as above described. But when the bile does not flow in one, two or three days, the disease will perhaps run its course, and I keep up a gentle diarrhoea or diaphoresis[55] till the tongue becomes clean and nearly of healthy appearance, and when only jaundice remains, I prescribe bitters and taxations and exercise on horseback or in a carriage. When the villous coat of the intestine and portal system are both diseased and death in the ardent state or subsequently in the gangrenous state apprehended, I am not aware of any more effectual mode of practice than endeavouring to urge all the secretions by means of saline purgatives diluents and warm bathing. The saline medicines I chiefly use are Seidlitz Powders,[56] soda tartarisata,[57] Rochelle Salts, Cheltenham Salts,[58] Cream of Tartar,[59] Tamarinds, Cassia[60] or some other kind of fluid, pleasant purgative medicine. When the stools become merely the fluids drank (sic), I give a saline diaphoretic medicine[61] and frequently a small pill of compound cathartic extract[62] with each dose when I wish to keep up the purging and to bring away more solid dejections. When convalescence of a very severe compound gastric disease begins, grateful food and a small quantity of wine or porter with gentle alterative purging are employed. Persons who cannot or will not swallow medicines or whose stomachs will not retain them may be treated by purging injections, agreeable ptisans,[63] warm bathing, and poultices to the epigastrium,[64] and some of my most successful cases have been treated in that simple manner.

When the vomiting is very harassing and when the stomach is very tender, the patient complaining that fluids passing down the oesophagus are to the sensation like balls of fire, then I use drinks of the blander kind, tepid or cold water, tea, lemon grass tea, spruce beer, rice water, barley water, toast and water, cider and lemonade, and prescribe the hot feet and hands baths or the warm bath, and purging injections, but do not annoy the patient with purgative medicines except those of the mildest kind and that are pleasant to the taste and to the stomach. I shall conclude this report by introducing some cases illustrative of my practice and varieties of the epidemic.

Cases of Patients Who Vomited Matter Similar to China Ink and Recovered:

Thomas Evans, gunners mate of the *Pyramus*, forty-two years of age, a stout-made man, was admitted on 22 November at 6:00 p.m. into the Naval Hospital. He was in a state of violent delirium, which came on that day at 2:00 p.m. His pulse was 140, and he had hiccough and constant jactitations and vomited almost incessantly with great straining and loud moaning. He reported that in the execution of his duty, the foul air in the magazine frequently made him vomit and extinguished a candle in the space of two minutes and that his assistants were often obliged to run up into the gun room or main deck to breathe fresh air and prevent themselves from fainting. The fluid he vomited on the 22nd, 23rd and 24th was like a solution of gunpowder or rather of China ink. The whole of the fluid was dark blue. There was some sediment at the bottom of it, the matter was not flaky and floating in separate portions of various sizes, and therefore, was easily to be distinguished from black vomit. He vomited yellow bile on the

26th and, from that period, gradually recovered, but his stomach continued irritable for several weeks. And when convalescing, he got rheumatism in the shoulders and lower extremities. He is now in hospital waiting an opportunity to join his vessel. The treatment was by Seidlitz Powders purging injections and warm bathing. When the vomiting and hiccough were distressing, tincture of opium was exhibited. The matter vomited was vitiated bile.[65] His tongue had never the slimy ceraty[66] crust and the scarlet edges which indicate approaching gangrene of the villous tunic.

John Pitty John, a blacksmith Barrack Department, was another of these cases. On the first attack, he was yellow and mad and had compound gastric disease. On the second attack, he was not mad but slightly yellow, but he vomited great quantities of a fluid like China ink, his tongue immediately after a fit of vomiting appeared as if he had applied ink to it. He recovered and is now doing his duty.

These cases are given as examples of the ink-like fluid vomited, which may be mistaken for the real black vomit. The prognosis in such cases is favourable, but the convalescence may be tedious for the liver is diseased in function. When the patient vomits, vitiated bile appearing like China ink, the alvine evacuations have a similar colour.

Cases of Patients Who Vomited Flaky Brown Blood and Recovered:

Mrs Thompson, aged twenty-four, wife to a sailor of the *Pyramus*, a stout plethoric woman, was admitted at 6:00 p.m., 25 November 1821, into the Naval Hospital. No account of her case was sent with her, but she stated that at 10:00 a.m. on Friday the 16th inst., she was seized with pain of her head and loins, succeeded alternately by cold chills and burning heat. She was bled on the 19th. She had on admission the brown ceraty tongue with red edges and the irritability of stomach, which marked the tendency to gangrene of the villous tunic of the intestine and also slight yellowness of the eye, which proved the compound state of the disease. The eyes were not red. She was treated by saline purgatives, warm bathing and purging injections. On the night of the 27th, she vomited the flaky bloody fluid, which is usually the precursor of the real black vomit. She was remarkably jaundiced, and her disease was tedious. She was discharged on 9 January and was then slightly yellow.

Lieutenant Andrews, Royal Artillery, had compound gastric disease this season, and the most aggravated that I have seen recover. He was attended by Mr Sproule,[67] surgeon, Ordnance Department and myself. He was nursed by Mrs Andrews and a coloured woman named Rachael, one of the best nurses in the island. He was treated chiefly by mild purgatives, diaphoretics and diluents during the disease and by bitters and taxations during convalescence. As auxiliaries, the tepid bath and hot bath for the feet and hands were used, and a blister was applied to the epigastrium. He was not bled nor stimulated with strong liquors, nor did he use mercury or cold bathing or any remedy that could have injured a person in health. The purgatives he used were principally Seidlitz Powders and Rochelle Salts but given in small doses at short intervals that their action might be kept up without cessation. As he lived in the unhealthy range of huts to leeward of the Ordnance Hospital, he was removed on the morning of 9 December to Major Crittenden's quarters, offered to him by the major with his usual kindness. (He was taken ill on 8 December.) At noon on the 14th, the nurse told Mr Sproule and myself that Mr Andrews had vomited something black, which she had kept for us to look at. We found that the fluid vomited contained black flaky matter, exactly of the kind vomited in the first stage of black vomiting by a person of his habit. I was not surprised, for I had not ventured to expect any favourable crisis till the 8th day of the disease at soonest, and perhaps not till the 15th or 22nd, nor did I altogether despair of his recovery for Mrs Thompson whose case I have given had vomited similar flaky bloody fluid. He used the Rochelle salts and diluents with great diligence; they operated well, and he did not vomit any more of that flaky matter but had haemorrhage from his nose and mouth for two or three days. The following is a copy of proceedings of a medical board held on him at St Ann's on 18 February 1822.

The board, having minutely examined the state of health of Lieutenant Andrews Royal Artillery, find that he labours under visceral disease consequent to yellow fever, which attacked him on the 8th of last December and from which his life during three weeks was in extreme danger. He was yellow, had haemorrhages from the mouth and nose, and vomited that kind of black, flaky fluid which usually precedes the vomiting of what is called black vomit. He still continues jaundiced and weak and does not convalesce favourably. His constitution has received so severe a shock that the board is of the opinion the complete re-establishment of his health in this country is not to be expected and therefore recommends that he be allowed leave of absence for twelve months to return to England for recovery.

Signed
Hugh Bone, MD, Physician to the Forces
Elliott, Surgeon to the Forces
Sproule, Surgeon Ordnance Department

Cases of Persons Who Vomited the True Black Vomit and Recovered:

Mrs Andrews aged twenty-two, a thin woman, wife to a soldier of the 4th regiment, was admitted into the Naval Hospital at 4:00 p.m. on 19 November. She had been washing clothes in the forenoon and was seized with pain of her back and inferior extremities, succeeded by rigours and pain in her head. Her countenance was pale, her tongue covered with a white cerate-like crust, her eyes suffused and her pulse 100 and small. She lived in one of the small huts near the canteen, said she had fever in Grenada in September 1820 and had been two years and a half in the West Indies. Her head was shaved, and leaves applied to it. She was put into the warm bath, and solution of soda tartarisata was exhibited to her at intervals of two hours, which during the night produced most copious alvine evacuations. On the 20th, the pain of her head and limbs was the distressing symptom. She took the solution every third hour and had a warm bath. On the 21st, her eyes were charged with blood and opened imperfectly. Her pulse was 110. She vomited everything she swallowed. Her tongue was covered with a white crust. Her head was giddy but not painful. She took a Seidlitz Powder with six minims[68] of tincture of opium every third hour, had a warm bath at noon, and a blister was applied to her epigastrium. On the

22nd, the same symptoms continued but were aggravated in degree, and the edges of her tongue were very red. She used the hot hand bath and the hot foot bath and took a diaphoretic[69] medicine with a small quantity of Paregoric[70] in it. 23rd: The vomiting continued, and her neck, chest and eyes became yellow, and she became delirious. She took half doses of Seidlitz Powders, used the foot and hand-hot bath, and had an Amodyne[71] draught at bedtime. 24th: The symptoms were as on the 23rd, except that the delirium had decreased. The same treatment was continued, and an emollient poultice was applied to the region of the stomach. 25th: The tongue was red in the middle with white sides and red edges, and the yellowness was increasing. She became delirious in the afternoon. The same treatment was continued, and she received a purgative injection, which was followed by a very copious alvine evacuation. 26th: The symptoms were the same this morning, and the same treatment was continued. 27th: She had been very restless during the night and had brought up a large quantity of true black vomit. A great quantity of it was upon the sheets that had been removed from the bed previous to the morning visit. The same treatment was continued. In the evening, she felt herself much better, and she passed a good night. 28th: Did not vomit; her tongue was clean and moist, and she was tranquil and ate some soup for dinner, but in the evening became delirious, screamed and talked incoherently. The same treatment was continued. 29th: This morning, she was better in all respects. A small dose of c. tincture of Gentail[72] and of c. spirit of Lavender[73] was ordered every second hour. 6th December, she was sitting up in her bed at the visiting hour and had improved in strength but was yellow. She convalesced gradually, and the yellowness gradually disappeared. She was discharged to her hut on 28 December.

Mary Anne Carmichael aged six years, the daughter of a serjeant of the 4th regiment, was admitted into the Naval Hospital at noon on 10 January 1822. She lived with her parents in a hut near the new barracks. On the eight[h] instant, she was seized with pain of her head and back and general pain and vomiting. She had taken, previous to admission, a dose of castor oil and some powders given to her by Mr Wood, which were all instantly rejected. At 6 p.m., she began to bring up black vomit, which nurse kept in a white basin to show to me. It was the real flaky black vomit. The appearance of the child, except for the suffusion and half-shut state of the eyes, did not indicate much disease. While I was dictating the report at the morning visit of the 11th, she vomited a gill of black vomit. She was put into the tepid bath on admission and again in the evening. A purging injection was given every four hours, and a large emollient poultice was applied to her stomach. And she was directed to use tea as a common drink, and lest any neglect should occur in the nursing and administering the medicines, I admitted her mother into the hospital to nurse her. The two first injections brought away a very large quantity of fetid thin matter; her bowels had not been moved since the beginning of her illness. At 3 p.m. on the 11th, the child asked me if she would die. I thought her death very probable. However, I waved the question and replied, what makes you think so? She was then respiring forty times in a minute; her lips were of a vermilean (sic) colour, and her countenance pale. 12th, she had vomited black vomit during the whole of the night and had passed by stool a large quantity of matter very similar in appearance, not quite so black. Her eyes were slightly yellow, and she had constant jactitations.[74] The prescriptions were repeated. 13th, she passed a very restless night and vomited and passed by stool large quantities of black vomit. At 7:00 last evening, she passed blood by stool during the day. She was delirious.

What she vomited was very similar to what she passed by stool; only the flakes in the vomit were larger than in the stools. The vomited fluid was very similar to the tea leaves suspended in water. The injections, warm baths, poultices, and diluents were continued. 14th About 1:00 a.m. Mr Campbell was called to see her. She was then screaming and tossing herself in bed, and her mother and the nurse thought she was dying. The vomiting of black vomit and the passing of black stools continued. Her eyes were yellow. The prescription was yesterday, 15th. She was less restless during the night. When I was dictating the report of her case at 7:00 a.m., she vomited about two ounces of black vomit. Her stools this day became less black. The same prescription was repeated. 16th Had not vomited since the morning of the 15th, and her stools were not very black. 17th She had passed a very restless night and was occasionally delirious and, after an injection, passed a large quantity of consistent offensive faeces. During this day she appeared evidently to have had a favourable crisis. She did not vomit. The same prescriptions were repeated.

18th She had passed a good night, did not vomit, her stools were of natural appearance, and she ate breakfast and dinner with a good appetite. From that period, she gradually convalesced and on 12 February, was discharged cured. This is probably the best-authenticated case of a person having vomited real black vomit and having recovered that is on record. She continued vomiting flaky black vomit from 6:00 p.m. on the 10th to 7:00 a.m. on 15 January. That is during 109 hours or four days and a half. Mr Sproull, Ordnance Department. Mr Lainsworth, staff surgeon; Mr Stuart,[75] hospital assistant, as well as Mr Campbell and myself are evidence that she vomited the true black vomit. And on Saturday, 12 January 1822 when Sir Henry Warde[76] was visiting the women's ward in the Naval Hospital, I mentioned her case to His Excellency and his staff.

A specimen of the black fluid she vomited is preserved for the Barbados Garrison Medical Museum. The girl now enjoys good health, and her mother, who nursed her, did not catch any disease in hospital or since. I might add to this report further illustrations of practice and numerous reports of dissections, but the length to which it has already extended, induces me to bring it to a conclusion.

Signed
Hugh Bone
Physician to the Forces

Extract of Half-Yearly Medical Report by Dr Bone, Physician to the Forces, Barbados, 20 February 1822

The contagion of yellow fever became the order of the day, and in this gloomy, agitated state of mind of the garrison, the weather being also hot and dry and the air stagnant, or any feeble breeze that blew being from the south, gastric disease appeared first sporadically in the Bay. Epidemically among, the military quartered in the low ground west of the parade and finally produced some mortality in the 21st Regiment.

The first cases that I heard of were two bakers discharged soldiers who lived opposite the commandant of St Ann's but during the day worked in the bay with Mr Maurey, a French baker. One was taken ill on 27 July, the other on the 28th, and both died yellow after a short illness of gastric disease. These men were in the habit of bathing in the sea after leaving their work. Both were drunken characters.

The locality of Maurey's house is most unhealthy and into the yard between the bake-house and dwelling house. Spouting from neighbouring houses conveyed water, which stagnated and mixed with foul water from these houses and Maurey's, and formed a foul stagnant pool from the effluvia [which] was most offensive. Maurey's House, too, was unhealthily constructed – the front room to the east, though very hot, was well-ventilated, but two rooms to the west were small, ill-ventilated and not in the English style of cleanness. The house I know well and Mr Maurey's premises after the death of his two bakers and of a female lodger who died in one of the small rooms described, but I attended in his house Mr Harrier of the Storekeeper General's Department gastric disease in 1820, and again in 1821. He recovered both times and now enjoys good health. Mr Maurey assured me that neither these men nor his female lodger had been near any person affected with gastric disease. He attributed the disease of the men to drunkenness and bathing in the sea when exhausted and perspiring. I attribute blame to these causes but also to the suffocating heat of his bakehouse and the pestilent smells in his premises. The death of the female he attributes to a broken heart caused by misfortunes. I allow very much to that cause, but the small, untidy, suffocating room in which she slept, and the local nuisances described appear to me to be more blameable. In that part of the Bay and, indeed, generally in the Bay and Bridgetown, the houses on each side of the street are one continued line without intervals between them for ventilation. The cellars under them are not ventilated.

The next two cases I heard of were two gentlemen clerks to Mr Alleyne. They lived in the Bay, which was not far from Mr Maurey's house. Both were young men and newcomers. One of them, Horatio Warder, was taken ill on 30 July at Mr Chas: F. Alleyne in St James's parish, where he had gone to spend a few days, and died on 2 August. He was taken ill in the country and died there and had not been near any person affected with yellow fever, nor did any person in the house where he died catch his disease. The other young man, John Calometi, hearing of the fate of his companion, became alarmed and, on 6 August, was taken ill at Mr Alleyne's house in the bay and died there on the 9th after an illness of 65 hours. He had not been near any person affected with gastric disease, nor was any person in the house where he died afterwards affected with it.

Concerning these two cases, I have the following correspondence:

Naval Hospital
21st August

Dear Catheart,
You were kind enough to say that you would procure for me any information I wished relative to the two young men who lately died of yellow fever, the one at St James's, the other at Mr Alleyne's house in the bay. As it is surmised that [these men caught the disease] from some person affected with yellow fever and lately landed in Barbados from Tobago or Demerara, and that these gave their disease to two bakers discharged soldiers of the 63rd regiment and these again, the same disease to others – will you procure for me any information you can obtain relative to this subject.

Yours truly
Signed
Hugh Bone

Mr Catheart
Purveyor to the Forces
In reply to this letter, I received the following schedule and letter.

Table 4.5: Schedule for Horatio Warder and John Calometi

Name	Horatio Warder	John Calometi
Age	18	18
Arrived in West Indies	At Barbados on 10 February last	At Barbados on 5 January 1820
Period in West Indies	Near 6 months	Seven months
When attacked with chillings	At no period of his illness being first served with an acute headache about noon on 30 July	The evening of the 6 August when he also felt a slight pain in his back but rose and went out as usual early next morning
When became yellow	The colour of his complexion did not materially change till about 18 hours before death, tho' his eyes were previously affected	After being blooded on the 7th in the morning about 11:00
When began to vomit	He had 3 or 4 vomits the second morning of his illness – 31 July, but none afterward. Everything to last remained on his stomach well	He had only one slight vomit about 14 hours before death. He retained his medicine afterwards well and never complained of nausea
Colour of the body after death	Pale yellow	A little tinged with yellow but not so much as the above (sic) patient
How many hours ill	From the period of being seized with a pain in his head to the time he expired was 68 hours, say from noon on 30 July to 8:00 on morning of 2 August 1820	From about 8:00 in the morning of the 7 August till 11 on the 9th at night when he died. Perhaps the period may be from 6:00 p.m. the 6th to 11:00 am the 9th – 65 hours
Where taken ill	At Mr C.F. Alleyne's	At Mr C. Alleyne's house
Where died	In the parish of St James, in a well-ventilated chamber	In Bridgetown, in an extremely cool chamber
Whether he had been near a person affected with yellow fever	No	No
Whether any in the house had since had it	No	No
Who attended him	Dr Hinkson Dr Caddle, as Physician	Dr Baycroft three times each day
Who can prove these statements	Charles F. Alleyne	Charles F. Alleyne

Reports from Barbados

Bridgetown
Tuesday, 28 August 1821

My Dear Sir

I have filled up the schedule sent me yesterday as accurately as I am able to do and hope it will answer the purpose of destroying any idea that these two poor young men were the means of infecting each other or anyone else with the direful malady which so quickly consume them.

Yours truly
Signed
C. Alleyne

Mr Catheart Esq.

As these were the first persons who were this season attacked in Barbados with the disease called yellow fever, I have demonstrated that their disease originated sporadically from assignable causes. Neither was received nor communicated by personal communication.

The first military person attacked with gastric disease in 1820 was the wife of Gunner John Carson, Ordnance Department, who was taken ill at Ricketts Battery, a post westward of Bridgetown about half a mile, and where the family had been stationed about a year. She had lately been brought to bed. The abdominal viscera were consequently in a weak state, she and her infant died of gastric disease. Her husband was brought to St Ann's and put under observation but continued well and is now alive. Mr Bradley Surgeon Ordnance Department, inspected the quarters of this family. It acquainted me that the state of the premises and the mode of life the family had been following fully accounted for the gastric disease of the female and her child. At least no contagionist cause could be given, for there was no proof whatever that she [died] of gastric disease.

There came to this country in 1819 – twenty-eight men, six women and four children belonging to the storekeeper general's department. The men were civilians receiving wages, rations and lodgings from government. They were generally quartered in the dockyard or the low flat ground near it, in Crabtown or Bay Street. The whole of the low ground between the parade and the sea has for many years been known to every officer in the garrison of St Ann's to be unhealthy during the sickly season. And on that opinion proved by melancholy experience to be true. The huts in Crabtown were condemned by a medical board in 1817. Doctor Menzies was a member of that board. These storekeepers suffered severely; fourteen of them were taken ill during the season, and nine of them died. As these people were all in the same employment, came from England in the same vessel, were unseasoned to a tropical climate, lived in huts, lodgings or quarters near each other on unhealthy ground, the contagionist could easily trace communication between sick and healthy individuals, and nothing could be more easy than in many of these cases to find that previous to being taken ill the sick person had touched, seen or approached some friend or acquaintance affected with gastric disease. This kind of proof, however, weighed nothing with those who denied the doctrine of contagion, for they saw that the situation, the quarters, the season, the climate caused the disease of those newcomers. Remove them to the 3rd or 4th Terrace to Windward. They will soon become healthy; keep them where they are. Of course, many of them will die. They were removed from the unhealthy situations in December but having lived in them during the hot and unhealthy months, their systems were predisposed to gastric disease.

From my own experience, I think an absence of a fortnight or three weeks from the sickly quarter or situation and residence in a healthy quarter or situation is requisite to give security against the explosion of gastric disease. I first observed this fact in St Ander [Santander] in 1813. The Royal Artillery and Royal Sappers and Miners suffered severely. On the quarters of these corps, I must offer some remarks. The artillery barracks are on the west side of the parade, immediately on the brink of a mural cliff which terminates it. The barrack faces eastward and now that the parade is completely drained, enjoys a pure and healthy breeze. Still, the upper storey requires a close gallery and to have jalousied windows or glass windows, for at present, the draught of air through these windows is frequently so strong that it must check perspiration and cause disease. The kitchen and guardhouse were objectionable, but a new guardhouse has been built, and the kitchen has been enlarged and properly fitted up. The engineer's yard, where some of the sappers and miners were quartered and where some of them constantly worked during the day, has the brow of a rock about twenty feet in height on the east and near the brink of that precipice a range of huts occupied by Ordnance officers; on the s and north are sheds and on the west a range of houses. To add to the comfort of the place during 1820, Roberts Drain discharged into a coral basin in the N.E. angle of the yard, the water from the parade. In that basin, the water was very quickly absorbed, for the rock is coral and indeed a dripstone, but when the fall of water was great as it was in October, the water was discharged from the drain faster than absorbed in the basin, and consequently overflowed the yard, and the floors of the houses and sheds.

But these were not the only medical objections to this yard in 1820. A covered drain passed from it under the houses to the sea, and the high tide caused a reflux of the putrid water through the drain into the yard. There is a trap door to the drain that opens east of the range of houses. Mr Bradley showed me this drain; we opened the door; the smell was putrid and most offensive. I examined it also with Dr McCreery, 1st W.I. Regiment, and we found the stench from it to be intolerable. The Benny family lived in the range of buildings on the west side of this yard and nearly over the drain. Had they *remained healthy,* there might have been *cause for wonder* that they should all have become sickly as they did, *was to have been expected,* yet this is the family to which the tracers referred for *proof* of the *personal propagation of gastric disease.*

Some men of the Ordnance Department lived in huts, some in quarters, some in the lower arsenal, all objectionable quarters, as being either on the low unhealthy ground or on the brow of the hill immediately to eastward of it. The range of huts occupied by the officers of the Ordnance Department are on the brow of the precipice eastward of the engineer's yard and are prevented from the breeze by the Ordnance Hospital directly to the east of them. This range of huts is decidedly unhealthy. In the sickly season of last year, I advised Mr Eyre to leave it, so soon as he recovered from an attack of sickness, he experienced it – and he did so. Mrs Graham died there. Mrs Andrews was ill there and removed from it. Several of the men who were quartered there were taken ill and died. Relative to the Ordnance Hospital, I shall not make any observations till I come down to the present year. The new barracks occupied in 1820 by the 21st Regiment are excellently planned for this climate. The lower house requires jalousied windows and a jalousied gallery to windward. The lower barracks occupied by the 1st W.I. Regiment [are] on the low ground under the parade, but they are in such excellent repair and so well galleried and jalousied that for black troops who cannot bear a keen wind, they are excellent and by some officers preferred to the more splendid new barracks on the parade.

At an inspection of these barracks the comfortable state of the married people of the 1st W.I. Regiment has frequently astonished and delighted me. They are in one large room. Each pair has a good bedstead and clean bedding. The room is clean and has an air of comfort seldom seen, I am afraid, in the quarters of a white soldier.

The parade was formerly during wet weather a marsh, and I have myself seen very good plover shooting on it. The first attempt to drain it was by Major Crittenden, who, in 1816, with a fatigue party, made an open drain from the parade to the covered drain of the military hospital. This drain although it prevented the parade from remaining long at any time, an open lake, yet had not sufficient declivity for draining the lowest parts of the parade completely.

In 1817, Captain Roberts, commanding the Royal Engineers, planned the draining of the parade in an effectual manner and being enthusiastic in carrying his plan into execution, he commenced in 1818. It is a covered drain four feet and half deep and two feet wide; the sides are built of calcareous sandstone or Coralline rocks. The roof is arched. It runs from the well east of the new barracks in a direction nearly west of the sea; from the barrack to the west boundary of the parade, the drain has been covered in long ago, but it has not yet crossed the low ground between the parade and the sea. This drain answers the original intention. The parade is now never a lake nor a fen for plover shooting. The drain runs between the two pavilions which form the new barracks. It was part of Captain Roberts's plan to build two ranges of water closets or privies for the soldiers over the drain between the pavilions and to have a tank of water from which water was to play occasionally thro' the drain under the water closets or privies and to have a covered gallery leading to them from each pavilion. This plan, it is to be hoped, will be put into execution for the present privy of the barrack is distant from the S. Corner of the new barracks about three hundred yards. It is situated on the roadside, and the contents never taken away. The sight of it is unpleasant, the smell to Leeward offensive, the distance from the barracks inconvenient and for weakly or sick men dangerous to life.

The soldier's wife in this command has half a soldier's ration, but without rum and without the indulgence of having fresh meat when the men have it, frequently she cannot find a quarter in the barrack huts or buildings and is obliged to hire a hut which usually in this island costs two dollars a month. To defray the expense, she washes for a certain number of men – ten or perhaps a dozen at four dollars a week each and her husband gives her what money he can spare. From this statement, it is evident that a soldier's wife suffers great hardships in this country. In fact, the mortality of these poor creatures, even in this island, is very great and, in some other islands, still greater. Nor is it to themselves only that they bring misery and death but to their husbands and children. When the proportion of women in a corps is more than six to a hundred men, supernumeraries have no rations except the share they receive from the allowance to the number of women allowed rations by His Majesty's Regulations. Hence, to save the supernumeraries from starvation, those allowed rations by His Majesty's Regulations are deprived of part of the food necessary for their support. The officers of the garrison who were attacked with the gastric epidemic were Mr Donnelly, assistant surgeon of Royal Artillery, Captain Roberts, Commanding Royal Engineers, Mr Bradley, Mr Caverhill hospital assistant surgeon, and Lieutenant Palmer 63rd Regiment in charge of the military labourers.

The whole of these officers lived in the low ground west of the parade. They all except Mr Donnelly dined at home and he generally three or four days a week. Mr Donnelly, a few days previous to his being taken ill resided in one of the rooms of Mr Bradley's quarters. There, he was taken ill and died. Mr Bradley, Doctor McCreery[77] and myself attended him but he followed principally his own plan. He tried to affect his mouth with mercury, and once he thought he had succeeded, but he became yellow and brought up immense quantities of black vomit. To use his own expression, "a pint produced a quart in no time". His sangfroid immediately previous to death was, as is usual in this disease, very remarkable. He wrote in a distinct hand a letter to his relations, and an hour after, he was dead. As he was a medical man and the corps to which he belonged very sickly, there can be no difficulty in tracing his having touched or approached some sick person. But he was a newcomer, lived in the hospital, a building now condemned as unhealthy by a board of officers, took little exercise, did not live regularly at the mess, had some belief in the doctrine of contagion and had been much fatigued with duty.

Captain Roberts, Commanding Royal Engineers, lived in Shot Hall. On Monday, 13 November 1820, he went to Bridgetown to order stock and arrange some business, for he was next day to have left Barbados for Trinidad on duty. He walked and fatigued himself in town. The heat was insufferable. He came home very much fatigued and, in the evening was seized with shivering and general pains. He attempted to relieve those symptoms by taking Sangaree, but he continued during the whole night. Next morning, Mr Bradley saw him and reported to the inspector. At noon, Mr Bradley and I saw Captain Roberts. He was evidently in the greatest danger, although he did not think so himself. His manner hurried, his breathing frequent, his tongue thickly covered with a crust, his face purple, his pulse soft and without force. He became yellow on Thursday and died on Friday morning at 7:00 a.m.

On Tuesday evening, Mr Bradley was taken ill, and during Wednesday and Thursday, Dr McCreery and I attended him. Although, at that time, the order for the black servants was in force, it was truly gratifying to see the manly and humane attention of Major Crittenden Royal Artillery and Captain Smith Royal Engineers to their friend Roberts on his deathbed. They were with him almost constantly during his illness, shook hands with him, talked to him, sat on a chair beside him, and both were in the room with him when he died. Yet neither were taken ill, neither were put under quarantine. This was a terrible upset to the doctrine of contagion.

Mr Carey,[78] surgeon of the 21st Regiment, saw Captain Roberts during his illness. Mr Green and Doctor Arthur also saw him, as did Mr Lancy Royal Engineers, Commissary General Turquand, and many other officers, all with impunity. Mr Bradley was attended by myself and Dr McCreery, so as soon as he could be removed, he went to the country to convalesce, and part of his furniture was burnt in conformity to the wish of the inspector. Although Mr Bradley believed nothing of the doctrine of contagion, if he had, I think it probable he should have died. Mr Palmer lived with this family in the dockyard in a house decidedly unhealthy from the situation and construction. His successor, Lieutenant McHewzie, lost one child in the same house last spring, and the other was very sickly. I condemned the quarter as a residence during the sickly season and advised him to leave it. He did so, got a quarter in the stone barrack, his sickly child soon recovered, and the family are all in good health. He went back to his old quarter at the beginning of the New Year, and as the obstructing partitions of the upper storey are removed and, Beckles Swamp, which is near it, filled up. I calculate that he may live there safely till next July.

I did not attend to Mr Palmer during his last illness, nor did I see him, but the situation and construction of his quarters, his anxiety and fatigue in attending to his sickly family and his military duties may be assigned as sufficient causes for his illness.

Mr and Mrs Ford and Mr Harmer, who lived in a low, damp, ill-ventilated house in the dockyard, were all taken ill. Mr and Mrs Ford were removed to the Quarantine Hospital; they both died. Mr Harmer was removed to Mr Maurey's house in the Bay; he recovered. Mr Caverhill lived principally in the lane leading from Shot Hall past the garrison privy. He had become a great contagionist. He was in charge of the military labourers and was labouring under mental distress consequent to an occurrence at Colonel Popham on the evening of 3 December. He was taken ill on Wednesday the 6th and died on 10 December at 11:00 a.m. The cause assigned for his death by those who argued for contagion was his having touched some patients affected with yellow fever. I, who do not believe the possibility of that mode of communicating gastric disease, ascribe his death to his full habit, his mode of life. It was also reported that he had been bitten by a mad dog about twelve days before he was taken ill. He complained of pain in his throat, but that symptom is usual in gastric disease. I did not attend him professionally, but I saw him several times during his illness.

Captain Roberts, Mr Donnelly, Mr Caverhill and Mr Palmer were the only officers belonging to the garrison of St Ann's who died during 1820. I think the causes of their death have been accounted for and that personal communication had no part in the production or propagation of their respective diseases. Colonel Popham's family went to St Lucia on a visit to the governor, Sir John Heane, on 1 August 1820 and did not return until 13 November. Mr Green had been some months the medical attendant of the family. They had left a serjeant in their quarter, Collymore House, to take care of it. The serjeant was seized with fever on the ...[79] was removed from it to a hut near the [Quartermaster] General's Office on 9 November, where he died on 15 November. Collymore['s] house was fumigated and purified by Mr Green himself, and when he judged it to be pure, he allowed the family to come to it, which they did on 22 November. On Monday, 27 November, when dining at the artillery mess, I received the following note.

My dear sir,
I will thank you to call on me after dinner to go see the youngest of Colonel Popham's daughters, who had a very smart attack of fever this morning and was going on at one o'clock.

Signed
R. Green

The family were taken ill in the following order of time: –

Emily Popham at 6:00 a.m.	27 November 1820 – Recovered
Catherine Popham at 6:00 p.m.	27 November 1820 – Recovered
Harriet, A servant at 6:00 p.m.	27 November 1820 – Recovered
Miss Popham at 11:00 a.m.	28 November 1820 – Recovered
Mrs Popham at 11:00 p.m.	28 November 1820 – Recovered

Miss Honora Popham at 7:00 p.m.	29 November 1820 – Died at 8:00 a.m. on 3 December 1820
Mrs Powell, the launderess, daughter to Harriet at 8:00 p.m.	12 December 1820 – Died at 8:00 p.m. on 19 December

They were attended by Mr Green and myself.

Dr Caddell joined us in consultation on 5 December. Mr Green's plan of gastric disease accorded exactly with my own. There was no jarring nor arguing concerning indications and the means of effecting them. There were no proposals of desperate remedies, but the plan of treatment so frequently recommended in my reports to the medical board was adopted. I do not think the success was very bad. The convalescence of the ladies was tedious, and they went home last August. With respect to the causes of the sickness in this family, I understood that those who maintain the doctrine of contagion suppose that the serjeant must have slept in some of Colonel Popham's beds and that some of the black vomit of the serjeant had remained on a chair when the family came into the house. With respect to the serjeant having slept in one of Colonel Popham's beds, I argue that the fact is not proved, and though it were, his having communicated any principle to the bedding capable of communicating gastric disease to the family is not proved, and cannot be proved, or made to appear possible. This possibility is one of the subjects relative to which the contagionist and non-contagionist is (sic) at issue. And therefore, assumptions are not to be admitted on either part of the question.

With regard to the black vomit on the chair, there is no proof that the man did vomit black vomit till he was removed to the hut, and altho' these were, there is no proof that black vomit is capable of communicating gastric disease. On the contrary that it cannot communicate gastric disease, I know by numerous proofs and the possibility of communicating gastric disease by the means of black vomit is one of the subjects at issue between the contagionist and non-contagionist and is not to be taken as an assumption. It is to be proved, not assumed.

During the convalescence of the family and till the return of the ladies to England, they stayed in Highgate House, which is two terraces more elevated than Collymore House. Part of their furniture was destroyed, and the colonel has been allowed for it by the government. The causes which I venture to assign for the sickness of this family are their residence in St Lucia and return to this island during the sickly season. It is a common occurrence for a person arriving from an aguish island or colony to be taken ill on arrival at Barbados.

Mr Jeffson, son of Sir R. Jeffson Bart, came from St Lucia, where he usually resided to Barbados, and had a very severe attack of general disease of the gastric kind, although without obstruction of the gall duct. He was attended by Mr Green and myself at the house of Mr Cavan and was supposed to have had a narrow escape with life. On coming from Trinidad, I had an attack of ague and the fact of there being danger in changing from one island to another, is established. Hence, the propriety of changing the stations of the troops in this command is, in a medical point of view, at least problematical. The offices of Colonel Popham's house wanted jalousied windows; the yard was not raised and gravelled. There was a foul drain that passed under the washhouse and which received the suds and foul water from the yard. One of the small rooms having suffocators was the lodging house of eight or ten military labourers; several of these people were taken ill with gastric disease, and some of them died. Colonel Popham's butler, who slept in the next room to these Congos, told me that during the night, they shut the windows, and the offensive smell and foul air of their rooms came through the lattice partition that divided his room from theirs and obliged him to get up to make them open their windows.

The foul air from the drain and Congos and the suffocators in place of jalousies I blame for the sickness of the Congos laundress and coachman and perhaps partly of the ladies, for the laundry was most unhealthy and the whole yard frequently a pond of water and smelling offensively. Having mentioned to Colonel Popham these probable causes of disease in his offices he allowed me to improve them on my own plan. I did so, and they have since continued healthy.[80]

The drought of 1820 continued during the spring months of 1821. In the summer months, the west coast of the flat district continued to be parched with drought, the ponds became generally dry, cattle were driven five or six miles from the country to water at Beckles Pond, the canes withered, and the ground provisions partially failed. On 2 September, however there was a heavy fall of rain over the whole island accompanied by thunder and lightning. The fall of rain was the greatest that had occurred since the hurricane of 1819. During September, October, November and December, the rain on the coast of the calcareous district was sufficient for the planter. Still, in the interior, the rain was scantier (and the [cane] crop on many estates totally failed). The weather, particularly in September, was remarkably hot and oppressive. The wind was frequently S or SW, and frequently, there was a perfect calm. October and November were also very hot and oppressive months. December was cooler but the atmosphere did not become perfectly pure and cool and circulate strongly until the beginning of February, the harvest time of the guinea corn. I think it probable that the cessation of sickness in St Ann's may have some connection with the reaping of the guinea corn, for it grows to the height of ten or twelve feet, and the greater part of the coast between St Ann's and Oistins is covered with it. It makes the field where it grows an artificial bog and weakens the force of the breeze. When the corn is cut down to Windward of my quarter, the breeze becomes stronger and more pleasant. This may be supposition for I have only observed the fact five years. But should it prove true, the calculation for the commencement of the healthy season should be when the harvest of guinea corn commences and without regard to the period of the year.

This season, the guinea corn harvest to windward of the naval hospital only began in the beginning of February. In 1820, every part of the surface of the island was scorched, and vegetation did not commence in the neighbourhood of St Ann's till the beginning of July. In 1821, the drought was not much felt on the flat coast between Oistins and Bridgetown. From 21 May till next February, grass was plentiful for cattle, and the produce of provisions was an average crop. This part of the coast is too sterile for the cane. In the interior, however, the drought was distressing till September, and the worm destroyed the cane. In 1820, the maximum heat was 86 degrees at the naval hospital. In 1821, 89 degrees.

In 1820, there was great mortality among dogs in the neighbourhood; in 1821, there was no mortality. In 1820, there was greater drought; in 1821, there was greater heat, more rain and more luxurious vegetation. The first fatal case of gastric disease I heard of this season was that of a Mr ..., who came to Barbados in the same vessel with Mr Tegart. He arrived in Barbados in June and died in July at Miss Betsy Austin's hotel. The next I heard of was that of a young man, a painter in the service of Mr Cavan. He had been only ten months in the island. I saw his body after death. It was very yellow, and his stomach had been irritable during his illness. He was taken ill on Wednesday, 28 August and died on the morning of Monday, 3 September. Another young European in the employ of Mr Cavan died a few days after. They both lived in Bay Street in a house in the enclosure on the slaughterhouse, which is on the south side of Beckles Spring.

Mrs Haversatt, wife of Deputy A.C. General Haversatt, was seized with gastric symptoms on the night of 11 September and died at 1:00 p.m. on the morning of the 19th. She was yellow and, previous to death, had profuse haemorrhages and delirium. Mr Elliott attended her. My assistant, Dr Bain, was much with her during her illness, and I saw her in consultation with Mr Elliott. On looking to my half-yearly report for 1817, I find that Mr Pitman died in the same house on 18 October, at twenty-five minutes to 11:00 a.m. he was taken ill on 12 October 1817, and she on 10 October 1821. Last year, Mrs Haversatt had been much with the people of the storekeeper general's department when they were affected with gastric disease. This year, she had not been near or seen any sick person. On 20 August, Mr Turner's storekeeper general's department was seized with gastric disease of the Spicus[81] that has its first seat in the intestines and colon. He was very ill in this hospital but recovered. He had gastric disease in October 1820.

Alex McCash, storekeeper general's department, was in hospital this year for gastric disease and also last year. He is now alive. Mr Harmer Conductor was taken ill on 31 October 1821 at Maurey's House in Bay Street, where he had continued to lodge since his illness in 1820. He was much alarmed since he was taken ill on the same day of the month last year and predicted that he was to die on 5 November. My assistant, Dr Bain and I attended him. He had true gastric disease, which continued about a week; the principal peculiarity was the swelling of his face, which occurred both years without any assignable cause. He was treated on the plan usually recommended for gastric disease during the epidemic season. He was remarkably well-nursed by Mr Maurey and recovered in spite of his prediction. I have received from Mr Haversatt, assistant storekeeper general, the following return. I insert it in this report.

Report of the Storekeeper General's Department showing the dates of their arrival at Barbados, sickness deaths, recoveries, etc.

Table 4.6: Onset of Yellow Fever among Military Personnel by Age, Rank and Arrival Date

Name	Age	Rank	Date of Arrival	When Taken Ill
Walter Ford	23	Conductor	January 1819	30 October 1820
Mrs Ford	28	———	——"——	1 November 1820
E. Harner	23	Conductor	18 January 1820	1 November 1820
——"——	"	———	——"——	31 October 1821
H. Clarke	25	Cooper	——"——	10 December 1820
Mrs Clarke	23	———	——"——	———
Louisa Clarke	2	———	——"——	———
Francis Catchlore	43	Carpenter	——"——	23 October 1820
Mrs Catchlore	43	———	——"——	28 October 1820
Henry Catchlore	6	———	——"——	28 October 1820
A. McAsh	27	Carpenter	——"——	18 October 1820
——"——	"	———	——"——	27 October 1821
Mrs McAsh	27	———	——"——	19 October 1820
Mr Turner	42	Packer	——"——	2 October 1820
——"——	"	———	——"——	23 August 1821
Mrs Turner	34	———	——"——	3 October 1820
Mr Hussey	27	Packer	——"——	10 December 1820
F. Hussey	7	———	——"——	10 December 1820
Mrs Hussey	30	———	——"——	———
Chs. Trueman	32	Packer	——"——	8 November 1820
Mrs Trueman	24	———	——"——	5 November 1820
G.F. Haversatt	38	Ass. Store General	6 February 1820	———
Mrs Haversatt	29	———	6 February 1820	11 September 1821

Table 4.7: Sickness Outcomes and Residence of Affected Military Personnel

Died	Recovered	Sickness	Residence
5 November 1820		Fever	Dock Yard
4 November 1820		Fever	Dock Yard
		Fever	Bay at Mr Maurey's
	Recovered	Fever	Bay at Mr Maurey's
14 December 1820		Fever	Dock Yard and Collymore Rock
		None	——"—— Returned to Europe
		None	——"—— Returned to Europe
27 October 1820		Fever	Cottages in Crabtown
2 November 1820		Fever	Cottages in Crabtown
7 November 1820		Fever	Cottages in Crabtown
	Recovered	Fever	Cottages in Crabtown
	Recovered	Fever	Cottages in Crabtown
	Recovered	Fever	Cottages in Crabtown
	Recovered	Fever	Cottages in Crabtown
	Recovered	Fever	Cottages in Crabtown
11 October 1820		Fever	Cottages in Crabtown
12 December 1820		Fever	Dock Yard and Collymore Rock
	Recovered	Fever	Dock Yard and Collymore Rock
		Fever	Dock Yard and Collymore Rock
12 November 1820		Fever	Cottages in Crabtown
	Recovered	Fever	——"—— Returned to Europe
		Fever	—— Bay ——
19 September 1821		Fever	——"——

G.F. Haversatt
Assistant Storekeeper General

Return of the storekeeper general's arrival at Barbados

The progress of the epidemic as it occurred to me in the naval hospital is endeavoured to be shown by the tabular statement which I annex. The first table is relative to convalescents of the 4th Regiment. They were generally stout, healthy men; none of them were yellow, and none of them relapsed or caught gastric disease in the naval hospital. The second table gives an account of the officers and men of the *Pyramus*. The third table is relative to men from the departments which usually supply patients from the garrison of St Ann's to this hospital. These men were treated by myself from the commencement of their illness, and except A. Rourke, who continued to stay in his hut in Crabtown till his recovery was an impossibility, they all recovered.

The fourth table is relative to the women.

Bone's Letter to Monsieur Chevrin dated 14 June 1822 Naval Hospital Barbados

Dear Sir,
In reply to your letter dated Bridgetown 4th inst. requesting me to state the result of my experience on the contagious or non-contagious nature of yellow fever and to give in support of my opinion some of the most striking facts that have fallen under my observation, I beg leave to state to you that I have treated the disease or various diseases commonly called yellow fever in 1813 at Santander in Spain and annually in the British West Indies for the last five years. Never having seen it propagated from one person to another, [I] am consequently of opinion it is not contagious. But an opinion is only an assent of the mind to an uncertain proposition and, when not proven, is to be disregarded in philosophical investigations. I shall, therefore, submit to your consideration the premises on which is founded my opinion that yellow fever is not contagious.

In the autumn of 1813, sporadic cases of yellow fever appeared in the British hospitals at Santander and, after the Christmas holidays, became numerous. The barrack of the depot was inspected and supposed from the state of the privies and sewers to be unhealthy. The troops were moved from it to moveable hospitals, which were placed in a healthy situation and soon became healthy. But the removal of the depot attracted the attention of the Spanish authorities. Their Board of Health inspected the British hospitals and pronounced the disease to be the yellow fever and contagious. The English medical officers were without exception of opinion that the disease was not contagious. However, the yellow [fever] cases were selected from our hospital and put in quarantine in moveable hospitals in healthy situations. I was then surgeon to the forces and had charge of the quarantine hospitals. The yellow cases were in number fifty-four, of whom eleven died and were all carefully dissected by myself and my assistants. None of the medical officers, hospital servants or washerwomen caught yellow fever nor any of the patients in the hospitals from which the yellow cases were selected. I calculated at the time that not less than seven hundred persons were fairly exposed to the influence of the disease, and none of them caught it.

The depot which furnished the yellow cases was not put under quarantine. The men from the depot mixed with the inhabitants as usual, and none of the inhabitants caught yellow fever. Although the cordons of troops surrounding the yellow cases did their duty – the British strictly, the Spanish with ferocity – yet they could not prevent all intercourse with the Quarantine Hospital, for one evening when my assistant Mr Williams,[82] assistant surgeon 23rd Regiment, made his visit to the female ward, he found one of the females with her sweetheart, "a serjeant from the depot", in bed with her. She was then yellow as an orange – the disease running its course, and the serjeant did not catch yellow fever. There was also in the same ward another female who continued to see her sweetheart while she was affected with the disease, and he also did not catch yellow fever.

In the Casa Blomeo, a hospital where two hundred patients were then under my charge, six or eight yellow cases having the utmost dread of being dragged to Quarantine Hospital from the comfortable one where they were treated, continued by covering their faces, lying on their sides pretending to be asleep or quite well to escape being taken to quarantine. They were put into a room partitioned off from one of the upper wards when the Spanish board inspected the hospital, which they did regularly every morning. The door of this ward was shut, and when the board left the hospital, it was thrown open, and the communication with the ward restored. None of those patients died. No person in the hospital caught any disease from them, and the number of patients was about two hundred. The president of the Board of Health had been a professor in one of the Spanish universities. He was a man of learning and for a Spaniard, liberal and not bigoted. Having repeatedly and minutely examined the cases of yellow fever in the British Quarantine Hospital, he changed his opinion. He declared the disease as not contagious or little contagious. The junta fined him for altering his opinion. He entered into a paper war with them. The argument was on his side, but the power on theirs, and they levied the fine. The English officers at Santander holding in abhorrence this illiberal act of the junta and thinking it unjust that the professor should suffer for avowing truth according to his conscience made up by subscription among themselves the sum he had been fined and presented it to him with a flattering address from Doctor Erly,[83] principal medical officer, which compensated for the persecution of his bigoted countrymen. The sum I subscribed was four dollars.

Sir James McGrigor,[84] the present director general of the Army Medical Department of the British Army, was then the inspector of the Duke of Wellington. He subscribed eight dollars.

In 1817, I saw and treated several sporadic cases of yellow fever in Barbados; some of them had black vomit, and none of them propagated the disease to the relations, medical attendants or those who visited them in their illness. In 1818, I was sent to Trinidad, where yellow fever was then destructive to the troops, and as Physician to the Forces had charge of the sick in hospital at Orange Grove near Port of Spain. The barracks at Orange Grove were supposed to be unhealthy partly on account of situation being on the bank of a dry river and too near the base of a hill to windward but principally owing to being crowded and in a ruinous state. Consequently, the troops were removed except the artillery, partly to St Joseph and partly Fort George. Both stations soon became healthy and did not communicate disease to any of the inhabitants in the neighbourhood of these stations. Neither the troops in the barracks at Orange Grove nor the patients in the hospital were under quarantine, and the disease was not communicated to the inhabitants of Port of Spain. They continued very healthy while the disease was producing great mortality within the pale of the garrison.

There were quartered in Trinidad in 1818 34 officers of the Royal York Rangers and 438 serjeants drummers rank and file. Of the officers, none died, but of the serjeant's drummers rank and file, chiefly of yellow fever 130. I calculate that had the disease been contagious, the immunity from it of thirty-four officers living in the same barracks but better accommodated, altho' badly, had been [an] impossibility.

In a barrack room at Orange Grove were quartered the band of the Royal York Rangers and a detachment of the Royal Artillery. A partition wall of boards separated them. The band in the windward end of the room continued healthy while the artillery in the leeward end were sickly, and from 26 November, six died from yellow fever. The band was then moved from the windward room and the artillery put into it, and there they immediately became healthy. Still, the women and children succeeded the artillery in the leeward room, and there they also in a few days, became sickly. These circumstances I represented to the commandant, and on 8 December, the partition wall was knocked down. Mark the consequences. On 11 December, all the women and children were well!!! And from that period, the room, altho' not white-washed, continued to be as healthy as any room in the barracks of Orange Grove.

The slight cases I sent from Orange Grove to St Joseph and treated only the severe cases at Orange Grove. The total number of these was sixty. The fatal cases, in number fourteen, were all except two opened by myself and assistants, and none of us caught yellow fever in consequence of these examinations, altho' each of us were inoculated while making them, and one of my assistants, Mr Sermon[85] assistant surgeon 3rd Regiment twice. The parts inoculated inflamed slightly, but no symptom of yellow fever followed.

The sickness in that garrison I attributed to crowding and, badness of quarters and want of ventilation. As an example of the grounds on which I form this conclusion, the history of the room in Orange Grove has been given, and I shall add another. In the summer of 1818, there were quartered in small rooms in Seafort Battery, thirty-two persons. In one of these room[s], a miserable shed, fifteen by sixteen feet and the height of the wall seven feet were quartered.

four men, of who three died

four women, of whom three died

six children, of whom two died

A total of fourteen persons became sick, of which eight died

In 1818, only three fatal cases of yellow fever occurred in the garrison of St Ann's, Barbados, and none of them were accused of being contagious. In 1819, I was sent to Tobago in consequence of the mortality of the troops stationed in it, the doctrine of contagion was believed there by every person except myself and Major Hetcher. The buildings were unfinished and badly constructed, and the season was most unhealthy. The troops were encamped on ground, selected by myself as the best in the neighbourhood of the garrison, and the admissions diminished greatly, as did the deaths. But the troops were under quarantine, and my anti-contagion plans were deemed heterodox. I had medical charge of the patients for forty-three days. The number treated in hospital was twenty-six, of whom thirteen died. I was not confined to the fort but mixed daily with the inhabitants. I opened and examined minutely all the fatal cases, except one, although assisted by a coloured surgery man. I did not catch the disease, and the inhabitants continued healthy, while the mortality in the pale of the garrison was most alarming. For seventeen months, only 45 from 144 persons were alive, notwithstanding strict quarantine regulations, and from 6 officers, Major Hetcher the only survivor.

In this year only one case of yellow fever occurred in the garrison of St Ann's. The Naval Hospital in Barbados is healthily situated for the West Indies, and in good order and well regulated. In 1821, yellow fever prevailed in the garrison of St Ann's and the *Pyramus*, a frigate on this station. The Naval Hospital was under my charge.

The total number of patients treated in it from June 1821 to February 1822 was 243. Of these, 101 were fever cases and 38 convalescents from fever. None of the patients under treatment for other diseases caught yellow fever. None of the fever patients or convalescents from fever relapsed or suffered a re-attack of yellow fever. None of the servants or persons employed about the hospital caught yellow fever. The former were in number thirty-eight, all white people, and the latter were in number fifty-eight, principally coloured people. The fatal cases were in number twenty-two. Post-mortem examinations were made in every case with one or two exceptions, and very carefully by myself and assistants, and with perfect impunity.

The hospital was not under quarantine. Disease was not communicated from it to the inhabitants, but the inhabitants of Bridgetown were themselves unhealthy. I have passed over 1820, altho' an epidemic prevailed in the garrison that year, for quarantine and contagion were then the order of the day, both of which, in my opinion, were absurd and pernicious. I shall state that the mortality in the troops in 1820 was 103. In 1821, when contagion was not believed nor quarantine introduced, the mortality of the troops amounted only to eighty-eight, and that the epidemic in both years terminated at the usual period, the beginning of February.

I have seen frequently orderlies attacked with yellow fever, but only in hospitals unhealthily situated or unhealthily constituted or crowded or badly managed. I have often observed that crowding, want of ventilation and cleanliness vitiate the atmosphere of a hospital barracks and cause persons who breathe the foul air to become sick. But I have not observed that crowding sick people is more dangerous than crowding those in health. I have never, in the course of my experience, seen a single instance of propagation of yellow fever from one person to another, nor have I met with any contagionist who can tell me in what manner it is possible to propagate it from one person to another. I every year see in Barbados sporadic cases of yellow fever originating without the possibility of suspicion of contagion. I have seen mothers ill of yellow fever nursing their children, the children continuing healthy, and vice versa, children having yellow fever, the mothers nursing them and continuing healthy. I have seen husbands nurse their sick wives and wives their sick husbands without catching yellow fever and having never seen a single instance of the communication of the disease from one person to another, altho' my opportunities for observing such communication existed have been at least equal to those of any physician at present employed in the British army, I think I may conclude that yellow fever is not contagious. If not contagious, how is it produced? I have a recipe for producing it, the reading of which amused you, you perused it, you shall have it. Take of soldiers lately arrived in the West Indies any number, place them in a barrack in a low, wet situation, or in the mouth of a gully, or on the bank of a dry river, or on the summit of a mountain, or to the leeward of a swamp, or of uncleared land, or where there is no water, or only bad water, give them each only twenty-two inches of wall in their barrack room, let this barrack be built of boards or of a sash and plaister and have neither galleries nor jalousied windows, but close window shutters, and a hole or cellar underneath the flooring to contain mud and stagnant water and holes in the roof for the admission of rain and the windows only eighteen inches from the floor that the soldiers may be obliged to sleep in the current of air and let them have drills on every morning on wet ground when fasting, and guard mounting and all kinds of fatigue not in the morning or evening but during the hottest hour of the day, when on sentry no shed to keep off the direct rays of the sun, and let them have bad bread, putrid meat, few vegetables, plenty of new rum, especially in the morning, discipline enforced by terror, not by mind and prevention, a hospital similar to the barrack room without officers, always crowded and plentifully supplied with rum, scantily with water, and under quarantine, and so ill regulated that the sick dread to enter it, a firm belief in the doctrine of contagion and a horror of approaching any one afflicted with yellow fever. Let these directions be attended to in the West Indies, America or Spain where the air is stagnant or charged with noxious vapours, subsequent long drought. The soldiers will soon die, some of them yellow, some of them with black vomit, and those first in the Ordnance where my directions have been most carefully observed.

With this recipe, I conclude my statement. May the Divine Being long preserve your life and give you health to enable you to complete your philanthropic undertaking.

I remain your servant.

Signed
Hugh Bone
Physician

Report of Observations to Accompany the Annual Report of the Sick in the 52nd Regiment at Barbados, 6 November 1838 to 31 March 1839 by Thomas Spence,[86] Assistant Surgeon, 52nd Regiment

The 52nd Regiment embarked on board HMS *Hercules* at Gibraltar on 12 October and disembarked at Barbados on 6 November, when they were immediately quartered in the Brick Barracks at St Ann's.

• • •

The average strength of the 52nd Regiment for the period here alluded to has been 530, which comprises 474 from Gibraltar, 68 arrived in October and 80 in February

• • •

Observations on the Epidemic Fever – The 52nd Regiment disembarked at Barbados on 6 November previously, to which date there had recurred well-marked cases of yellow fever. The officers took up their quarters vacated by the officers of the 36th Regiment, and the men were accommodated in a barrack within fifty paces and standing at an obtuse angle to the officers' range of buildings. Rain began to fall on the evening of the 6th and continued nearly the whole of the following day, the atmosphere being close and hot and the sun occasionally shining, with great power under which circumstances the fatigue duties incidental to recent arrival were to be performed and in consequence, the men were admitted into hospital. Soldiers landing from a sea voyage may be considered under peculiar circumstances. There has been a lack of sufficient exercise and generally some irregularity of bowels added to which there is a degree to unsettledness, which conduces to considerable drinking. The officers, too, are in like manner affected. The method of living is on board ship, different to their usual habit and in the *Hercules*, the sea being unpalatable, very many took Porter for breakfast and on arrival in a strange garrison, a great deal of hospitality was passing so that officers and men on arriving at Barbados might be considered in a highly inflammable state, requiring only the quick match to render the whole a blaze; as it happened that the torch was quickly lighted, on 10 November. A man of the 36th Regiment died in hospital of Yellow Fever. On the 14th, Major Cross of the 36th died, having embarked with his Regiment on board the *Hercules* on the eleventh. On the 15th, Ensign Gough of the 52nd was attacked and died on the 19th. Then Lieutenant Murray and, on the following day, Lieutenant Jarvis, with three officers who lived in the adjoining rooms [were attacked]. One of the mess waiters was admitted into hospital on the 20th and died on the 24th. Paymaster Winterbottom and his family were affected on the 22nd. He died on the 25th and Mrs Winterbottom on the 28th. Corporal Chas: Rose, the other mess waiter, was admitted on the 28th and died on 2 December. Private Loote, who had acted as servant to Lieutenant Jarvis, was admitted and died in four days.

Eight persons were successively attacked from the orderly room (an officers quarter adjoining Mr Winterbottom's), of whom three died, the Paymaster Serjeant, who had been employed a great deal in writing in those quarters, died, the quartermaster and his serjeant, who had been engaged in the Quartermasters Store (also an officer's quarter) were both severely affected, Lieutenant Pocklington, the adjutant having been much in the Orderly Room narrowly escaped death. Lieutenant Surties, who performed the duties of the last officers, died. Various other officers were attacked but less severely, and lastly, Captain Sigors was affected with the most violent form of the disease; all this happened to men freshly arrived in the country, but a Serjeant of the 69th who had been several years in this command was lent by Colonel Morius to the officers who [w]as suddenly called upon to perform the duties of paymaster. This man only wrote in Captain French's room two days, when he was taken ill as was at first thought by intermittent fever to which he was liable; the disease, however, assumed the peculiar epidemic character, and he died on the fifth day.

In his detail, I have passed over the occurrences of seven weeks to the 31 December, up to which time there had been many cases admitted into hospital, but not one had proved fatal, where the individual had not been immediately connected with the officers' quarters, and whilst considering this part of the subject, it may be well to remark that it has been reported that every officer of HMS *Hercules* who had dined at the mess of the 52nd was more or less affected with fever on the voyage to Halifax. This detail of facts will, there is no doubt, be considered by many persons satisfactorily to prove that some contagion existed in or about the officers' quarters. There have been many speculations offered as to the origin of this phantom, this will o' the wisp, this shade without a substance, one class of persons being satisfied that the seeds of the disease were brought from Gibraltar and another believing that it had been brought by the *Columbia* Steamship from St Lucia; but time does not permit me to attempt a refutation of these imaginings, for in a truth, bringing fever to Barbados would be like taking coals to Newcastle.

The influence of this fever was so peculiarly confined to the 52nd Regiment that His Excellency the Lieutenant General commanding ordered the assembly of a board of officers for the purpose of investigating and reporting upon the state of the barracks, as well as the drains in the neighbourhood. Still, after a patient survey, no tangible cause of disease could be observed, no circumstance appeared to exist which had not been in a similar condition during periods of the greatest immunity from sickness. Whence then came the poison? I know not and am willing to shelter any ignorance under a quotation from Dr Baueruff, who says, "The causes of this epidemic are still involved in so much obscurity and placed so little within our power, that neither human ingenuity, nor patriotic zeal with their most persevering efforts have as yet been able to hinder its appearance, or perhaps materially to check its ravages".

Symptoms – the disease generally set in with headache, giddiness, pain in the back, weariness of the limbs and aching of the knees and ankles combined with thirst, restlessness, oppression of the system, absence of sleep and irritability of stomach; the tongue being foul and yellow or brown in the centre with bright red tip and edges. The pulse, in many cases, being full, hard bounding, and quick, but in others, not less severe, this function seemed but little severe. The eyes were almost invariably injected, and the eyelids swelled and heavy, which caused a furious yet stupid expression of countenance; the skin generally was heated but conveying to the touch a peculiar pungency over the abdomen and on the forehead. Profuse perspiration was more than once observed at the commencement of cases which ultimately proved fatal. The bowels were easily acted upon, but the stools were almost invariably dark brown and liquid. Urine was scanty, high coloured and at first passed frequently and in small quantities and entirely suppressed in some cases towards the termination of the disease.

These symptoms were usually but not invariably preceded by rigours, and the attacks were, for the most part, sudden in their invasion. In some cases, the attack was, in the first instance, most insidious, and the patient merely complained of indisposition with loss of appetite and weariness, so remarkably was this example.

Some cases assumed the character of Phrenitis,[87] some of the delirium tremors (sic) – and others have appeared as cases of acute gastritis. The symptoms delignating (sic) the particular affections were again occasionally so amalgamated as to render it difficult to pronounce which organ bore the greatest pressure. Such were the cases on admission and the symptoms in the progress of the disease were generally modified by the treatment adopted or by the functions of the organs implicated. In the enumeration of the symptoms, it may be proper to remark that although the excitement in some cases ran extremely high, there never was any power to sustain the abstraction of a large quantity of blood. The patient soon either became faint or the stream of blood, vigorous at first, shortly began to flag however large the orifice might be. Further the blood taken was invariably dark coloured, never but twice buffed, and but rarely duly separating its serum. On the second or third day, the eye became yellow, and the skin soon after changed its colour, and the colouring elements of the bile became so generally diffused throughout the circulation that in more than one instance, the sheets were actually stained by the perspiration.

In the more severe cases, a considerable depression of the powers of the constitution became apparent on the third day, the heat of surface except of the abdomen or head fell considerably, the thirst, irritability of stomach and distention of the abdomen became intolerable, incessant sighing and hiccough were exceedingly distressing and haemorrhages from the nose, gums or bowels marked too generally the condition of the patient. In cases where the head was not pre-eminently affected, the grand climacteric was marked by the substance ejected in vomiting consisting of a glary fluid like the white of an egg tinged slightly yellow and striated with bloody points which looked like small portions of capillary vessels. These ejecta increased in sanguineous matter as the patient approached the final struggle and generally terminated in the black vomit, specifically so-called. When the cerebral symptoms were more conspicuous, it sometimes happened that the black vomit was not ejected till almost the last convulsive expiration, where it was literally jetted from the mouth. In one or two cases, the patient never vomited this peculiar fluid, but the stomach was found full of it after death. It frequently happened that the intellect was unimpaired 'till the very last hour, nay moment of existence. Occasionally, there was delirium of a low typhoid form and once or twice of an active talking character. The termination of the disease by death was usually on the fourth or fifth day.

On Dissection – the brain in those cases where morbid changes might have been expected exhibited high degrees of vascular congestion with a small quantity of serum in the lateral ventricles. The stomach and intestines were generally exceedingly distended and usually contained the matter termed black vomit. In one case, a large quantity of blood was formed in the ileum, and others, a quantity of black bloody substance adhered like paint to the walls of the intestines. Without exception, the mucous membrane of the stomach, as well as of the ileum, prescribed marks of inflammation to a greater or less degree. In the man who died after having been twenty-eight days under treatment, it was literally as black as possible throughout the whole of the stomach. Ulceration was frequently observed in the mucous membrane of the ileum but I think never in the stomach. The liver was invariably so far as my observation extended of a nutmeg colour and granular consistence – easily broken down by the finger, usually much engorged with blood, and in one case of an old soldier, modulated throughout the whole structure. The gall bladder was, for the most part, entirely empty and collapsed. In one case, it contained some bile of the colour of an egg's yolk, in which case the coats of the viscus were at least a quarter of an inch thick. In another it was full of very dark bile, its duct rendered quite impervious by the pressure of the head of the pancreas, in a shrivelled state.

These, I think, are the prominent features in morbid anatomy which I observed during the progress of the epidemic, but a man was admitted on 2 February and, after struggling with the disease to an extraordinary degree, died on 2 March. For a fortnight previously to death, he had no pulse perceptible at the wrist of the right arm. He was affected also with Paroxysms of Dyspnoea[88] of a most severe character, and therefore, my attention was directed particularly to the heart. The tenderous part of the mitral valve of [the heart] exhibited a most extensive ulceration, being more than an inch in length and nearly half an inch in depth, apparently as if the part had sloughed. This I considered merely in the light of an extraordinary coincidence being no part or parcel of the disease so-called yellow fever, but in all probability having influenced the struggle of the constitution with the epidemic.

This heart was preserved and shown to Dr Evans, a Civil Practitioner in Barbados, the author of an excellent practical work on the yellow fever. He admitted that a similar case had never come under his observation, but as it agreed with his theory of inflammation of the lining membrane of the heart being part of the pathology of yellow fever, he looked upon the preparation as valuable.

The next case of yellow fever, which proved fatal, was a man of the 69th Regiment, an invalid waiting for transport to England. He was admitted into hospital after a debauch, and therefore, the symptoms were, in some degree, equivocal at first. However, he died on the fifth day, and more from curiosity than from an expectation to find the morbid change, I opened the left ventricle when, to my astonishment, I found precisely the same disease or appearance.

The third fatal case which occurred since my first discovery occurred in a Serjeant of the 76th who died of apoplexy twenty-four hours after admission – that is to say, he had a fit of a mixed character between apoplexy and epilepsy succeeded by delirium ... [His brain] was highly inflamed. [Is] it then too much to presume that if the disease had been protracted, he might have had black vomit – or in other words, is it unphilosophical to suppose that the case was one of yellow fever?

But at all events there was the same disease in the mitral valve as occurred in the two former instances. It is far from my desire to jump hastily at conclusions or to build up theories on slender grounds, but it is not a little remarkable that a precisely similar morbid appearance should be found in this form of disease in three consecutive cases. It may be enquired if this appearance did not exist in any of the cases previously examined during the epidemic. In stating that it was not observed, I either do away with the supposition of this being a part of the pathology of fever or stamp myself a careless observer. But in justification, I must observe that during the prevalence of an epidemic, a single medical officer in charge of a Regiment has such a pressure of duty his mind and body are so exhausted that it is only [a] wonder he is able to examine bodies at all, much less to spend an hour or two over a subject putrefying in a temperature [often] far above eighty. The disease of the mitral valve consists of a series of depositions fringing the margin of the *catura tendinea*,[89] which depositions vary in size from a millet to a small pea and then appear to ulcerate or slough.

The nature or pathology then of yellow fever as it occurred epidemically at Barbados within the period now alluded to is certainly Muco Gastro Enteritis (i.e.) inflammation of the muc[o]us membrane of the stomach and bowels, with a chemical change in the blood and invariably structural disorganization of the liver with or without cerebral congestion, which being determined, there remains but to consider the most appropriate treatment

On my arrival in this country, I determined to cast off all previously entertained opinions of the nature of fever learned elsewhere, resolving that in the event of such cases being prevalent, I should submit my judgement entirely to that of others of experience in the country and under these circumstances, it was my peculiar good fortune to meet with the counsel, the assistance and support of staff Surgeon Franklin[90] for which I can never be sufficiently grateful, the method of treatment which he recommended followed – of course modifying the principles to particular cases. It consisted in the abstraction of blood to the amount of sixteen, twenty or thirty ounces at the onset of the disease to administer a full dose of Calomel ten or twenty grains and use freely Enemata, with the application of blisters to the stomach, head and neck according to circumstances, which practice may be said to have been far from unsuccessful. For out of fifty-six cases of men and officers of the 52nd, we lost twelve. In this particular, I may explain that in returning the number of cases admitted, I have acted to the best of my judgement as far as possible. Honesty to designate each case under its proper terms, though after all, it is subject to error because, as is well remarked in an article on yellow fever by Dr Gillkress in the *Cyclopaedia of Practical Medicine*, "In no disease do symptoms take a wider range than in yellow fever",[91] and therefore to have excluded all the cases except the most severe would have been injustice to myself and an unphilosophical proceeding.

Signed
Thomas Spence
Assistant Surgeon, 52nd Regiment

Extract of Annual Report of Sickness and Mortality in 52nd Regiment Barbados from 1 April 1839 to 15 February 1840 by Mr William Robinson,[92] MD, Assistant Surgeon, 52nd Regiment

Febris Communis Icterodes[93] – I shall preface the observations I have to make on this disease by a few remarks relative to the circumstances under which it appeared in the Regiment with its progress and decline. The weather during the last ten days of October was very changeable – frequent heavy showers with a powerful sun in the intervals and variable winds prevailed. The low ground before mentioned was partially flooded, particularly about the hospital.

The disease first appeared in the hospital about 1 November, the serjeant and three orderlies being taken ill in a day or two of each other, two of the latter died. It next appeared among the married families on the east and western sides of the barracks. Then, in the huts opposite the officers' quarters and soon afterwards in the barrack rooms both upper and lower, but principally in the windward building. The officer's quarters then became the seat of it. The quartermaster's wife, two officers and two mess waiters were taken ill. The quartermaster occupied the lower rooms in the centre of the building and the two officers those above. Remarkably, those rooms have always been particularly unhealthy in the various epidemics that have appeared in these barracks. The great mortality among the women rendered it necessary to remove them from the huts, and they were encamped on a higher position near the sea at the end of November. But the increasing severity of the disease in the barracks obliged the same step to be adopted with the whole regiment. Accordingly, it was encamped about 4 December on an elevated position, formerly the site of the Naval Hospital and to windward of the barrack and all the low swampy ground previously mentioned. The beneficial effects of this measure were very soon apparent. The number of cases rapidly diminished but the few that did occur were among the most severe I have witnessed and generally fatal. As all communication could not be cut off with the barrack, I was unable to trace clearly any of the cases among the men to their new position, but two women took the disease after they had been encamped upwards of a week and died.

The barracks were reoccupied the first week in January since which time scarcely a case has occurred. They have been some heavy showers but no other obvious atmosphere phenomena worthy of notice on the decline of the disease. In conclusion, I may say that the men did not suffer more from other diseases while encamped than might have been expected at the season. The manifest advantage of the change clearly points out the course to be adopted in future epidemics.

The following table shows the extent of the disease and fatality among the different classes of patients.

Table 4.8: Admissions, Deaths and Mortality Ratios by Type of Resident

	Admitted	Died	Proportion of Deaths to Disease
Officers	2	1	½
Officers' Wives	1	1	1 to 1
Men	70	21	1 in 3 1/3
Women	15	7	½
Children	8	2	¼
Total	96	32	1 to 3

Symptoms:

Slight rigours, weakness, and darting pains through the limbs coming on suddenly were the usual precursors of the disease. Those were soon followed by headaches chiefly in the forehead and orbits. Most frequently, there is suffusion of the eyes, hot, dry skin, flushed countenance, quick but generally a small compressible pulse, and irritability of the stomach. As the disease proceeded the eyes became more suffused and yellow, the skin hotter and more pungent with a bilious tinge of different degrees of intensity, the pulse quicker and often irregular. Mild delirium set in, the vomiting became more distressing, consisting at first of the contents of the stomach, then a clear, glowing fluid and finally either a thick greyish fluid, blood or black vomit. The tongue became dry and pasty giving the finger the sensation of its being covered with thick mucilage and of a fiery red colour, the mouth parched, teeth covered with sores and thirst urgent. The alvine[94] evacuations were copious fluid and of a brown colour. The urine, at first high coloured, was soon either suppressed or only a small quantity tinged with bile was secreted, although the desire to make water was urgent in others where no such symptom existed. The bladder has been found distended, but in those the cerebral system was prominently affected. Haemorrhage from the mouth, nose, urethra and blistered surfaces also occurred in a few cases.

Instead of the active form of the affection here delineated, a few cases occurred in persons addicted to drink, where no reaction took place from the commencement. They sank rapidly into a state of collapse as if the powers of life were overwhelmed by the intensity of the malady. I need scarcely say that most of the recoveries were of a milder form than either of those mentioned. Still, in all, either the peculiar appearance of the eyes, skin or headache and the matter ejected from the stomach were sufficient to denote the character of the disease.

Recovery took place in two instances, both addicted to drinking, although they had black vomit and haemorrhage from the mucous surfaces. Death has occurred from the third to the eighth day, most frequently about the fifth or sixth. Symptoms of amendment usually appeared on the third or fourth though some have continued in a precarious state until the eighth or ninth day. Only one man was admitted who suffered in the epidemic of the previous year, and his case was very mild.

Head – On cadaveric inspection,[95] the brain exhibited no disease except where the nervous system had been prominently affected. In those, the arachnoid membrane was thickened and opaque, the pia mater very vascular, the ventricles, base of the brain and spinal canal contained an increased quantity of fluid and the cerebral structure rather vascular but, in some instances, soft and blanched.

Thorax – The lungs presented no morbid change of structure peculiar to the disease. The head was invariably soft, pale and flabby, the fat around it as well as the valves tinged yellow. With reference to the inflammation of the mitral valves found in a few instances last season by Staff Surgeon Spence, I have not observed it in this epidemic, but we both lately saw it in the heart of a man who died of chronic catarrh and could therefore have been but accidental to the fever. Its true nature is yet to be ascertained. The blood was always dark, either fluid or imperfectly coagulated. In the few cases that I tested it, I did not detect acidity, but that state has been satisfactorily ascertained by others.

Abdomen – The mucous membrane of the stomach and intestinal canal exhibited various grades of vascularity. After approaching a dark purple hue, rather soft but [with] scarcely any thickening, the vascularity resembled the atonic distention in chronic ophthalmia more than that in acute inflammation. I have not observed ulceration of the mucous membrane, but the glands have been frequently enlarged. The contents of the alimentary canal were either blood, the greyish fluid before mentioned or black vomit by which I mean a substance like coffee grounds floating in a clear glary fluid and not tinging white paper. This latter was always acid, effervescent with the alkaline carbonate. Carbonate of potash caused a somewhat sanguineous appearance and precipitated a fibrinous deposit. Curiously, nitric acid changed the greyish fluid above mentioned into one closely resembling black vomit.

The liver was soft, of a mottled nutmeg appearance and full of blood; the gall bladder generally empty but, in some instances, contained a little viscid bile. The pancreas, kidneys and urinary bladder presented no disease; the latter was generally empty and contracted. In one case, mortification of the skin of the penis scrotum and lower part of the parietis of the abdomen occurred connected with an abscess around the bulb of the urethra into which there were several openings. A nearly similar case is recorded by Dr Chisholm in a note to his observations on the malignant pestilential fever (page 181)

Signed
William Robinson, MD
Assistant Surgeon, 52nd Regiment

Report of Observations to Accompany the Annual Report of the Sick Treated in the Garrison of St Ann's Barbados between 1 April 1839 and 31 March 1840 by Thomas Spence, Surgeon to the Forces

•••

Section 8th Epidemics

Rain began to fall towards the end of October when, at intervals, the heat of the sun's rays was very powerful, the wind blowing sometimes in violent gusts and at others being still, and the atmosphere close and oppressive. On the first of November, the hospital serjeant of the 52nd became affected with a severe form of bilious fever. About the same time three orderlies of the same regiment were attacked. Then it appeared amongst the married people and non-commissioned officers occupying quarters and huts on the east of the Brick Barracks and from this, in regular progression to the rooms occupied by the soldiers of the 52nd Light Infantry so that its course was directly with the wind in a straight line from the north wall of the hospital across a swamp to the east wall of the Brick Barracks. At this time, the wall of the hospital of which the serjeant's house forms part was more than three feet deep in water. It is most important to observe that the huts and serjeants' quarters where the pestilence raged with the greatest malignity are immediately opposite and parallel to the officers' quarters, the locality where, during the epidemic of last year, death did seem to hold his court in the very centre of this range of buildings. There resided in the upper part, Captain Vigors and Captain Palmes and on the ground floor, the quartermaster and his family. One of the captains had the fever last year and so had the quartermaster and his family, except his wife, and strange to say, she and the other captain were the only individuals attacked, and they both died. An officer who occupied the quarters to the south of Captain Palmes had an attack of fever of a milder form. I may mention that the room below this last officer's was used as the Paymaster's Office, and the clerk was the only person occupying it, but alas, he died. The room next to this, the one which last year was occupied as an orderly room and which seemed so evidently to contain the focus of disease, was most fortunately unoccupied this year. The pavilion, usually appropriated as quarters to the officers of the medical staff, being near the hospital and forming the south boundary of the before mentioned swamp, seemed to be within the malarious range, and three officers recently arrived from England were all seriously affected, and one died. But during this period, there were only three cases from the barracks occupied by the other troops in the garrison. Therefore, upon these facts, it was evident that from some unknown cause, this was the tainted circle. This knowledge induced the inspector general of hospitals to recommend to His Excellency the Lieutenant General commanding the expediency of removing the 52nd Regiment into camp, which was immediately carried into execution with the happiest effect. The disease seemed to be stopped as if by magic, and for a fortnight after the encampment, not one case occurred. After this, however, there were three or four fatal cases, but they only show the evacuation of the barracks should have been more strictly enforced than was really the case, for the officers' mess being still kept up and certain stores, etc., not being moveable without great inconvenience were still retained in the barracks. This entailed some going backwards and forwards and, to my conviction fully accounted for the few cases before alluded to.

It has been my lot to witness this form of yellow fever two successive years, being the former in actual charges and the latter in immediate superintendence of the medical concerns of this devoted regiment, and I have no hesitation in stating that the malignancy of the disease was infinitely greater during this than the previous year. The disease usually set in with intense headache, pain in the back and weariness of the limbs, with fever preceded by shivering deep pain and burning within the eyeballs and fiery redness of the conjunctiva, the tongue being coated with a thick, brownish yellow fur in the centre and red on the edges and tip, and in many cases, there was a remarkable degree of mental excitement and despondency.

The usual measure of evacuations, etc; having been adopted, the patient either became very considerably relieved with a subsidence of fever or the train of symptoms set in which indicated a case of the severe type. These symptoms are continued pain over the orbits, burning heat of the forehead, injection and yellowish of the eye, thirst with irritability of stomach, brown watery evacuations and pungency over the abdomen, which terminated in black vomit, retention of urine sloughing the scrotum. [There were also] haemorrhages, hiccoughs, delirium, coma and death. Some cases occurred when the symptoms were of an apparently mild character. Yet, the termination was fatal, which leads me to observe that during the prevalence of an epidemic form of yellow fever no individual having certain peculiar symptoms characteristic of the disease should ever be pronounced in safety so long as the slightest sign of illness continued. Drunkards frequently escape entirely but should one of this class be attacked, his chance of recovery is very small. The functions of the brain become, in such cases, peculiarly disturbed, the powers of the constitution are sunk, and the wretched man dies in the most extreme exhaustion.

In the epidemic of 1839, very few fatal cases existed beyond the fifth day, but this year, some lasted 'till the eighth or ninth. Remarkably, only one man was admitted into hospital with anything like a feverish attack this year who had fever last, and in this case, it was very mild on both occasions. The investigations in the morbid anatomy of this form of fever have not added anything to our previous knowledge except that further examinations have failed to corroborate suppositions which were entertained respecting the influence of the state of the mitral valve, the state of this membrane described in the last report having been since detected in diseases unconnected with yellow fever. I have this year had an opportunity of instituting and witnessing several chemical experiments upon the fluid termed black vomit ejected from the stomach, as well as upon the contents of the alimentary canal and blood contained in the veins after death. They are minutely detailed in the accompanying report of Assistant Surgeon Robinson of the 52nd Light Infantry, a young officer whose praises I should be glad to sound did I not think that I have too lately emerged from the situation of a subordinate officer to entitle me to assume the privilege of judging others.

On his report, however, I beg to refer as the best means of bringing to light his zeal and high professional qualifications. He has left me little to say further than a general summary of this epidemic. It is but honest to state that bleeding generally was more extensive[ly] had recourse to in the last year than this year, and the mortality was less, but in admitting thus far, I must also urge that the generality of cases in this epidemic was nearly on a par with the worst of last year. So far as I have seen, I am satisfied that the principal chance which any individual has on being attacked with the yellow fever is a strong and sound constitution. If such a person be attacked, the chances are greatly in his favour, whereas if any organ be tainted, the danger is considerable, and I, therefore, am of opinion that in this fever, palliation or mitigation of symptoms is all we can achieve. And he will be the most successful, who having fixed principles to guide him steers to the right or left according to peculiarities of the case and the existing symptoms. My views are then to reduce the fever with the least possible reduction of strength by diuretics purgatives and ablutions[96] and after evacuating the alimentary canal and having alleviated by cold lotions to the shaved head or fomentations to the stomach and abdomen, the local uneasiness. I then place my full dependence on the alkaline salts administered in such a variety of forms as may at the time, appear to be most expedient. Stimuli with Laudanum[97] and nutritious soups are commonly indicated in these cases wherein there is in the symptoms a close resemblance to delirium tremors (sic).

During October and November, seventy-three seamen were admitted into the hospital of the 67th Regiment. These cases occurred in Her Majesty's Ship *Satellite* from Jamaica and the *Vestal* and Steam Ship *Pluto* from Antigua. It is stated by Assistant Surgeon Blakeney[98] in his quarterly report for this period that whilst the *Vestal* was at Trinidad in October, a quantity of fresh cut unbarked wood had been taken on board and stowed away in the fore and after holds of the ship and from which a most noxious and disgusting smell arose and that the men on board attributed to this cause the origin of the fever. Whether or not this was the case, it is certain that the disease closely resembled the fever common in this island, cases of which had occurred in Bridgetown previous to the arrival of the *Satellite* on 1 October. The plan of treatment which had been adopted by the naval surgeons before the sailors came on shore seemed to have been general bleeding, and the free exhibition of mercury and the greater number of cases admitted from the *Vestal* were in a state of bloody ptyalism and Mr Blackeney remarks that "little else was left for him than smoothing the way to a better world".

I am particularly desirous of attracting attention to this circumstance as I believe the practice to be injudicious, and yet there are practitioners of great merit who think it indispensable. The common continued fever occurring in this island is almost invariably depending upon inflammation or ulceration of the mucous membrane of the ileum and prevail[s] at all seasons. But except in particular habits [it] is not very unmanageable, and the proportion of deaths is very small, being in the white soldiers 1 to 24 2/5 but in the blacks 1 in 8.

• • •

Section 9th – Relating to the influence of age and length of service in the country upon the mortality

Respecting the first portion of this section, my information is very inaccurate, and there have not hitherto been any returns sent into my office showing the strength classified according to ages, but of the eighty-eight fatal cases, two have been under twenty; twenty-six between twenty and twenty-five; twenty-eight between twenty-five and thirty; twenty between thirty and thirty-five; eleven between thirty-five and forty; and one only has been beyond forty relative to the second division of the section. I may extract the following table from the Sanitary Report.

Table 4.9: Yellow Fever Admissions and Deaths by Period of Residence and Class Strength

Period of Residence	Strength of Each Class	Admission of Each Class	Deaths of Each Class
Under 1 year	1556	986	26
1 to 2 years	634	639	38
2 to 3 years	25	177	3
3 to 4 years	49	126	1
4 to 5 years	35	51	2
5 to 6 years	120	67	2
6 to 7 years	101	391	15
Above 7 years	3	3	1

• • •

Signed
Thomas Spence
Surgeon to the Forces

Extract of Annual Report of Steamers, Royal Navy at Barbados 31 March 1842 by A. Mackintosh MD, Assistant Surgeon, 33rd Regiment

From my ignorance of all the duties, dieting punishment, etc, of men afloat, it is evidently impossible for me to make out a report for the Royal Navy according to the prescribed form.

The class of ships that have sent almost all the cases to hospital are the steamers, and both in the want of accommodation for the men and the arduous duties of coaling, etc; to which they are exposed. There is no doubt a good deal of the comparative unhealthiness of that class of vessels is to be attributed; there is also another subject which seems to be overlooked by the naval authorities – the great danger of sending ships to have their flooring rip[ped] up and thoroughly cleansed in such an unhealthy harbour as English Harbour, Antigua. This operation is not altogether in production of fever in more temperate climates. In one steamer, the *Maegaera*, the endemic having disappeared, she went down there to be thoroughly cleansed. The four first men that went down the hold were seized with malignant fever; two died in forty-eight hours, and the other two very nearly shared the same fate. What should prevent ships running down to Bermuda for this purpose? The *Heela, Maegaera,* and *Firefly* were the ships that suffered most. Of 109 admissions, 83 were cases of malignant remittent fever (four cases of febrile consumption and twenty cases of other diseases; of this number, 22 have died). The type of the fever was of the worst description, accompanied in the fatal cases by black vomit and a deep yellow tinge of the surface. Tho' the proposition of deaths seems so large it can easily be accounted for; slight cases were treated on board ship, and in one-quarter alone, five out of nine fatal cases of fever were landed – in the last stage of the disease, fatal symptoms having set in before the patients left the ship.

The *Heela* had just returned from Jamaica, where the disease was raging. A few days after leaving the island, the commander was attacked and recovered. The assistant surgeon, two engineers and two or three men died on board the ship. After this, with the exception of four, every man on board was attacked, and even after the crew had become perfectly healthy, of one engineer and six men drafted to the ship, everyone was seized with fever. There was a report about the pumps of this ship being out of order, and an officer of the *Blazer* steamer who went on board with a mechanic to repair them was seized with the prevailing fever and died in this hospital.

The *Maegaera* is stated not to have had any fever on board till she conveyed an officer of the 92nd from Dominica to St Thomas's labouring under remittent of the most aggravated form [so] that after this, the commander took fever and died. The disease spread rapidly among the crew. Though this may look like contagion, there are sufficient grounds for maintaining that a local cause existed in the ship. She had been five years in commission, the boilers much out of repair and leaky when the flooring was ripped up in English

Harbour. Two lighters full of the most offensive and putrid filth were removed from the hold, and as already stated, the first four men that went down were seized with fever of the most malignant type, being partially asphyxiated when brought on deck. Lights would not burn below for some hours. These facts are mentioned on the ....[99]

A. Mackintosh,[100] MD
Assistant Surgeon, 33rd Regiment

Extract of Annual Report of the Medical Occurrences in the 92nd Highlanders at Barbados from 1 April 1842 to 31 March 1843 by C.J. Palmer, Surgeon, 92nd Highlanders

•••

Febris Continua Icterodes

This fatal variety of febrile disease has not prevailed so extensively as at former periods of the service of the Regiment in the command, and although the aggregate appearing on the numerical return as having been treated in the year amounted to thirty-nine it may be proper to remark that twenty-six of the number remained at the end of the preceding in a convalescent state and were eventually discharged free from complaint. Thirteen recent cases were admitted during the present. One of these occurred in the first mentioned and the other twelve during the last four months of the year. December being the period of its greatest prevalence, in the course of which eight cases took place and four in January, February and March. They were derived from various sources – seven from the Brick Barrack, one (an officer's servant) from a part of the town called The Bay, two were hospital orderlies, and three patients in hospital who had been originally admitted with bowel complaints, of the three last mentioned two had a fatal termination accompanied with black vomit. The three men attacked in hospital were all taken ill in the lower ward. It was also in this ward that one of the fatal cases under the head of *febris cont: communis* was attacking. Cases of fever of an aggravated type appear to have taken place at former periods in the same ward and another on the same flat on the opposite side of the passage in which no less than thirteen cases of yellow fever of a highly aggravated character lately occurred amongst the patients of the 46th Regiment. The two hospital orderlies were attached to this ward, but they had committed previous excess in liquor [and] had lain in the open air a whole night. The men admitted from the barrack were some from the upper and some from the lower flat of the building and had been employed in their ordinary military duties. The febrile excitement was generally preceded by the usual premonitory indications and the heat of surface in most instances of a very ardent character. In two of the number the disease was attended with slight cough and pain and oppression in the chest. In a third, with marked derangement in the hepatic system; and a fourth, with the last mentioned together with severe enteric irritation, delirium with a strong marked typhoid diathesis, foul and parched tongue and incrustation or sores about the teeth. Indeed, the typhoid diathesis was a constant accompaniment in all generally attended with a great degree of lethargy and apathy during the continuance of the acute symptoms and followed on remission by much depression of strength and a peculiarly slow, languid and sluggish pulse. Yellowness of the surface was also a constant attendant, though not in general. Except in two cases, and these, it subsided slowly.

C.J. Palmer
Surgeon, 92nd Highlanders

Windward Islands
Barbados
25 November 1848

My Lord,
It is with much concern that I have occasion to report to your Lordship the prevalence of yellow fever with greater or less intensity in the garrison of St Ann's since December 1847. From the mortality which occurred about the period of my arrival in the beginning of September last, it was deemed advisable to remove the 66th Regiment from their barracks and to encamp them on the savannah. Shortly afterwards

the detachment of the Royal Artillery was encamped, and this change appeared for a time to have a beneficial effect in checking the disorder. Recently the fever has broken out in the 72nd Regiment, who have also been encamped in the neighbourhood of the garrison on the side of the old naval hospital.

The mortality to the present time, including that which occurred in the early part of the year in the 88th Regiment, has amounted to nine commissioned officers and 105 rank and file. As the fever has prevailed through all seasons, and as some cases have occurred in Bridgetown, it is impossible to foresee when it may altogether subside.

It has been satisfactory to find that the removal of the troops has been found to arrest the progress of the disease. As it has been in contemplation to form a convalescent station at Gun Hill, an elevated position situated about eight miles distant from the garrison, and to which a company of artillery who have recently arrived have been removed, I hope that this intention may be carried out, as it is the opinion of all medical practitioners of experience in the West Indies, that the early removal of those who are attacked with yellow fever, whether in its effects on the minds of the patients or on the disease itself, conduces to their ultimate recovery.

I have the honour to be,
My Lord,
Your Lordship's
Most obedient servant,
The Right Honourable Earl Gray.

5. Reports from British Guiana

Preview: The reports that are transcribed in this chapter bear some commonalities with the previous reports. However, there is one point of contrast to the earlier transcriptions in that the British Guiana reports begin in the 1830s and continue into the 1840s. One possible explanation for the later dating of the initial reports here is that the former Dutch colonies of Demerara and Berbice do not officially become part of the British Empire, as one colony, until 1831. Thus, although the Royal Navy would have been active in this region following British incursions in the earlier nineteenth century, these two colonies would not have come under the jurisdiction of British medical military authorities in the earlier period. One useful point to be made here is that the dating of these reports does permit us to see if there had been significant medical developments since the 1820s. As it is, some of the medical philosophies operating in the earlier period continue to be present in the commentaries of the doctors whose observations are made available to us here.

Extract of Annual Report of Diseases Prevailed at Detachment Hospital 69th and 1st West India Regiments of Capory from 1 January to 31 December 1835 by Assistant Staff Surgeon R.G. Webb,[1] Demerara

Fevers
Fevers formed a very large proportion of the diseases treated. They amounted altogether to sixty-nine, but of this number, twenty-nine were admitted for ague.

These agues generally appeared as quotidians[2] and were probably, for the most part, owing to derangement of the biliary system. For after the patient's bowels had been well moved, the paroxysms ceased to return, and the men were sent back to their barracks until some further excesses produced a recurrence of the disease. None of these cases were severe, with the exception of one, in which the disease assumed a remittent form and proved fatal. In all the rest, an emetic, with purgatives and some quinine, put a temporary check to the disease. Under the head of remittent and continued fever, forty cases were admitted. These forms of disease so strongly resemble each other in this climate that it is sometimes very difficult to distinguish between them during the first day or two. However, most of the cases admitted for continued fever were convalescent on the second day. A purgative and foot bath with rest and low diet being all that was required to remove the febrile symptoms. But such simple measures did not suffice when the disease assumed the remittent form; for them, all the judgement energy and discrimination which the practitioner possessed were required to struggle against the danger or to guide the disease to a happy termination. Remittent fever as it appears among the troops in this climate, presents itself to the notice of the medical officer under two very opposite states. Both of them depend upon the promptitude or tardiness with which the patient reports his indisposition. It is a matter of the deepest regret that the soldier cannot be sufficiently impressed with a notion of the vital importance of applying for medical aid without loss of time and that in place of doing so, he too frequently goes to the canteen and attempts to relieve the depression of mind (one of the earliest symptoms of the disease) under which he labours by the use or rather abuse of ardent spirits.

The Bilious Remittent of tropical climates may be considered as a fever of nine days' duration. I scarcely recollect an instance in which the disease proved fatal after that period. In the periodical returns of casualties, it often appears that the patients have been under treatment for only two, five or seven days, but I believe this *apparently* rapid progress of the fever is owing either to the negligence of the patient in reporting himself sick or *possibly* to some mismanagement on the part of the medical officer which soon cuts off the unfortunate sufferer from every chance of escape. The type of this fever is distinguished from that of all others by [being] Apyrexious.[3] Remissions occurring at irregular intervals. The shorter and the less distinct these intervals are, the more dangerous will the disease be found. In very bad cases, the remissions disappear altogether. The skin becoming mauvish and clammy, and the patient falling into a state of coma, the forerunner of death. During a remission, the heat of the surface diminishes, the skin becomes soft and perspirable, the pulse likewise becomes softer and fuller. Thirst abates, and the mind is tranquillized, but there is no cessation of fever. After an interval of from two or three to twelve or fourteen hours, symptoms of intense excitement ensue, and thus, the fever runs on in alternate remissions and exacerbations. The remissions, however, in some cases, are so distinct as to deceive the medical attendant and induce him to suppose the patient is convalescent.

The early delirium which attends the exacerbations seems, in general to be confined to some one particular object, for the mind is sound and acute enough upon other points. This delirium may be said to result from a depressed state of the nervous system and from the derangement of the digestive canal (which always produces deep despondency and even mental illusions) rather than from cerebral congestion, for bleeding in such cases only aggravated the disease and hastens the occurrence of coma, a still more dangerous symptom than the delirium itself.

About the end of March many of the 69th people began to lose the healthy look and florid appearance which they had brought from St Vincent. Those who complained of illness had generally a livid or cadaverous complexion and seemed to be overpowered with debility and despondence. They first complained of headache and sometimes of a slight rigour, which was more generally the case when they came off guard. The pulse ranged from 90 to 120 but had little force and was easily compressed. The skin was hard and dry, the tongue was either based with cream-coloured mucus or it was black and dry in the centre. The secretion of saliva was scanty. Nausea and thirst most distressing, and the irritability of stomach very difficult to be relieved. The patient was soon so much reduced in strength as to be unable to move from his bed without aid. If the remedies employed were inefficient, the remissions became daily less distinct. The disease assumed a typhoid character. The skin was marked by a yellow tinge and appeared as if flea bitten from the rupture of its minute capillaries. Finally, a cold moisture bedewed the surface. Respiration became more and more impeded either from some change taking place in the nature of the circulating fluid or from the pectoral muscles becoming incapable of fully expanding the chest.

Coma, with involuntary dejections, closed the scene. With respect to the remedies employed, general bleeding did not appear to retard the progress of the disease. It should never be resorted to without the utmost caution and at an early period. The strongest men have nearly fainted or become convulsed on losing six or eight ounces of blood. But sometimes, even this small quantity, if abstracted in the hot stage, will induce perspiration and unload the stomach by means of the sudden sickness excited in that organ when it sympathizes with a diminished circulation in the brain. The blood never showed a buffy surface. It scarcely afforded any serum and remained fluid for many hours. Indeed, the very nature of the blood itself appeared to have undergone some morbid alteration, owing probably to the derangement of the functions of nutrition and of the chylopoietic[4] organs. A purgative of Calomel[5] and Jalap or the extract of Colocynth[6] was early exhibited for the purpose of unloading the colon and liver. If copious draughts of tepid water did not allay the vomiting, a few drops of Laudanum[7] were given or a blister applied to the epigastrium. The head was shaved, and a tendency to delirium and coma was resisted by blisters to the neck and occiput.

But as the cerebral disturbance is generally preceded and kept up by disorder of the abdominal viscera, the great invocation was to restore the healthy secretions of the liver and other glands and to remove the torpid state of the canal. The patient cannot be considered out of danger until the most desirable object is attained and no medicines appear to answer this purpose so well as Mercurial Purgatives. After the intestines are relieved from their feculent contents, a pill of six grains[8] of Calomel made up with some soft bread and repeated every four hours will, if given before coma has set in, be found to restore the secretions to a healthy state and remove the torpidity of the canal. Calomel also seems to exercise some influence upon that copious extrication of gaseous matter, which is sometimes generated in the intestines and gives the patient so much distress.

During the continuance of fever, the diet should be restricted to the use of mild fluids or acidulated drinks alone; and no stimuli should be given unless where cold, clammy sweats prevail. Quinine in full doses, either alone or in combination with Calomel Blue Pill or Epsom salts, has been found a highly valuable remedy. It has now retained its character as a febrifuge sufficiently long to entitle it to the high reputation it has acquired, and I only regret that the supplies of it to this Post have been scanty.

Quinine seems to produce a sedative effect upon the *sensorium*[9] and on the nervous system. I do not pretend to say what influence it may exert in the prevention or removal of coma or in restoration of warmth on the surface in place of the cold, clammy sweats, but it is certain that it may be given in very large doses with safety and advantage. When exhibited to prevent relapses in fever, its use should be continued until it has produced temporary deafness.

It rarely, if ever, causes headache, but it is *apt to nauseate* if given before the bowels are evacuated and the stomach and liver have resumed their healthy action. When these points have been properly attended to it may then be given in conjunction with almost every other remedy. It has been recommended by some medical men to give the Anti-periodic Remedies such as bark, Quinine, Arsenic during the remissions, but a high authority condemns this practice as one likely to invest the disease with a more continued and dangerous character.

With regard to necroscopic examinations,[10] I regret to say that I have not been able to inspect the head for want of proper instruments, but the appearances presented by the abdominal viscera were amply sufficient to account for every fatality.

The coats of the stomach were always found diseased. Its mucous membranes being marked by florid patches, so much softened as to be easily detached by the fingernail. In some cases, it contained a fluid resembling coffee ground or grumous[11] blood. There was likewise a partial thickening of its muscular tunic. The peritoneal surface of both small and large intestines were, in many cases, marked by patches of a deep red colour. The urinary bladder was almost invariably empty and contracted. The liver, in some instances, was pale and firm and in others, it was of a deep red and so soft as to permit the finger to penetrate it without resistance. The spleen, in every case, was converted into a soft black semi-fluid mass resembling grumous blood. Adhesions of the great peritoneum to the adjoining viscera occasionally existed.

Signed
R.G. Webb
Assistant Staff Surgeon

Extract of Annual Medical Report of the Service Company's 67th Regiment for the Year Ending 31 March 1838 by E. H. Blakeney,[12] A.J. 67th

In reporting upon the medical occurrences of the Service Companies 67th Regiment for the past year, I have to promise that it was not until February 1838 that I relieved Staff Assistant Surgeon Nicoll[13] in medical charge of headquarters stationed at Berbice and where they had been removed by order of Lieutenant General Sir Sanford Whittingham R.C.B at the suggestion of Staff Surgeon Scott[14] P.M.O. Demerara and Assistant Surgeon Smith[15] 67th Regiment, through the major general commanding on account of their having suffered so severely in Demerara during the sickly season of 1837. Annexed is the abstract report of Assistant Surgeon Smith, then in medical charge of the regiment to the officer commanding on 12 December 1837.

That the disease in the Regimental Hospital still prevails to an alarming extent, and no remedial agent seems to arrest its progress and the despondency of the troops, which later acts as I presume as a predisposing cause and thereby renders the likelihood of disease and approaching mortality now frequent. He further states that at this time, there were fifty-six men in hospital, of which number two men were dying and a third died this morning. Under these circumstances, he felt it is his duty to recommend, if practicable, a change of air for the regiment.

The weather about the end of April was disagreeably wet. The rain chiefly from the land in heavy showers and squalls with close sultriness and scorching sunbursts. It appears that in the latter part of this quarter, five cases of remittent fever and one placed under the head of *Febris Intermittens* proved fatal. I apprehend this was the commencement of that unfortunate sickly season which deprived the 67th Regiment of three most excellent officers and fifty men in the short period of nine months, showing a proportion of deaths of one in twenty-nine.

The remittent type, with some degree of excitement, was the form assumed by the disease at the outset but soon followed a state of prostration and collapse, which defied all remedial agents and terminated fatally in many cases on the third day.

Black vomit occurred in the greater number of the fatal cases. The loss sustained by the 69th Regiment, who were stationed in the same barracks compared with the 67th, was most trifling.

I need scarcely observe that the barracks are well situated within half a mile of the sea and that the supply of water and rations for the men were excellent, besides the admirable precautions adopted by the Officer Commanding Major Orange to prevent, if possible, the spread of disease and afford to the sick soldier immediate medical attention.

The disease, I am informed, first made its appearance among the seamen in the numerous shipping frequenting this port. A good deal of sickness also prevailed among the white population for the first five weeks, chiefly confined, however, to newcomers from Europe. Great numbers of whom died before any classes began to suffer, but about the termination of the first quarter, the disease attacked the seasoned as well as the fresh arrivals.

The regiment previous to 7 June had enjoyed a comparative exemption from disease. Under the different heads of diseases will be found more detailed information of the various cases, the post-mortem appearances of those which proved fatal, and other general matters of interest. In accordance with the directions of Staff Surgeon Scott P.M.O. Demerara, who was then in medical charge of the regiment, the annual return was made up to and for 31 December 1837 in consequence of headquarters being ordered to Berbice where they have enjoyed a remarkable exemption from disease showing at once the beneficial effects of change of air and scene. Doctor Riach[16] from his unremitting exertions in attendance on the sick, not only on his regiment but likewise the staff, fell sick and was ordered home by the recommendation of a medical board and carried on board ship in a state of extreme danger.

A. Surgeon Smith, 67th Regiment, Staff Assistant Surgeon Irwin,[17] and Staff Surgeon Scott were the medical officers who succeeded Dr Riach one after another in charge of the regiment on 24 January 1838. A draft consisting of one captain, one subaltern, one staff, one serjeant and fifty-four rank-and-file joined the service companies. One captain, one serjeant and twenty-eight rank-and-file of the above were landed at Berbice from the *Horatio* transport. The remainder are at present at headquarters, Demerara. The number of relapses that occurred in the different diseases amounted to ninety.

Febris Quot: Intern: The different cases of Intermittent Fever up to the commencement of June went on favourably and yielded readily to the usual plan of treatment. The exhibition of large doses of Quinine after the sweating stage had subsided. The bowels freely evacuated until about the middle of the month when many of them verged into Remittent of a bad character, and fears were entertained that unless some favourable change in the atmosphere took place, a severe sickly season would ensue and which opinion was too truly verified.

Febris Remittens: Sixty-one treated, eighteen recovered, and forty-three died. The first case that presented itself under this head occurred about 3 June in a lad belonging to the band, recently arrived from Europe. He was received into hospital with the usual febrile symptoms, which assumed a remittent character and, after exhibiting yellowness of surface and black vomit, terminated fatally on the fifth day.

Sectio Cadaveris[18]: Twelve hours after death body plump, joints rigid, skin somewhat yellow, patches of livid discoloration all over lower limbs. Cranium considerable congestion of the vessels of the meninges and brain, a little serous fluid under the arachnoid, a considerable quantity in the cerebral ventricles and the base of the cranium.

Thorax: Lungs and heart quite healthy; about two and a half ounces of deep yellow serum in the pericardium.

Abdomen: Nearly eight ounces of yellow serous fluid in this cavity. Stomach inflated, its inner surface coated with deep slimy matter, and the mucous tunic showing numerous round red patches consisting of dots of extravasations and minute arborescent[19] vessels.

Intestines: Distended with gas, their inner surface is at least that of the small lined with dark shiny matter similar to that found in the stomach and their outer showing more red vessels than usual.

Liver: Paler externally than usual, but its substance containing much blood; vesicular fill is distended with very black fluid bile.

The 8th furnished no fewer than three fatal cases. Of two of these, the subjects, Charles Holloway and John Gray, musicians and of very drunken habits, walked together to hospital about 11:00 a.m. The first complained of cough and the last of fever. And there seemed nothing in common between them excepting habits of extreme intemperance and having been much in town, where a very fatal form of fever was at the time raging. The former was reported on the morning of the 10th to have been delirious in the night. He now seemed quite composed, but symptoms of collapse came on, and he expired at 6:45 p.m. The latter became delirious on the night of the 10th, and the case ran a course exactly similar to the other, terminating on the 11th at 9:00 p.m. These cases were considered modifications of delirium tremens and treated as such. Still, it must be very evident that in a course of such rapidity, no remedial means could have availed much.

The third fatal case of that unhappy day, Private Henry Bass, age thirty-three, presented an Intermittent character and was met in the usual way by Quinine with seemingly all the success that could be wished. On the 9th, he was quite apyretic.[20] On the 10th, he felt rather sick in his inside and had seven or eight dark, thin stools. On the 11th, he complained of slight sore throat and pain in his legs, and he was somewhat feverish. On the 12th, at about 7:00 a.m., he fainted on the night chair. On recovering, he complained of feeling weak in getting up and of not having the proper use of his legs. He had a heaviness in his forehead, a dimness of vision. The pulse was 110, the skin hot dry, eyes heavy looking, and the conjunctival capillaries injected with red blood. From this time, the velocity and force of the circulation varied. The heart diminished and increased again in the extremities, but at 11:00 p.m., he said he had some nice sleeps and felt much better. The pulse was vigorous, the skin warm and moist all over. On the 13th at 1:00 p.m., he was found muttering and turning incoherently. His face red and tinged, the pulse one hundred, pretty full but undulating, the carotids acting strongly. He was throwing his arms about, eyes partially closed, highly icteric[21] and bloodshot, and the surface of the body was now very yellow. At 2:00 p.m., the justitation[22] was increased; he had convulsions, jerking of the trunk and limbs and flushed cheeks and forehead. He soon after became insensible and died at 3:00 p.m.

On 10 June another unfortunate case was received into Hospital Private James Tugwell. This man came from the contract baking where he had been employed for some time in the very centre of the prevailing disease in the town. He had turned ill on the preceding night at 10:00, remained feverish all night and was prescribed for by a private practitioner. He said he felt now pretty well, but weak and lightheaded, and pain in his back with bad taste in his mouth and thirst. He fainted in coming up to the hospital steps. The pulse was moderate, skin cool, the tongue whitish and moist, and he had no headache. On the 11th, he was found to have had [a] sleepless night but had been quite cool. He still had some pain of back, a dry, harsh, not hot skin, a dry, rough tongue and a pulse at fifty-four. The skin and eyes rather yellow. In the evening, he felt pretty well, had sweated pretty well from 1:00 p.m., his tongue was improved, the pulse at seventy-two, and he was quite cool. On the 12th, he was reported to have been raving a little. In the morning, he had taken twenty-four grains of Quinine, looked ill, features rather shrunk. He said he did not seem easier and had still some pain in his back, pulse seventy, small, heat rather low, some tenderness at epigastrium on pressure, 13th died at 6:30 a.m. The rapid succession of these untoward cases could scarcely fail to excite considerable alarm, and indeed, a sweeping mortality was confidently expected.

Many of the cases presented a somewhat sinister aspect, but most agreeably disappointed me, and the usual monotony of professional practice in this part of British Guiana remained perfectly unbroken in upon till 29th June when another case proved fatal within seven hours and a half from the time of admission.

The subject of this case, Private Christopher King, age forty-seven years, admitted at 8:45 a.m. in sweating stage of fever, having had a paroxysm coming on at 6:00 a.m. The cold and hot stages each lasted an hour. The former was attended by bilious vomiting, the latter by frontal headache and pain in the small of his back and legs. The pains continued, and he had thirst and a bad taste in his mouth. He had a strong smell of ... studded with red spots of minute arborescent vessels and dots of extravasation. Liver very large, weighing six pounds three ounces, pale externally as well as internally, containing little blood, unusually dense yet particularly about its back part, remarkably easily penetrated by the finger. Its outer surface of a mottled greyish and white appearance with a deceitful look of inequality. Spleen large, weighing one and quarter pounds, but its structure not particularly deranged. *Vesica fellea* distended with deep green bile of a treacly consistency. The symptoms of the remaining cases of the endemic varied considerably in the different individuals but the morbid appearances were much alike. The plan of treatment naturally varied according to symptoms. Venesection (a most doubtful remedy) was by some had recourse to. Artonotomy[23] cupping, purgatives, cold effusion, Calomel, blistering, effervescing draughts to relieve that peculiar irritability of stomach either conjoined with or without Opium and wine were the means employed.

Signed
E.H. Blakeney
Assistant Surgeon 67th Regiment

Extract of Annual Report on the Diseases That Were Treated in the Hospital of 76th Regiment at Demerara from 1 April to 12 November 1838, by W. Birrell,[24] MD, Surgeon, 76th Regiment

Febris Remittens   76th Regiment: 7 cases
69th Regiment: 1 case
Total: 8 cases

These cases were of a severe description of a low type with obstinate gastric irritability and occurred in constitutions impaired by former illness. Private Thomas May, of a slender, weakly constitution, was attacked on 5 July with rigours and, when admitted, complained only of pain of forehead, but gastric irritability soon made its appearance. The usual remedies were employed, no remission took place. Ol: Tiglu[25] was had recourse to simply and combined with other remedies. Blisters to the nape of neck. *Pediluv Call*[26], etc., but the surface remained hot and dry, although the headache subsided after the cathartic effects of the medicine. A warm bath was ordered with a view to promote perspiration. Two hours after its employment, the report was: "perspired freely after the bath, is now extremely weak, pulse 80, small and feeble, eyes dull and heavy". Stimuli were now employed with Quinine and so on, but next morning, the symptoms of "sinking" were more evident, which continued rapidly to increase, and he died the same evening being, fifty hours after admission into hospital.

The morbid appearances were vascularity of the vessels of the brain, serous fluid in the ventricles, the liver was partially indurated, and there was lymph on the upper part of the right lobe; spleen was large and soft.

Regiment 8 Folio 91. The other fatal case occurred in a man of good character and of steady habits. Sergeant William Bree was admitted into hospital on the evening of the 4th August in the hot stage of fever when the usual remedies were employed. On the following morning, there was apparently a complete remission, and Quinine was prescribed. In the afternoon, a sudden and strong Paroxysin[27] of fever came on, which soon terminated in a copious but cold perspiration and at 6:00 p.m., the report was "great debility, inability to raise himself in bed, the whole body is covered with cold, clammy sweat, the extremities are cold. Pulse, ninety, feeble; Blisters were then applied to head, neck, *inter scapulas,* and to lower extremities and various cordial and stimulating remedies were employed internally, but all without any permanent beneficial effect. The "sinking" symptoms rapidly increased, gastric irritability supervened, and he died on the third day. The matter ejected from the stomach was dark brown. The principal morbid appearances were detected in the brain, the lateral ventricles of which were literally filled with serous fluid and there was lymph here and there on the surface of the brain. This man had only been a short time previous to the attack discharged from hospital and, from the nature of his duty, had been exposed to the sun.

Signed
William Birrell, MD
Surgeon, 76th Regiment

Extract of Annual Report of the Medical Occurrences of the 67th Regiment from 1 April 1838 to 31 March 1839, Stationed at George Town, Demerara by E.H. Blakeney, Assistant Surgeon, 67th

I am sorry I can offer no remark on the probable cause that has led to the sweeping mortality by which we have been and continue to be visited. Intermittents and remittents appear to be Indigenous to the place and, but few escape the former disease whilst the latter will, in one period, prevail amongst the shipping and in the town. The garrison remaining perfectly healthy and, unfortunately, vice versa, for of late, the terms I'll die, "sure I must die", and of late, that prophetic language has been too truly verified for some of the finest fellows in the Regiment have gone to their long homes.

Frequent consultations have been held at the hospital with some of the most respectable and oldest practitioners in this colony. Minute post-mortem examinations were also made in their presence, but no suggestions or remedial measures appeared to have the slightest effect in arresting the disease.

About 17 February, fever of a malignant remittent type first made its appearance in this garrison and continued without any cessation the entire quarter. The duration of the disease has varied, of course, according to the age, temperament, length of residence in the tropics and previous habits of the patients. I cannot again help remarking that the greater number of the cases which proved fatal occurred to men of the most intemperate habits.

The morbid appearances varied but little in the different cases that peculiar icteric tinge on dissection appeared to have permeated in many; every structure. The vessels of the brain were much congested with effused lymph between the *Tunica Arachnoidea* and the Pia

Mater[28] also effusion into the ventricles and base of the brain. In the chest were found occasional adhesions between the *Pleura Pulmonalis et costalis*.[29] The liver was sufficient to account for death.

The following tabular found consider the best to answer this query instead of entering into lengthened detailed observation.

Table 5.1: Summary of Strength, Admissions, and Deaths of Military Ranks by Period of Residence

Strengths, Admissions, and Deaths of Military Ranks by Period of Residence	Strength of Each Class	Admissions of Each Class	Deaths of Each Class
Under one year	130	149	16
1 to 2 years	98	206	6
2 to 3 years	62	110	5
3 to 4 years	38	35	1
4 to 5 years	36	76	2
5 to 6 years	374	528	28
Upwards	7	1	0

Table 5.2: Ages of the Fatal Cases

	Corps			Totals
	Royal Artillery	67th Regiment	76th Regiment	
From 20 to 25	4	17	4	25
From 25 to 30	0	15	2	17
From 30 to 35	0	11	1	12
From 35 to 40	0	3	0	3
Upwards	0	0	0	1
Total	4	46	7	58

Signed
E.H. Blakeney
Assistant Surgeon 67th Regiment

NB: Pages 2, 4 and 6 are missing from document.

Extract of Annual Report of Medical Occurrences in the 76th Regimental Hospital from 1 April 1839 to 26 March 1840 by Leigh MD,[30] Assistant Surgeon, 76th Regiment, dated Demerara

Febris Remittens

Table 5.3: Yellow Fever Cases and Fatalities among Military Units

	Treated	Died
Royal Artillery	13	2
67th Regiment	4	3
16th Regiment	167	48
1st W.I.	13	0
General Department	1	0
Total	**198**	**53**

This disease presented itself in various grades of intensity, from the mild remittent to the malignant and adynamic. The symptoms differed so much in different cases that the disease might be subdivided into three or four different species owing to its assuming different types, difference of constitution and habit, duration of disease previous to admission into hospital, age, length of service in the West Indies, whether complicated with other diseases (as delirium tremens) or not and of course required so many different modes of treatment.

With reference to the malignant adynamic[31] form of the disease, I will say little as I only arrived in George Town on 6 September when the epidemic was on the decline. But under the head of the epidemic, I shall give its history from the books left by my predecessors. The principal symptoms were severe pain [in] the head, heat of skin and the other symptoms of inflammatory fever, which was soon followed by excessive debility as if the whole nervous system were implicated. The urine considerably decreased in quantity (in one case, there was a total suppression of urine till the patient showed symptoms of getting under the influence of mercury), skin and eyes yellow, frequent vomiting of a dark fluid but not black.

Signed
Leigh MD
Assistant Surgeon, 76 Regiment

Signed
C. Maclean[32] *MD*
Staff Surgeon

Extract of Annual Medical Report of the Diseases of the Troops, etc., from 1 April 1841 to 31 March 1842 by A. Melvin,[33] Surgeon to the Forces

The average strength of the white troops during the year has been 533, that of the black, 282.

The total admissions during the year from the white troops were 1796, total treated 1,831, of which number 51 died; 994 cases of intermittent fever have been treated, and 362 under the head of remittent and continued fevers of these 39 died. Two hundred and seventy-seven of the above were cases of malignant or "yellow fever", of which 30 of the above 39 died.

It may be remarked that the whole under these two heads would have been considered by the civil practitioners as cases of "yellow fever", and from what I can learn and have been told in the Public Establishments of the Colony, all such cases are called and returned as cases of "yellow fever".

• • •

The cases of intermittent fever chiefly prevailed at Berbice; very few in comparison took place at Demerara. They were particularly frequent during the third quarter and the relapses were many. Those who once had experienced an attack during wet or damp weather were certain of a relapse from it. The cases returned under the head of remittent fever occurred for the most part at Demerara, and almost all the cases returned under the head of continued fever were treated at Berbice, but they were all of the same character as the remittents, and I think ought to have been returned as such as every case of fever which I have observed in this colony has been of the intermittent or remittent type.

Fever of an epidemic and malignant character made its appearance in the garrison at Demerara early in August last and continued with more or less severity until December. During this period, 277 cases were admitted and treated of which number 30 died. The admissions and fatal cases would have been awfully increased had not nearly the whole of the white troops been sent to Berbice without delay, at which station the troops were healthy. These cases have been returned under the head of remittent fever but, in reality, were true cases of *Febris Icterodes*[34] and were almost always of a very insidious nature being after the commencement apparently very slight and trifling but becoming afterwards of a most malignant character.

Many more cases of the above might with propriety have been added. For the cause of this fever, it would be impossible to assign any particular or specific local origin about the barracks or hospital and their localities as these were the same as during the former year through which the troops passed without any serious sickness and during which only two cases proved fatal – the subjects of both were drunken characters.

But this was not the case at Berbice. Here, the serious cases came from Eve Leary Barracks while the men stationed at Kingston were healthy. Many cases commenced in the hospital with men who were there under treatment for other complaints and had been so for some length of time previous and died. Three or four hospital attendants were also attacked and died.

At the time the epidemic commenced, the winds prevailed chiefly at night from the Southward and Westward over the land. When it was from this quarter, the fever cases were greatly influenced by it, the cases under treatment and when it was dry, the weather was sultry and close, and the heat of the sun great. At night, when the wind prevailed from the Southward, the atmosphere became exceedingly oppressive and was accompanied by a very disagreeable smell. The wind no doubt passing over such extensive marshy grounds had a baneful influence, and close to the Windward of these barracks, there is a large cane field which at that period had had the canes cut down, leaving the surface more exposed to the influence of the sun. This field was then covered with the [remains] of the cut canes in a decaying state and was intersected with various trenches filled with fresh water for the purpose of keeping the ground wet to produce vegetation. This also must have had its effects in the production of the fever, as it was well calculated to produce an abundance of malaria. I believe the principal cause of these malignant fevers in this colony is also of the intermittents.

The general symptoms attending the epidemic fever were rigours more or less severe. At the commencement, much headache especially about the forepart, heaviness about the eyes, the vessels of the conjunctiva of which were sometimes infected and pain in the loins. Tongue of dirty white colour and very greatly loaded ... pulse generally full, strong and varying from 80 to 100 and upwards. Much thirst, sometimes urgent. Frequently, there was much irritability of stomach at the commencement, with dark bilious vomiting which, towards the close of the disease, became the true "black vomit".

In some cases, which proved fatal if this particular appearance did not show itself before death. The stomach was found to contain much of it after death. In many of the fatal cases, there was a suppression of urine for three or four days, sometimes before death. This was always a bad symptom, but the most sure and certain symptom of a fatal termination was the "black vomit" with a yellow tinge of the conjunctiva and skin. Also, haemorrhage from the nose. When these took place, every hope was gone and no [person]; fatal without them and no case recovered which had them.

I have seen cases with the black vomit only recover; in all the severe cases, there was also a great want of sleep which could scarcely ever be procured, and if obtained, it was unrefreshing. These patients were also exceedingly restless, wishing their position or bed to be changed every few minutes. Relapses were frequent, and many of them were fatal. Indeed, in many of the fatal cases, the subjects of them appeared perfectly convalescent for days, being perfectly cool with a very good pulse, regular functions and with some appetite, and were able to take nourishment with relish.

Generally, there was but occasional vomiting. Delirium seldom made its appearance until the latter end of the disease. When it took place, it was sometimes violent, attended with great frequency of pulse, which was generally full and strong. In other cases, the patients became perfectly comatose and insensible to everything. In these cases, the skin was often covered with a clammy perspiration, but the pulse until nearly the last kept of a moderate strength, soft and regular. *Singultus*[35] frequently occurred and was always an unfavourable symptom.

• • •

At the post-mortem examinations the morbid appearances were formed to be almost uniformly the same in all. The vessels on the surface of the brain were full and congested in some; these were marks of inflammation of the membranes and general effusion of serum under the membranes as also in the ventricles and at the base of the brains.

Thoracic viscera always healthy. In the abdominals the liver was generally a good deal enlarged and much congested and sometimes appeared inflamed. The stomach externally was, in some instances, inflamed. Internally, the mucous membrane was either inflamed over the whole surface or in patches and always contained a good deal of the "black vomit". The mucous membrane was softened and easily scraped off. Only in one instance were the kidneys disorganized.

• • •

During the year, four officers have died of fever during the epidemic but three of these decidedly might have been saved had they been more prudent. The 4th case, viz Lieutenant Lycters Royal Engineers, was one of the most perfect cases of "yellow fever" which occurred during the epidemic. There was haemorrhage from the gums for several days. Little or no sleep was obtained during the whole illness, and there was very great restlessness. The conjunctiva and skin became yellow, and there was the black vomit. He was perfectly sensible till within a few hours of his death, of which he was quite aware.

Signed
A. Melvin
Surgeon to the Forces

Extract of Annual Report and Observations on the Diseases, etc, Which Have Occurred among the Troops from 1 April 1842 to 31 March 1843 by A. Melvin, Surgeon to the Forces. P.M.O.

British Guiana

During the year, there has been a very marked difference between the cases of fever admitted at Demerara and those at Berbice.

At Berbice, the cases of intermittent fever have prevailed greatly over those under the heads of remittent and continued fevers, and none of the remittents there have assumed the malignant type of yellow fever. At this station the intermittent fevers have been as [many as] two to one to the other forms. The relapses also have been very many, and out of the whole number stationed there not 30 have escaped an attack of fever of some form or other, and many have had from six to eight attacks of fever.

At Demerara the nature of the fever has been very different, and very few cases of the intermittent type have occurred. During the three first quarters, the whole of the fever cases except for two or three trifling ones were of the remittent type, and almost every one was of a severe character or a malignant form of the true yellow fever (prominent symptoms of fatal cases). Out of the thirteen who died with fever, ten had black vomit, six of whom had suppression of urine for two or three days before death, and the same number had considerable haemorrhage from the mouth and nose. These cases have occurred during every month to the 31st December last, which shows that this season has been throughout sickly. Indeed, what is properly considered the sickliest period of the year, the second quarter did not prove more so than either of the others but even less sickly. More fatal cases occurred during the first quarter than during the following two. Four of the fatal cases were taken ill about the hospital and had the most severe and regular symptoms of the yellow fever.

Many of the cases which recovered were cases of yellow fever although not of so malignant a form as the others. One case, however, which recovered had very malignant symptoms, viz the black vomit, to a great extent haemorrhage from the gums for seven days; also, an extremely disagreeable cadaverous smell was emitted from the body for several days.

Another case had haemorrhage only. Some other cases, although they had not the black vomit, yet they passed by stool quantities of matter in every way resembling it. Several of the cases which recovered were attended with delirium to a considerable extent and appeared quite hopeless. At Demerara, it would appear the causes producing the fevers were of a much more powerful and malignant nature than at Berbice otherwise, more of the fevers would have been of the mild intermittent type.

(*Cause of the fever at Demerara more malignant than at Berbice*)

From the character of the fevers at Demerara for the three first quarters it would clearly appear that the two types of yellow fever may take place at any time of the year. The cause seems always to exist and, according [to] the circumstances, may produce that malignant form of fever, the common remittent or intermittent.

It is greatly influenced by the habits of men attacked, then exposure to the influence of malaria and exposure to heat of the sun, which I think is very predisposing. Few subjects of the fourteen fatal cases were drunken characters. The state of the mind has also great influence in the result, which unfortunately very often becomes much alarmed when labouring under fever in this colony and is frequently much prejudiced against a hospital, which was the case with the men of the 47th Regiment with regard to the hospital at Eve Leary. After the sick were removed for treatment to the barracks and fumigation they felt at ease and were satisfied.

(*Locality of Eve Leary Hospital unhealthy*)

It is difficult to say how far the locality of the hospital is at fault, but it would appear certain that it is so from what has occurred during the present and last years by the number of attendants which were taken ill with the worst symptoms of yellow fever and died.

The symptoms and character of the Fevers which prevailed during the three first quarters of the year have been in every respect the same as those which have so frequently occurred at various periods in this colony, and which have been as frequently described, especially when so fatal in 1828 or at other periods when prevailing as an epidemic with this exception that until the present and previous year I have not observed haemorrhage from the nose, gums or mouth taken notice of as a prominent and dangerous symptom.

The post-mortem appearances have also been the same as in former years.

Signed
A. Melvin
Surgeon to the Forces P.M.O.

Extract of Annual Report with Observations on the Forces Prevalent in British Guiana from 1st April 1843 to 31 March 1844 by Staff Surgeon C. Maclean, MD,[36] and Containing a Letter to him by J.B. Beresford,[37] Dated Berbice, 5 January 1844

The troops in this colony are liable to attack of remittent fever at all seasons but assuming a malignant character more generally in the autumn and severe according to the intensity of the cause producing it, which as yet appears to be but obscurely understood beyond conjecture in anything except the influence of malaria. The climate of Demerara is, in general, more the source of this malady – in this year, however, the greater number occurred at Berbice.

About the end of August 1843, remittent fever of a most malignant type attacked the troops quartered at Berbice, and although the troops (consisting of two companies, 33rd Regiment) were removed as soon as I became aware of the nature of the malady, yet the mortality was great; the moves consequent on this state of things. I stated fully in my Quarterly Summary ending September 1843 and need not be repeated here. One company sent from Mahaica from Berbice lost in the first ten days twelve men but none afterwards.

A few days prior to the arrival of the white troops from Berbice at Demerara (15 September), several cases of fever of the same formidable character occurred at Demerara. Most of those cases occurred in the Eve Leary Hospital among patients under treatment for other diseases and the servants in the hospital. The disease continuing to increase and proving in many instances fatal among the new attacked in hospital (few cases having been admitted from the barracks). I deemed it advisable to remove the whole of the patients to Kingston Barrack, formerly the old hospital; this change was attended with the happiest result: only one man having died. Indeed, so marked was the change that the soldiers already began to look less desponding, and the sick convalesced rapidly, and the hospital was no longer dreaded as a pest house.

Having entered fully into the causes, symptoms and progress with the treatment adopted in this disease in my quarterly Reports, I have only to refer to them. But as it may be interesting to have the opinion of the private medical practitioner who attended the troops at Berbice through nearly the whole of the attack I shall transcribe a communication received from him on his subject.

Berbice 5 January 1844
Staff Surgeon Dr Maclean, Demerara

Sir
In conformity with Dr Bones' wish for an account of the disease which lately prevailed at the garrison at Berbice, the causes of death and my particular treatment, I beg to subjoin the following explanation, which, although a mere sketch of the disease, is in substance what I wrote to Dr Murray on the occasion on 31st October last, without notes of reference which the number under active treatment and the time I was obliged to devote to them in noting their most particular symptoms as a guide to me, at my next visit, in cupping and other requisite operations entirely precluded, it is impossible for me at this date to give anything like an accurate account of matters. This, however, I may state confidently that the fever at the outset was that peculiar form of Typhoid insidious in its origin and progress and not infrequently fatal in its termination; that has for several years past

since the year 1836 I think, been the epidemic of British Guiana of this country at least that during the first eight or ten days the disease, except in certain persons of very depraved habits did not assume any peculiar feature that could have induced me to consider it otherwise than fever of a continued type wherein symptoms of a typhoid character were very prominent but that suddenly it assumed a most formidable aspect. Ten to eighteen being daily admitted to hospitals, the characteristics of fever being then, much general excitement, hot and dry skin, full bounding pulse of 120, very soon followed by corresponding depression and terminating in many instances on third and fourth day, baffling all treatment suggested by myself or Assistant Surgeon Andrews[38] with whom I subsequently for a fortnight at least, acted in concert without remuneration as you well know.

The prostration of strength was very great and immediate (in the first 24 hours) when the tongue became Typhoid, and the secretions generally arrested, quickly followed by vomiting that defied the catalogue of remedies employed for its relief. Suffused eyes with injected capillaries, yellow tinge of surface becoming very intense, black vomit, delirium, coma and death either on the third or fourth day or on the seventh. I saw very few of the post-mortem appearances having too much to attend to. To admit of such examinations prior to Assistant Surgeon Andrews' arrival both in the garrison and my private practice, and taking of course less responsibility to myself on his assumption of garrison duty, and am therefore hardly able to offer any correct ideas on the subject.

The liver was, however in almost every instance in which I had an opportunity of viewing the body, pale, and the gall bladder colourless and quite empty. The stomach and continuous mucous membrane highly vascular to all appearance but, in reality, degenerated and of a soft, puffy consistency, with considerable bloody exudation even when black vomit had not occurred (and this was frequently a symptom)

Signed
John B. Beresford

P.S. The average in 1842 was two and a fraction per cent; in 1843, not quite two per cent. The habits of each of the men being perhaps the nearest to that of soldiers, I have thought proper to make the above allusion, leaving Dr Bone to draw his inference from it and thinking it may serve to show that something beyond miasm and the common epidemic of the country had effect in the late and awful situation at the garrison.

Signed
J.B.B.

Signed
C. Maclean MD
Staff Surgeon

Extract of Annual Report on the Diseases of the Troops in British Guiana from 1st April 1846 to 31 March 1847 by J. Millar,[39] Staff Surgeon, 1st Class Principal Medical Officer

The proportion of sick to well daily has averaged 9 per cent. This altho' a large proportion, does not much exceed that of other years in which there was no extraordinary visitation of epidemic disease. Fevers, of course, constitute the most numerous and the most important class of disease. They are the prevailing disease of British Guiana, but altho' the cause everywhere abounds, some stations are unhealthier than others. During the past year Fort Canje Berbice has been the sickliest and the most fatal and has been so for several years past. The following will show the relative health of the three military stations, as far as the prevalence of fever and mortality therefrom is concerned.

Table 5.4: Incidence and Mortality of Yellow Fever by Military Unit Strength

	Strength	Fevers	Ratio Per cent	Died	Ratio of Deaths Per cent to Strengths
George Town	131	136	104	4	3
Berbice	119	178	150	8	6.7
Mahaica	13	36	276	0	0

[It was occupied] for a short time by white troops and by a company from Berbice sent there as a sanitary measure with all the convalescents so that no conclusion can be drawn as regards the relative health of this Post from the occurrences of the past year. But as regards Berbice, the contrast between the health of the troops stationed there and those at George Town is striking, not only in the proportionate increase in the number of cases of fever, occurring at the former as also in the severity of the disease as shown by the rate of mortality. At Berbice, the number of fevers was at the rate of 50 per 100 mean strength, more than at George Town, [and the death rate was twice as high, the former at 6.7 per cent].

As has already been remarked it is difficult to account satisfactorily for the disproportionate health of these two posts, but that such is the case would seem to be established by the occurrences of several years past. Eve Leary Barracks has been comparatively exempt from fevers of a severe grade. Several of those that did occur were in men who had arrived but a short time previous from that Post.

Early in October, remittent fever made its appearance amongst the white Troops composing the garrison at Fort Canje, Berbice, composed of the 19th Regiment and a small detachment of the Royal Artillery and from that time continued to increase in number and severity so that by the end of the month 51 cases had been treated in hospital. During the following one, there was no appearance of disease, although the wet or generally considered healthy season had set in. On the recommendation of Dr Knox,[40] Surgeon of the 1st Royals, then in medical charge of the Post, half the number of troops were removed to Mahaica on 14 November. The fever continued to prevail for some time among the remainder. It had not altogether subsided when all the white Troops were removed to George Town on the 12 January at the recommendation of the inspector-general of hospitals. The men composing the detachment first moved to Mahaica appear to have recovered their health in an extraordinarily short space of time – the disease having in most assumed the distinct intermittent form. Those moved to George Town did not recover so rapidly. Several very aggravated cases occurred immediately after their arrival, two of which died, and relapses were frequent.

The general health of the whole appeared to have been re-established before they left the district on 24 March. Lieutenant Hughes, a young and athletic officer of the Royal Artillery, fell a sacrifice to an attack of the fever at Berbice on 29 November. The cause of his attack was attributed to shooting in the neighbourhood swamp during the heat of the day. There can scarcely be a difference of opinion as to the character of the endemic fever of the colony, and such as prevailed during the past year. Intermittent and remittent fever are but grades of the same disease, assuming one form or other perhaps from some latent and unknown cause, but often traced to circumstances of constitution, habit, locality or intemperance. They are decidedly "marsh" or "malaric" fevers, whatever may be the theory attached to the name, such as prevail in all marshy districts in every cline (sic) and rendered more common and dangerous in British Guiana from the concentrated nature of the cause, and the tropical position of the country.

First attacks have generally, but not always, been in the remitting form, the remission more or less distinct according to the severity of the disease, but they and the exacerbations could be detected even in the worst cases once in twenty-four hours but in many the tendency to the tertiary "periodicity" or forty-eight hours was evident every alternate day, an exacerbation of symptoms, the other alternate days a diminution, the patient being moved one day and better the next and so on.

The termination was very frequently in a quotidian or tertian. Relapses or second or third attacks most generally assumed the distinct intermittent, and the tertian form was by far the most common. Altho' not practically conversant with the subject, it is the opinion of several of the leading civil practitioners of the colony that relapses have an invariable tendency to recur at stated intervals and with as much regularity as the Paroxysin[41] of the intermittent. These two intervals are distinguished by the "paroxysmal interval or period".

• • •

Dr Blair, surgeon general of British Guiana, writes as follows: "Altho' the important doctrine of relapse periods has not much if at all in a practical point of view engaged the attention of authors it is as familiar to the Colonists of British Guiana as the ordinary paroxysmal intermissions. The visitations of intermittent fever arrive to some here with the regularity of the packet". He states also that "little more than the existence of the law can be pointed out" and "that at present it is necessary that two paroxysms and one relapse should occur before the future intervals can be predicted". It is scarcely necessary to add that should this be established as an invariable law in the progress of this disease, it would be of great practical importance.

● ● ●

Before concluding these remarks, I have to observe that amongst the most rapidly fatal cases, not a single one presented the character of yellow fever. This last disease does not appear to have visited Demerara since the year 1842 and Berbice the following year. It has fallen to my lot to see a great deal of yellow fever and I cannot trace out the slightest resemblance between it and the most aggravated case of the Remitting Fevers of this colony.

Yellow fever is a fever of but one paroxysm ending in death or recovery but never in an Intermittent. It has appeared occasionally in places when remittent and intermittent fevers are unknown, and there does not appear, therefore, to be either identity of disease or identity of cause. When yellow fever is superadded to the fevers of this colony all forms would be found in the same hospital. It would be natural to conclude from this circumstance that they were all so many varieties of the same disease, and hence the distinction of "mild remittent", "protracted remittent", and "concentrated remittent" than which, in my humble opinion, a greater mistake could not be committed, although adopted by such high authorities as Jackson, Bancroft, Masley, Lind, Johnson and others.[42]

Arguments founded on well-established facts of the present day are in favour of considering yellow fever as a distinct and separate disease and that it has no alliance whatever with that known by the name of "bilious remittent" or "marsh fever" that it is regulated by peculiar laws of its own, and that it is not indigenous to this colony, or any of the West India Islands, and that when it does appear, it is introduced from without and assumed all the characters of a highly contagious and fatal disease.

Signed
J. Millar
Staff Surgeon 1st Class
Principal Medical Officer

6. Reports from Dominica

Preview: As in the reports previously transcribed from Antigua and Barbados, some of the doctors who authored those documents also appear here. In that context, some of the musings about the cause and treatment of yellow fever that we have seen before, continue to reappear here. The Dominica reports begin in the 1820s and continue into the 1840s, which also gives us some view of what changes, if any, might have taken place between the earlier and later years. One feature that run through the Dominica reports that follow relates to the fairly detailed commentary on environmental factors, which reflects that these doctors had observed some correlation between the outbreak of yellow fever and the geographical/environmental features of the various islands. In some cases, the environmental features speculated on by the various doctors might be location-specific, even in some cases traced to conditions on a specific ship.

Remarks on the Lately Prevailing Fever at Dominica by John Arthur, MD[1]

Roseau 10 February 1818
I regret not being able to offer remarks from my own personal observation on the lately prevailing fever in this island having only arrived here on 10 December having been then ordered here as principal medical officer in consequence of the much to be lamented death of Staff Surgeon Woulfe.[2] But from the returns before me and every account that I have heard, it appears that a fever of unusual malignity prevailed last season both among the inhabitants of the town of Roseau and its environs and the military on Morne Bruce and

more lately extending even to the most distant parts of the island. Dr Clarke, the oldest practitioner in the island who in the year 1797 wrote a treatise on the disease of the West Indies then after an experience of twenty-five years in it, told me that he never witnessed anything like it, but in 1794–95 and 96 and again in that of about 1805, and that the fever which raged in these periods exactly corresponded with that of last season, only that in 1805 it appeared rather slighter as being less destructive, perhaps as I should be inclined to think in consequence of the number of the survivors from the sickness of the preceding period that then remained. The extreme mortality caused by it and that nearly equal under very great diversity of treatment with or without bleeding as far as I have been able to ascertain manifests a malignity characteristic of the disease and of a difference in it from the ordinary endemics of the country.

The proportion of deaths to those attacked by it amongst the military at Morne Bruce according to the return is as one to two and a half and amongst the civilians and town I have reason to think has been at least equally great and, in this respect, has been by no means singular in this island. For previous to being ordered here desirous of gaining information concerning the fever prevalent the preceding year in some of the other islands, I made every enquiry on the subject and from all I could learn was led to the very same conclusion. In the 2nd or Queens Regiment at Barbados, from 1 to 28 December 1816, the number attacked was sixty-nine, that of deaths twenty-seven. The proportion about the same one to two and a half. I take this month in preference as during it the malignant fever seemed principally to have prevailed unmixed with those of the common ardent kind of which previous to it as was to be expected. In a newly arrived regiment, there were a considerable number of cases but mild and easily yielding to the usual mode of treatment so that according to Mr Ralph's table out of one hundred and twelve cases in the months of June, July and August, not one died.

Table 6.1: Attacks with Fever and Deaths in the Queens, June–August by Mr Ralph

Periods		No. Attacked	Died	Proportion
From	To			
June, July and August		112	0	112 to 0
1st Sept	7th Sept	22	0	79 to 13 (about 1/5)
8th Sept	14th Sept	26	7	
15th Sept	21st Sept	16	2	
22nd Sept	28th Sept	15	4	
29 Sept	5th Oct	20	3	70 to 7 (nearly 1/7)
6th Oct	12th Oct	21	1	
13th Oct	19th Oct	9	1	
20th Oct	26th Oct	20	2	
27th Oct	2nd Nov	24	6	135 to 33 (about 1/4)
3rd Nov	9th Nov	30	7	
10th Nov	16th Nov	32	8	
17th Nov	23rd Nov	25	7	
24th Nov	30th Nov	24	5	
1st Dec	6th Dec	24	9	69 to 27
7th Dec	13th Dec	22	9	
14th Dec	20th Dec	9	4	
21st Dec	28th Dec	14	5	
29th Dec	4th Jan	14	2	34 to 9 (about 1/4)
5th Jan	11th Jan	6	3	
12th Jan	18th Jan	6	1	
19th Jan	25th Jan	3	1	
26th Jan	1st Feb	5	2	

But after the arrival on 26 or 27 August of the *Childers* Brig of War in the sickly state already well known and whose sick were received into the military hospital ashore, the mortality commenced early in September and gradually increased to the extent above stated thus indicating a wide difference in the fever then prevailing from that of the preceding months. According to the annexed report from

Reports from Dominica

Artillery Hospital Barbados, of sixty-three attacked, twenty-one died and of thirty-nine of those from whom no blood had been taken, the proportion of deaths to recoveries was exactly in the same ratio as thirteen to twenty-six.

Table 6.2: Incident Report: Cases and Outcomes

Cases	No. Attacked	Recovered	Died	Total Attacked
In which no blood was taken	39	26	13	39
In which small bleedings were used but not exceeding twenty ounces	5	2	3	5
In which from 20 to eighty ounces were removed from the system	15	11	4	15
In which eighty to 118 ounces were taken away	4	3	1	4
General Total	63	42	21	63

Ordnance Hospital, St Ann's Barbados, 25 May 1817, Signed J. Homor, Assistant Surgeon, Royal Artillery

The *Childers* directly before her arrival at Barbados in a short period of twelve or fourteen days, between 14 and 26 August, by this fever lost twenty-one persons out of ninety, the total number on board, and of ten cases admitted from *the Antelope* into the General Hospital Barbados between 6 and 18 November 1816, five died – though they had been bled freely at the commencement of their illness on board previous to being sent ashore. While it is very remarkably deserving particular notice that out of forty-one cases from the *Tigris* Frigate admitted about the very same period between 28 October and 13 November, but one died, a Mr Moore, a midshipman showing a difference between the two kinds of fever occurring at the same time, in the same hospital, under the same medical officer, the late Dr May[3] – similar to what was observed in the Queens Regiment in the different times stated and that much difference was not caused by any change of season or weather. Indeed, many instances occurred, particularly in the newly arrived regiment. Of the two kinds of fever having successively attacked the same individual different periods of complete recovery from the one in different individuals having intervened before the attack of the subsequent one and which were considered by those not making any distinction as second attacks of the same disease. But as appears from the late Dr May's diaries, the first were usually mild and manageable, the latter malignant, intractable and fatal in a very great proportion.

That the cases from the admiral's ship, the *Antelope*, a fine two-decker, were not more numerous during the time above stated will not appear extraordinary when we consider the exact cleanliness usually observed on board such a vessel. The abundant room for the men, the free ventilation it is capable of from the numerous ports at each side, and the opportunities they enjoyed of immediately separating those taken ill with fever from the rest by sending them to hospital ashore at first at Antigua from whence they had just arrived and then to the one at Barbados, Advantages not always enjoyed in vessels of a smaller class and in one so small as the *Childers* circumstances of a contrary tendency may prevail.

The sudden appearance of the same fever in this island toward the latter end of June; its rapid progress both amongst the inhabitants of the town and the troops on the hill; its very general prevalence amongst all descriptions of persons not confined to the young and newcomers unassimilated to the climate but extending in numerous instances to those seasoned by long residence in the place. Even it is said, in some cases, to coloured people without any peculiarity of season or alteration in the state of the place to account for it, are circumstances widely different from anything that has been experienced in the West Indies for several years as I can myself testify. As far as my observation can go during the years 1812, 13, 14, 15 and part of 1816, that I before served in different islands of this command and during this period new regiments – the 4th Battalion, 60th Regiment and York Chasseurs and several batches of recruits (some of whom I have had under my own care) arrived without suffering materially.

Mr Woulfe himself was nearly two years [here] this last time and had been several years before in the West Indies. His wife, I understand, who died before him, was an East Indian. Lieutenant Langley, who fell an early victim, I had known in this very place three years ago, and he was not then a newcomer. The other two gentlemen of the detachment here that died, Mr Hood and Mr Hurst, had been also, I am told, some years in this climate. The older officers belonging to it were also attacked.

The same thing was to be observed at Barbados the preceding year. Of the artillery officers that died there, the greater number, if not all, had been some years on this station. Lieutenants Wood and Shaw I had known at Guadeloupe, the latter had escaped even that very fatal spot to Europeans Pointe-à-Pitre. Captain Crittenden, a major who was very severely attacked by it, had been six or seven years in the West Indies. The old servants that had been some years about the General Hospital there, the steward, under-steward, clerk, etc. were carried off by it. The resident mate, Mr Bateman, suffered so severely from it that his constitution never completely recovered and [he] was obliged to resign his situation to return to Europe, though he had previously for years enjoyed good health in that station and many other such instances too tedious to particularize.

The very acute nature of the disease, its extreme severity and the rapidity with which it extinguishes life appears from the list of deaths annexed to the quarterly returns according to which three-fourths of the deaths from it happened on or oftener within the fourth day. Though I cannot, at present, attempt to offer any specific symptoms as characteristic of this particular kind of fever, by which with certainty the milder cases of it might be discriminated from the more severe ones of the ordinary kind. Yet it cannot be considered as a valid objection to the actual existence of such a distinction when that very attentive observer, Dr Jackson,[4] after such long and extensive experience acknowledges the difficulty of giving discriminating characters for distinguishing cases of the contagion types of Europe from those of the endemic of Santo Domingo. Diseases so very distinct and different, speaking of them he says, "The causes of fever are thus fundamentally different and minutely examined will be found to originate hordes of action of a peculiar cast, yet the derangements exteriorly are so much alike that the discriminating characters cannot be delivered but with doubt and hesitation". And again page 213, "yet if two cases of those diseases be examined as they actually appear unconnected with collateral circumstances, it will not perhaps be an easy matter to say in what the difference consists". And the difficulty of distinguishing cases of intermittent fever whilst in the continued form which it not infrequently assumes before it, shows itself by a tendency to intermit from continued fever properly so-called [which] has been noticed by authors and must be well known to all persons conversant with the disease.

The milder and slighter ones pass under the common name of remittent or bilious remittent such is almost the only distinction I have known observed here. Opinions thus formed and confirmed by a continuance of similar events for a series of years are not easily to be shaken by any after occurrence. The opinions of the elders will, of course, have weight with the juniors of the profession, and the novelty of the doctrine will also have its attractions for those who suppose whatever is most modern must be the most approved. It is surprising how averse persons thus prejudiced by preconceived notions are to see things that happen to be unfavourable to their principles in their proper light.

The very circumstances that I have heard stated by them against contagion as the cause, on careful enquiry and examination of the facts themselves, I have found to be on the contrary strongly in proof of it. It has been asserted that it did not extend from the sick to their medical attendants or the servants waiting on them; that those in the same hospital or house with them were not usually affected by it, and that it did not spread through families. The very reverse of which from public documents, medical returns and hospital books as far as they go, I have found to be the case. Of the medical officers that served here, during the sickness, Staff Surgeon Woulfe,[5] Assistant Surgeon Allen,[6] Hospital Assistants Oakly[7] and Wilson,[8] were all attacked and but one, Mr Allen, recovered. Hospital Assistants Caverhill[9] and Williams[10] arrived more lately. The latter has been stationed at Prince Ruperts, where he has only suffered from intermittent fever, the constant disease of that post. The former, a strong, robust young man, has escaped altogether.

Of hospital orderlies at Morne Bruce, I find in the returns four as affected with fever; Mr Orman, Heaning, Harris and Samuel Holt. The two first died of it. The third recovered after a severe attack, and the fourth after having been returned in the expenditure and sick returns under the head fever, when on [the] eighteenth day from his admission he died, is stated to have died of dysentery from which and a communication from Mr Caverhill on the subject who attended him. It appears that he died of dysentery supervening on fever as appears also to have been the case with Staff Surgeon Woulfe himself. Poor Dr Wray, when early in the sickness at Barbados, in his official report, [he] mentioned the escape then of himself and his two assistants, Hospital Assistants Colville[11] and Allen as a reason for supporting the fever to be non-contagious, had no idea that they were shortly about to prove melancholy instances of the reverse. Himself and the first mentioned one having died of it and the last who, though if not a Barbadian, was at least an old resident of the island, suffered a very severe attack of it. The resident mate Mr Bateman also as before mentioned suffered severally (sic). The two medical officers that were with the Queens were both attacked, and one of them, Mr Prendergast,[12] fell victim to it. An assistant surgeon of artillery, Mr Wales,[13] and one of the 3rd West India Regiment, Mr Payne,[14] also did. The long list of deaths amongst the medical officers throughout the command during the period of the late sickness tends towards confirming the same thing.

On my return from England after an absence of eleven months, I found not a single one of the old servants of the General Hospital remaining, and on enquiry heard nearly the same story of all that they were attacked with the fever of the preceding season and carried off by it.

I annex a list of the deaths of the General Hospital servants for that period. Military hospitals in this climate where ventilation and cleanliness must form a very principal object with the officers in charge of them cannot be supposed to be particularly favourable for the propagation of contagion.

In civil hospitals in Europe, where from the structure of the buildings and nature of the climate, ventilation to the same extent is not possible, how frequently we see cases of typhus fever intermixed with others without in general remarkably ill consequences ensuing. The one at Morne Bruce is particularly well-placed, for receiving the breeze pretty constantly blowing down a valley directly opposite to it, and there is no obstruction whatever to its passing freely through (there being not even jalousies to the windows) unless when it is shut up altogether by the window shutters being closed. Nor are patients ill with dysentery and under the influence of mercury, the most likely subjects for being affected with the contagion of fever.

Table 6.3: Return of Hospital Servants Who Were Successively Taken Ill of Fever between 18 September 1816 and 7 February 1817

Regiment	Names	Capacity	When Taken Ill	When Died
Queens	Josiah Marsden	Cutter	18 Jan 1817	21 Jan
Queens	William Fielding	Hospital clerk	8 Dec	9 Dec
Queens	Geo Smith	Hospital clerk	1 Feb	7 Feb
Royal York Rangers	James Scott	Hospital clerk	30 Nov	2 Dec
Artillery	Hendy Anderson	Steward	20 Nov	3 Dec
Queens	Serj. Jno. Puntin	Steward	29 Jan	1 Feb
25th Regiment	Phillip Carroll	Asst. Steward	18 Sept	21 Sept
Queens	John Teagers	Asst. Steward	9 Dec	12 Dec
Queens	John Benblidge	Cook	1 Oct	30 Nov
Queens	John Ashmore	Surgery Man	28 Nov	5 Dec
Queens	Benjamin Atkinson	Surgery Man	11 Jan	16 Jan
Queens	James Rogers	Surgery Man	30 Jan	6 Feb
4th Battalion 60th	Peter Divit	Orderly	6 Oct	7 Oct
4th Battalion 60th	Pierre Alexander	Orderly	6 Oct	8 Oct
Queens	Corporal Paradise	Orderly	5 Dec	8 Dec
Queens	Edward Colwell	Orderly	10 Dec	17 Dec

Such were those who principally occupied the hospital when the fever commenced, and during the height of its prevalence, there appears to have been very few of any other component in it. Of those that were dismissed and cured of dysentery, I find many to have returned after a short period ill with fever. And the following to have been actually attacked with it whilst in hospital. Private Morton admitted 26 September, 29th attacked with fever, 1 July delirium, coma and black vomit stated to have come on, which soon terminated in death. J. Mitchell, dysentery, admitted 14 September, 7 October reported to have been convalescent till two or three days before when he was attacked with fever. Black vomit and coma soon appeared, which carried him off. Charles Paterson, dysentery, admitted 15 September, 17 September [additional symptoms] supervened, 19th attended with vomiting, 20th dead. Holstein, who died of fever five days after his admission into hospital, which could not be accounted for by any appearance of the wound examination after death so that the man who wounded him escaped prosecution for murder.

Dysentery, as it usually appears here, and as I also witnessed it lately in the Queens Regiment, is of a chronic kind unattended with febrile symptoms protracted to a long period without affecting the skin or pulse, the seat of the disease being generally found to be in the large intestines. Several cases of it besides these, I have mentioned, I find by the reports in the diaries after having been some time in hospital to have been attended with fever, which not being in the usual course of the disease, would appear to have been contracted in the hospital. The assertion that it did not affect any two of a family at the same time is equally groundless. For of sixteen women that by the copies of the returns appear to have been accommodated in hospital, the names of eight of their husbands and some of their children are contained in the very same returns, and of the remaining eight some have been pointed out to me as having been then widows. There are others of whom I have only heard casually. No accounts having been kept of them, not being I suppose in hospital nor included in any return, and the medical officer that attended them perhaps dead who were affected at the same time with their husbands and children; as a Mrs Everit, ill along with her husband [and] a Mrs Pallet who died thereafter.

According to the Commissary papers, the number of women belonging to the West India Rangers on 25 July was nineteen married and five widows, total twenty-four; on 25 December 11 married and four widows, total fifteen; difference nine. Of children 25 July, nineteen; 25 December, fifteen; diminution four. Of the artillery of six women, one died; of thirteen children, six died. I have heard a vitiation of the atmosphere vaguely mentioned and a want of the usual thunder and lightning stated in attempting to account for the above sickness.

But on receiving the half-yearly return from Prince Rupert's, I was surprised to find in the meteorological observations annexed to it much thunder and lightning mentioned as having been observed in June. I supposed this at first to have been a mistake 'till on making further enquiries, I was assured of its correctness. The particular kind of vitiation was not attempted to be described nor any other cause assigned for it. As far as my own observation goes and that of several of whom I have enquired, the season has been a fine, mild, moderate one. No sensible variation in it from that of ordinary years nor any perceptible peculiarity whatever. The same heat and moisture as usual at the same time in every other year, neither to any excess. Indeed, while writing this, the weather has been for some days very wet, much rain having fallen. The thermometer occasionally high with temporary sunshine. Vegetation luxuriant. Yet no remarkable sickness prevails, on the contrary but twenty-six men in hospital at Morne Bruce, only one of them a slight fever from which he is recovering. The principal are cases of dysentery, a disease most likely to proceed from such a cause. Was any particular state of the atmosphere arising from the nature of the season the cause of the fever? It is but reasonable to suppose that the effect must have been as general and simultaneous as the cause. When the other islands, Barbados, Martinique, Guadeloupe and Antigua suffered so severely the year before, how on such a supposition could this one have then escaped and suffer solely this year. Islands so very contiguous and where the same trade wind blows so regularly must enjoy the same kind of seasons in the same years particularly the islands Martinique, Dominique and Guadeloupe, so adjacent to one another, separated only by very narrow channels of a few miles across, formed exactly alike, equally hilly, and their principal towns, St Pierre, Martinique, Roseau of this island and Basseterre of Guadeloupe similarly situated on the sea-coast to leeward under hills rising behind them.

In fact, the same kind of weather is known to prevail in these at the same time and the ravages that the yellow fever made in the two other islands the preceding year when this one escaped it are notorious, and while this one suffered the last year, there appears to have been no very remarkable sickness in the others. At least so I have been informed as to Martinique by a gentleman, Mr Ravarier, lately arrived from it; and I have heard no mention made of any particular sickness more than usual at Guadeloupe, which would be apt to be very generally known if it was the case.

To account for the escape of this island the year before when the adjoining ones were affected, supposing the fever to have been contagious and likely to be carried from one to the other, it is necessary to recollect that the others being in possession of the French, no regular trade is carried on with them from this and indeed but little communication with them or even the other islands but by very small vessels manned generally with coloured people even to whom, if taken ill, the vessels are too small to afford accommodation. If the sickness depended on so general and extensive a cause as the nature of the season, it ought to affect at least the different parts of one small island at the same time, but on the contrary, we find that it usually commences at the general sea port town. Its course from thence toward the more distant parts is gradual and progressive.

The first cases of it amongst the military were two of the artillery quartered in Fort Young, which I may say is actually in the town. D.M. Hinley admitted 26th June and died on the 29th. R. Richards attacked on the evening of 27 June and died early on the morning of 1 July. The only case of fever for a considerable time previous appears to have been that of I. Huck, Regiment West India Rangers, admitted 22 June which proved to be pure intermittent, which he told me himself he had suffered severely from at Guadeloupe and is apt to recur from slight causes.

The guardhouse for the town guard is in the fort and close to the artillery quarters, several of the West India Rangers are stated in their cases entered in the medical diaries to have been taken ill on the town guard or directly coming off it. The last cases in the island were in the most windward part of it, after it had ceased in the town and seems to have terminated there, but lately with the death of one of the most respectable inhabitants of the place, Mr Simpson, well-known and very universally regretted, when the fever raged here the other two military posts – Prince Rupert's at the northern extremity of the island and Scotshead Convalescent Post at the southern one, continued free from it and in a healthy state as noticed in the late Staff Surgeon Woulfe['s] letter of which I submit a copy.

20 August 1817

Sir,

The endemic fever which has for the last eight weeks prevailed at Roseau, its garrisons, and Morne Bruce becoming daily more general. The hospital containing many sicker (128) than there is proper accommodation for and each day bringing a considerable increase. I beg leave to suggest the expediency of removing the whole of the remaining European troops from this garrison to a healthier part of the island. At present, Prince Rupert's is particularly so as there is but one European there ill, now recovering, whose complaints can easily be traced to have originated here. It is possible the post of Scotshead may admit of more troops than are there at present. In that case, a boat would be required daily. A change of air as far as Point Michel may be advantageous. The very imminent dangers in which the whole of the white part of this garrison are now placed will, I trust, be deemed by you a proper motive for the opinion I here have the honour to submit to your consideration for the preservation of the troops.

I have used the word expedient above. In my mind, a removal is absolutely necessary, but should circumstances, which I am unacquainted with, render the measure improper, I look forward with the most anxious apprehension for the few who have escaped as yet. Annexed is a state of the admissions from this disease alone during that period together with the event.

I have the honour to be and remain

Signed

Robert Woulfe

The only cases that occurred at either of these posts at that time could be evidently traced to have had their origin here. The only one [at] Prince Rupert's was early in August, that of Captain Hyde, 1st West India Regiment, who directly after his return from this place where he had been to sit on a court martial was attacked so severely with fever that Staff Surgeon Woulfe was sent for to attend him and is the person alluded to in his letter in the following words "as there is but one European there ill, now recovering, whose complaint can easily be traced to have originated here". But as he was quartered in an airy attached quarter on top of the outer Cabrits distant from any other and the troops doing duty there being of a black regiment, it did not appear to have been then communicated to anybody else there. His fever, I am informed, did not terminate in intermittent as is usual with those at that post.

Again, early in December when the fever had almost entirely subsided here, Lieutenant Pilkin[g]ton, 1st West India Regiment and Mr Page, ordnance clerk, were carried off by fever there and which also happened to both of them directly after returning from this place. However, it is also right to mention that Mr Pilkin[g]ton, when he came up to this place, was only just recovered from an attack of the usual disease of that post, intermittent fever, and that Mr Page was represented to be of intemperate habits which are supposed to have contributed to his death. Mr Birmingham,[15] hospital assistant, also died just before, but whose cause I am not acquainted with the particulars of previously the place had been considered so healthy while the fever prevailed here that some sick of dysentery were removed there for the benefit of change of air.

But since then, there have been a few suspicious cases amongst the troops. The barrack serjeant having died there of fever rather suddenly and, as appears from the return, some few also of the 1st West India Regiment. When I was there myself, there were in hospital five fever cases, four of whom were of the same company, and the fifth had entered the hospital with pneumonia and when convalescent from that complaint was taken ill with fever whilst there. Four of them were convalescent there, and it is remarkable that not one of these was affected with intermittent as usual with the fevers of that part. The place projecting into the sea and being pretty generally exposed to a strong breeze of wind, I recommended them to avail themselves of it to air the men's barrack, necessaries, bedding and so on frequently, since when it seems to have extended no further.

When I visited Scottshead in answer to my enquiry whether they had suffered there from the fever, the serjeant who had been in charge of the post the entire time and who had there between twenty and thirty weakly and convalescent men principally from dysentery told me he only knew of two cases. One a boy, a son of a Serjeant James of the artillery, who when the rest of the family was lying ill of the fever, was brought there to be out of the way of it. But it also appeared on him a day or two after his arrival there. He was then sent home again; his father and mother had been ill together. It ran through the entire family. He lost two brothers by it and was communicated from him to the man that brought him to Scottshead, with whom he lived there and slept in the same bed with Private Frazer of the artillery, which was the second case and who died of it a day or two after being sent to hospital.

This spot is merely a high projecting rock in the sea connected with the main lands of the island by a narrow sandy isthmus commanding an extensive view of the coast of Martinique and the channel therefore useful as a look out post and on account of its salubrity receiving only the sea breeze as a convalescent one. On the very top of it is a small room usually allotted for two artillery men, in which were stated this man and another named Corbin, who of rather a disease habit subject to intermittent fever, was admitted into hospital since my arrival here, ill with fever of which he died. But the length of time since the death of the former man and the appearance of the fever in this case, which was a lingering one; As it appears that he had been ten days ill of it before his admission and did not die 'till the fifth day afterwards and of rather the intermittent type. I am inclined to think not connected with the former. The other men were quartered in a separate barracks about one-third down the rock on the windward side.

The separation and the free ventilation by the constant strong breeze were sufficient to account for their escape. The effect caused by the removal of the troops to Point Michel is also remarkable, a step recommended by the late Staff Surgeon Woulfe, with the hopes of checking the rapid progress that the fever was there making and which for the first week or two was attended with happiest effect as stated by the Commandant Major Cassidy in his letters to the Deputy Adjutant General Barbados extracts from which I annex.

Extracts of Letters from Major Cassidy, 1st West India Regiment Commanding the Troops in Dominica to Deputy Adjutant General Barbados

Morne Bruce Dominica
29 August 1817
Sir

Having in my letter of the 23rd instant had the honour to acquaint you with my intention to remove from the garrison such men of the Regiment West India Rangers as had not already been attacked with the fever now prevailing. It becomes my duty to report to you that this measure has been carried into effect and on the morning of the 25th instant those troops were marched to Point Michel where they are quartered for the present. As a proof of the good effect attending the change of quarters, I take the liberty herewith to enclose the daily state of sick on the 24th instant (the day previous to the change having taken place) and that of this day, and the only admission into hospital of men belonging to the Rangers is one man who had remained here as my groom.

From another dated 7 September 1817, it will be seen by my letter of 29 August that the sickness amongst the troops has considerably decreased, and I feel much pleasure in stating that it continues to do so. I am convinced that this change is chiefly, if not solely, to be attributed to the troops having been moved off the hill, as will appear by the daily status of the sick since that period as also from the fact of the greater number of those who were left there (chiefly women and children) having been lately attacked with fever which has even extended to the black troops. A man of 1st West India Regiment, having died yesterday with the usual black vomit, and others of that corps bring at this time ill with the same disease.

Remarks

The weekly and daily states having been forwarded to Barbados I could not get them so as to enable me to enclose copies of them. Nor could I learn other particulars of that period, the medical officer that then had charge, Hospital Assistant Wilson, being dead, nor do I find the cases of the W.I. Regiment entered. But I have been informed that it was afterward that some men joined from hospital with their clothing, necessaries and so on, that the fever renewed its violence amongst the troops at Point Michel.

But on account of the proximity of the place, not distant more than about three miles from Roseau and connected with it, I may say by a continued line of suburb with but short interruptions and the daily communications with it for provisions and so on, and the medical officer passing repeatedly between the hospital on the hill and the troops stationed there, it could not be expected that they would continue long exempt from it. And in consequence in a few weeks, they became as bad as ever when they were removed back again to the barracks on the hill.

It is to be observed that the communication had been carried on as far as possible by errand of the Black Pioneers and that the troops during the time that they were at Point Michel did no duty in the town. The benefit at first derived from the change; the return of sickness again among the troops though kept as close as possible to their new station.

The exemption of the other posts except in the instances stated and whose origin were to be traced to this place are circumstances that can hardly be accounted for on the supposition of so general a cause as vitiation of atmosphere or anything particular in the state of the weather or season having given rise to it though the explanation by means of contagion is so very plain and simple. How far with any degree of plausibility it could in this distance be ascribed to marsh miasma will appear at once evident from the fact before mentioned that Prince Rupert's, a place so notoriously fatal to white troops from an extensive marsh on the isthmus connecting it with the main land of the island, having so far escaped the fever, while Morne Bruce and Roseau, usually reckoned healthy, suffered so severely from it.

Staff Surgeon Hartle,[16] having a perfect knowledge of Morne Bruce from his long residence here and no particular doctrine to support, gave the following description of it. "To the east and immediately over the town are the military barracks on a hill 460 feet above the level of the sea called Morne Bruce. These barracks are all new, built of stone and brick. The situation is remarkably healthy and commands a full view of the harbour as well as from Scotshead to the projecting point of the saints. The part has no low grounds or stagnant water near it; therefore, nothing can be alleged against its local situation."

It may be conjectured that the time of the sickness being partly the rainy season, the swamp may have been covered with water and thus rendered harmless. This at the very first view of the place would appear to be totally impossible. The swamp is so completely intersected with drains. Main channels are cut directly across from the sea at one side to that at the other, from which I saw myself. The water running out regularly when it was not particularly wet, these are crossed again by other smaller ones so that the entire surface of it is divided into regular parallelograms, which drains though not effectual in draining the swamp completely must prevent water collecting on it to the extent above supposed. A small spot about the centre being, I believe rather below the level of the sea, might possibly be covered, but there must still remain a very large extent of it uncovered. No doubt the frequent fall of rain water may dilute and render less noxious that of the marsh before more stagnant, which I believe to be the case. This is but a supposition and would equally apply to swamps elsewhere and thus rather argue against their operating so powerfully at such a time as to cause so generally such a violent malignant fever.

That it certainly did not proceed in this distance from such is manifest from the very general course of the fever not exhibiting at any part of the period the intermittent form as is usual with those of Prince Rupert's and of every other place where I have known such a course to exist. The effect and course were equally visible and certain. However continued and severe such may have appeared at their commencement, they very generally terminated with those that in obstinate intermittents requiring the most patient persevering use of the bark for their removal and which, at such a station, would usually constitute the largest proportion of fevers at once in hospital, though it might not appear so from the returns, they being marked first as remittents or continued and not afterwards altered.

When I visited Prince Rupert's, of four officers stationed there I found two, Lieutenant Rice, 1st West India Regiment and Hospital Assistant Williams,[17] ill with intermittent fever. Of five artillery men, one was in hospital with the same disease, one came up with me for a change of air on account of it, and the others though endeavouring to do their duty were, I understand, also labouring under it. Those of them that I saw were of pale yellow sickly appearance, as if from visceral disease and one man of the York Rangers who had been sent there with dysentery of which he was then seasoned but suffering under obstinate intermittent, I also brought up with me, so that of all the white persons I knew of there, the only ones exempt from intermittents were Captain Hyde and his wife, quartered in the commanding officer's quarter on top of the outer Cabrits, reckoned the healthiest one in the garrison. Lieutenant Brown who in a variety of bad situations always maintained good health and the commissary who had been there but for a short time, while at the same time I did not know of a single case of intermittent here, but one that had been contracted there, a Mr Jameson, ordnance clerk, under my case with quarter ague, which he says he got by sleeping but one night at that post.

I have carefully looked through the hospital diaries of Morne Bruce for the last six months and could only find of fever cases, seven, that terminated in intermittent, most of which manifested that for from the commencement and as far as I could ascertain, they had before been affected with it. Indeed, I should have expected a much greater number knowing how very apt that disease is to return even after a long interval from slight causes, and that the West India Rangers had only arrived here the preceding year from Guadeloupe where they had suffered severely from it. The same remark holds good with respect to the cause of the fever when it prevailed at Barbados.

The cases of which treated in the upper General Hospital, there are fully detailed in Dr May's diaries, which I have taken pains in examining. I do not recollect a single case of intermittent throughout.

Dr Caddle, the most extensive private practitioner there in answer to my question whether he had ever known such kind of fever produced in that island answered in the most positive decided manner in presence of Assistant Surgeon Ralph[18] of the Queens, never in his life that he has treated them when brought from other islands but never knew one actually originate there. My own experience as far as it goes during the different periods that I have had charge of the medical patients in General Hospital most exactly corresponds with this, though I am inclined to think that others biased with notions of marsh miasma and mistaking the interval of ease too frequently delusive between the first and subsequent stage of the malignant fever for an intermission administered bark freely to which if the patient survived his recovery was attributed and his fever considered as an intermittent one.

I have also seen a few instances in hospital there of patients ill with some other complaint being attacked with ephemeral fever but of which there was no second paroxysm though no bark was given, which I purposely withheld in order to see the result. I have known such also mistaken for intermittent and treated accordingly those also that have been attacked with ague in other islands [who] may have a recurrence in that one from occasional causes and if the history of these be not particularly enquired into, they be supposed to have originated there. Such I believe to be the sole sources of intermittent at Barbados.

And this is only as might be expected from the nature of the country there which is known to be throughout well cleared and cultivated and in consequence to be usually healthful. On the parade ground in front and very generally in the vicinity of the barracks the rock presents its base surface. Every half dozen or dozen steps the intermediate parts lightly covered with thin black mould producing scanty pasturage usually dry and parched, but when the rain falls then from the unevenness of the surface the water may lodge while it continues to rain and supply it afresh, but it cannot stagnate to putrefy and produce noxious miasma. From the porous nature of the coral rock beneath the rapid evaporation caused by the heat of the sun, a great part of the day and the several channels that are cut to allow it to run off so that after the rain ceases it soon again becomes parched and dry. The small narrow patches adjacent to the seashore that in a few places here and there have a marshy appearance being in a sandy soil, and the water, I may say, circulating freely through the higher sands on one side draining through the porous coral rock and from the sea on the other, with which it is nearly on a level and being below and to leeward if (sic) the other parts of the island appear to be inoxious.

The principal one towards Oistins (in Barbados) also on account of its distance from the garrison of two or three miles can hardly be supposed to affect it. Other causes usually offered and assigned for such sickness in this case proved equally unsatisfactory.

The town of Roseau at the commencement or during the prevalence of it was not crowded with strangers nor the barracks with troops who were not sufficiently numerous even to occupy the entire of them. Duty was not severe or hard on them; quite the contrary very light and easy. Nor could it be considered a disease of nervousness when it affected some of the oldest inhabitants even creoles themselves, some of whom were carried off by it.

Though I am well convinced of the disease being contagious to ascertain at this late period in what manner the contagion of it was brought here is not so easy and where the persons concerned in bringing it must be interested in concealing the circumstance and no person having been particularly solicitous to discover it, it is likely to remain in obscurity. However, the following circumstance deserves notice. The disease appeared very early if not actually in the very first instance amongst the artillery. The men first attacked were but lately arrived from barracks where the disease was known to have existed, but four months before, and they had actually with them some articles of clothing that they bought there at auctions of the effects of deceased men who died of that fever. Serjeant Sawes, who suffered here as well as his entire family from it, had on him when he informed me of the circumstance, a white cotton waistcoat purchased there at one of these auctions. These are at least very suspicious circumstances.

I have before mentioned the mortality having commenced at Barbados so soon after the arrival of the *Childers* Brig of War there as to be by very many persons ascribed to it. In each of the ships of war that were affected with it as far as I have been able to learn, it could be traced to contagion brought on board.

When in June 1816 I was for a few days at Guadeloupe, I heard casually of some persons having been suddenly carried off by a severe suspicious kind of fever. We find that in the beginning of August the *Childers* and the *Scamander* Frigate were employed in removing troops from that island to others, I believe Grenada and St Vincent, that Lieutenant Nixon 6th West India Regiment was on board the former vessel ill with fever attended with black vomiting, of which he died a few hours after being landed. They then proceeded to the Gulf of Paria,[19] the station fixed on by the admiral for the ships of war during the hurricane months, and in both vessels, though at a considerable distance from each other, the very same time I am informed about a fortnight after the performance of the above service the fever commenced in the *Scamander* among the midshipmen so as speedily to carry off four or five of them and the servant that attended them. However, the captain, immediately taking the alarm, had all from that berth brought and kept upon deck in the free air the place below well-cleaned and purified and thus most successful, stopped it in his vessel. But in the other one, where from the smallness and closeness of it, every circumstance favoured the propagation. If contagion is spread in the manner before mentioned and that progressively forward from where the sick often must have been accommodated as thus stated in the late Dr May's report:

> Twenty-one died out of ninety persons, officers and men on board in the following progression – a boy servant in the gun room, a purser of the ship, a purser's clerk sent on board from the *Antelope* to fill the situation, were the first victims. Light marines whose berths were in the after part of the ship contiguous to the gun room and midshipmen's berths. Four midshipmen next died. I believe they had been imprudently shooting ashore when the vessel was at anchor there – three seamen and three women.

When the *Childers* arrived at Antigua from Barbados not having a sufficient number of persons onboard able to work to bring her to anchor – two transports, the *Lord Eldon* and *Walker* that were lying there were obliged to send men on board to assist and the captains of these vessels told me that directly afterwards their entire crews suffered severely from the same kind of fever and that they lost a considerable number of them. Captain Richardson of the *Lord Eldon* mentioned himself as the only instance on board his vessel of escape from an attack of it and that several years before he had been affected by it severely in the West Indies.

The *Brazen* continued healthy 'till 26th September when about to sail from Barbados for Antigua she received on board thirty-two recovered officers and men of the *Childers* from the General Hospital to join the vessel there; also a man of their own, James Bradberry who had been in hospital with slight fever from which he was then recovered but appears to have contracted the malignant one there with which he was seized a few days afterwards and on their arrival at Antigua on the 30th, was sent to hospital where he died, was told by the surgeon in two or three days. It then spread through the vessel rapidly so that I believe only six escaped and a considerable number died of it. It is to be remarked that she had been the entire of July and 'till 19th August in the Gulf of Paria, which was a longer time than I believe any other of the vessels staid there and yet continued healthy. So it is clear that the station there could not with any degree of reason be charged with having produced that fever. Indeed, I am told that vessels of any burthen cannot approach within a considerable distance of the shore from the shoalness of the water so as to be affected by any marshes that may be there. To account for this fever, thus appearing after so long an absence, successively in so many different places in such different situations and under such a variety of circumstances has puzzled the ingenuity of the non-contagionists more than a little. They are obliged to have recourse to different causes in almost every individual case. Secondary assisting and predisposing ones are ranked as the primary and principal and in order to adduce something analogous to marsh miasma, causes are stated that as far as I know were never before thought of, as the word they may have had on board for fuel. Mud collected in the hold as was said to be the case with the *Childers* and supposed to have contributed in causing the fever in her, and other supposed instances of neglects of cleanliness on board as in the midshippersons' berths of the *Scamander* are mentioned as productive of the fever though Dr Bancroft[20] in his essay on the yellow fever from page 103 to 156 produced a number of facts to disprove such a supposition. The bad smell, which was said to be so offensive in the *Childers* I am informed by a gentleman of the ship, was by no means perceptible 'till after the great accumulation of sick from which alone any that may have been processed as to the air in the hold on being first opened after having been some time closed extinguishing a light brought suddenly into it is only what might be expected, and I am told usually happens, and I can hardly ascribe much mischief merely to the mud that was stated to have been found in her hold on cleaning it out when I have repeatedly seen at the mouths of large rivers ballast for vessels dug out of their muddy bottoms without having ever before heard of ill consequences from it.

Thus, very dissimilar and unlikely causes are loudly proclaimed while the plain obvious one to which it could be traced in each of the instances I have mentioned is passed over in silence. Nearly all the facts and circumstances that I have stated in proof of its contagious nature and positive the weight and force of which against negative ones must be evident. Was it otherwise there is no disease whatever not even the plague small pox scarlatina or measles that might not be proved to be non-contagious from the numerous instances that could be brought forward of persons exposed to contagion of each without suffering there from and such negative cases must tell equally against any other general principle that they may assume as the cause and only prove the persons thus escaping to beat the time in a state not susceptible of it. From all which and the positive evidence I have formerly had of its contagious nature not a doubt exists in my own mind on the subject. So, few persons do I know now remaining that were here formerly when the malignant fever last prevailing as to afford but few opportunities of judging whether the constitution is liable to suffer more than once from it, but as far as they go, they form the idea that it is not.

Colonel Maxwell Governor of the island is one of the few that escaped, and he told me that about the year 1797 he had a severe fever in Jamaica. Dr Greenway who has been thirty-four years in this place suffered a severe attack of fever in 1792 and escaped it last year as did also I understand Drs Clark and Garroway, very old practitioners here. I may also instance myself having laboured under it in Gibraltar Bay 1810 and not at all affected by it here though soon after my arrival in assisting at the dissection of a Mr Taylor who appeared to have been carried off by it as he had been walking about his business on Friday and on Tuesday following his body was the subject of our examination, was very yellow throughout and his stomach contained the matter of black vomit. My finger was pricked deeply in replacing the integuments after examining the brain, so that I might consider myself fairly inoculated with his blood with which my fingers were covered at the time, but I am glad to say without any ill effects from it. When I hear mentioned frequent instances as having occurred of persons recovering from fever with black vomit and to have died of a second attack of the same disease attended with the same symptoms, it so ill accords with the experience of other old and extensive practitioners according to which recovery from fever after the appearance of that symptom is a very rare occurrence indeed. That I am strongly inclined to suspect some mistake and which when we consider how very possible it becomes the more probable. Coffee, which is one of the most common articles of diet, if taken before the patient happens to vomit, must give that appearance to whatever is thrown up. I have known Port Wine mixed with the contents of the stomach mistaken for black vomit. The mixture of some of the most usual medicines may produce the same appearance. Calomel, the one most frequently administered and ammonia, not infrequently given in the later stages when the patient is apt to be low and vomiting urgent if they should happen to be mixed even in the stomach, may have the same effect. That black vomit is not peculiar to this disease is noticed by Dr Bancroft in page 3, where he quotes instances of its occurring in other complaints, and I have myself known such cases and heard of others. Where every mode of treatment practised appears to have been so generally ineffectual, I can have little to offer on the subject of cure. Bleeding very generally formed part of it, and in several cases, to a considerable extent, which though I have to regret that it did not prove effectual. Yet I have no reason for concluding that it was actually injurious or detrimental. I have seen some recovered that had been bled largely and others that lost not blood at all. From which and the great benefit that I have seen derived from it in other fevers of this climate, I would still be inclined to try it in conjunction with and as an auxiliary to some other active means.

I have now in conclusion to lament that while in other diseases some advancement is daily making towards a more perfect knowledge and appropriate treatment of them by establishing nicer distinctions that may have hitherto escaped notice, in this one course is rather retrograde in neglecting distinctions long since noticed and handed down to us confounding all the fevers of this climate under one common head with the appellation of remittents as if derivable, but from one source alone marsh miasma certainly most incorrect and which must even prove a source of endless confusion and controversy.[21] Dr Jackson on the fevers of Jamaica marks a distinction between the fevers of Savanna-la-Mar, where he resided in that island for four years and those that fell under his observation afterwards in America, which I have found most exactly to apply to the ordinary fevers of the different islands of this command.

According to the diversity of local circumstances [on] page 5 "the paroxysms of the fevers of Jamaica are observed in many instances to terminate in more perfect remissions than the paroxysms of the endemic of North America which is known to be fundamentally an intermitting disease". Again, [on] some [other] page "yet I cannot help remarking that certain appearances incline one to be of opinion that there subsists between the endemic of Jamaica and the endemic of North America a difference in some degree fixed and essential". Page 6 [says] the common

> fever of Jamaica for instance was not only disposed to terminate of its own accord, but it was disposed to terminate on certain critical days, often at an early period, and by signs of crisis too clear to be mistaken. Neither did the Peruvian bark in the manner at least in which it was managed ever cut short its course with certainty. The endemic of America on the contrary often lasted long. It frequently indeed changed to another disease after a length of time, but no period could be assigned for its natural termination. The signs of crisis it may likewise be remarked were so obscure as scarcely to be distinguished with the closest attention. At least for my own part, I will own that after an experience of several years and the greatest care in noticing the minutest circumstances, I never yet was able to say with confidence that the endemic of America, particularly in the Northern provinces, was gone not to return again till the hour of its return was past, neither did the

Peruvian bark, though its effects were so equivocal in the fever of Jamaica scarcely ever fail of stopping the progress of this disease, to which may be added that the complaint which strictly speaking is called the intermittent or ague and fever can scarcely be said to belong to Jamaica. At least it was not known at Savana-la-Mar.

Page 9: "the fevers of the Aegean Sea as described by Hippocrates and of Minorca as described by the accurate Cleghorn bear the nearest resemblance to the endemic of Savanna-la-Mar. The fevers of Italy, of different part of the continent of Asia, as described by various writers, as well as the fever of America, of which I have personal experience. However, obscure remissions seem rather to be degenerate intermittents. Thus, the endemics of dry situations as Barbados, Saint Pierre Martinique and of this town as far as I have yet seen, corresponds with the first kind, have a tendency to terminate spontaneously, generally soon yielding to the free use of the Lancet and Calomel without any inclination to recurrent and in which bark is totally unnecessary at least as far as concerns the fever. While those of marshy or uncleared places or that have such in their vicinity to windward as Morne Fortune, St Lucia, Basseterre, Guadeloupe and Prince Rupert's of this island.

However, continued at first, [they] apt soon to assume the intermittent from proving tedious and obstinate and requiring the full and free use of the bark to overcome that strong aptitude to recurrence of paroxysm, remaining for a length of time. Such are the ordinary evidenced fevers of the West Indies and which do not usually manifest any strong appearance of contagion but rather generally seem to arise from some other obvious causes.

While that which lately prevailed here and which occasionally spreads with so much destruction through all the different islands, I have stated my reasons for believing to be altogether distinct and different and to be most highly contagious. I have now also good reasons for supposing the common typhus fever not to be so great a stranger at least in some of the islands as has been generally imagined. Dr Caddle of Barbados, whom I formerly mentioned, has been in the habit of speaking of this disease as one of the most common occurrences amongst the negroes on the estates and kindly offered to show us some cases of it. I, accordingly, for the sake of seeing such, accompanied him to an estate on which it had just commenced. He expected to find two, but it had then extended to two others. Also, those that had it the longest had certainly all the appearance of the complaints. Along with low fever, there was great general prostration of strength, the patients hardly able to sit up in the bed without support. Tremor of the tongue and limbs and on conversing with the gentleman that owned the estate, he spoke of it as a disease that they were most familiar and conversant with, mentioning different estates that it had passed through, affecting the negroes to a very considerable number, that it was a low-lingering disease usually protracted to three or four weeks duration, in a few instances extending even to the whites such as the bookkeepers who are usually the most amongst them, but mostly confined to the blacks themselves from their manner of living in their huts, which they usually keep closed to exclude the air for the sake of warmth, while the whites on the contrary admit it in every direction and do everything to promote free ventilation for personal comfort and are thus generally exempt from it. About two months afterwards when I met Dr Caddle again, he told me that about thirty or forty, to the best of my recollection, on that estate had been then attacked with it. I have been thus particular, I am afraid tediously, so from a desire of removing as far as possible doubts and uncertainties from fact of importance in opposition to doctrines of, I conceive, the most dangerous tendency".

Signed
John Arthur MD
Physician to the Forces

Extract of Half-Yearly Report of Prevailing Diseases in the Detachment Hospital on Morne Bruce Dominica from 21 June to 20 December 1821 by Edward Dow,[22] Surgeon to the Forces

Epidemic bilious remitting fever prevails amongst European troops more or less every year in the West India Islands. At Morne Bruce, its appearance is frequent and during some years is very fatal in its progress. The duties required of the detachment occupying the barracks on Morne Bruce must always be accounted as a powerful predisposing cause of epidemic fever – hitherto it has been usual to have six or eight sentries in town during the night and none during the day. They are marched down about sunset and their posts are so detached that there cannot be the smallest difficulty of procuring ardent spirits, and it is scarcely necessary to add that British soldiers are much addicted to the abuse of spirits and I am compelled to say that the present detachment have that vice, to a great extent.

The guardhouse is situated in Fort Young and is heated during the day to such a degree, that it is with difficulty the soldiers can be made to sleep inside but prefer the cooler situation afforded them under the gateway of the fort, where however they are exposed to sudden gusts of wind when the relief is marched out.

At daylight, the sentries are withdrawn and returned to Morne Bruce, where they are apt to get chilled suddenly after the fatigue of climbing the hill. The present detachment having come from an elevated dry windward situation in Antigua to Morne Bruce which is quite the reverse, must also be allowed to have a great effect on their health. In Dominica, this year, bilious remitting fever has been general throughout the island and the fatality of it has not been confined to European inhabitants or the soldiers, as a large proportion of deaths from this disease has occurred amongst the coloured population.

The weather during the month of June, July and August was without rain and hotter than has happened within the memory of the eldest inhabitant, and had an uncommon influence on the human body. The winds were from the south and west and very sultry during the day, whilst the true land breeze generally prevailed during the night time.

At this period, it was observed that vegetation was much impaired by it. Another source of malignant epidemic fever may be traced to the caverns and excavations all over the extent of Morne Bruce even under the barracks, where no doubt large quantities of rain lodge, saturated with vegetable remains which speedily pass into a state of putridity in this climate and exhale noxious vapours in great abundance.

The garrison, however, continued tolerable healthy till about the middle of September, when the admissions became daily more numerous, and the cases more aggravated, especially amongst such as had suffered previously from dysentery, the debility left by it was according to its degree proportionally fatal. Despondency has been general in all the cases and on that account a powerful assistant in swelling the list of fatal case[s].

The attack in most was sudden, commencing with some degree of coldness or shivering, succeeded by ardent and deep-seated heat, violent headache particularly over the orbits and in some, strong flushing of the face, acute pain across the loins stretching down the back part of the thighs as far as the calves of the legs, accompanied in some instances by spasms, nausea, and in most instances, violent, vomiting, the pulse in many full and often irregular, in some small and oppressed.

The action of the great arteries was very irregular, in some distressing throbbing in the temples in others in the carotids, the eyes were inflamed, watery and often suffused and of a yellowish cast. Bowels were generally costive, or the stools dark coloured and acrimonious. Tongue generally moist and covered toward the front with white fur, in a few it was red, glossy and parched.

When the irritability of the stomach proved obstinate, the matters ejected became as black as pitch. *Petechiae*[23] and livid spots occurred toward the latter end of the fever, and in many accompanied by violent haemorrhage from the nose and gums and anus. In most, the pain at the *praecordia*[24] was severe and communicated to the fingers or pressure a disagreeable sensation which remained for a considerable time.

The urine in small quantities and at first very pale but afterwards highly tinged and in a few, of a deep dark red colour and of a highly putrid smell, suppression not total, but even when partial an unfavourable symptom. Delirium was not a very general symptom and when it terminated in coma, always fatal. In some, where irritability of stomach did not prevail, the dejections were exactly similar to black vomit, but not necessarily a fatal symptom. Countenance in the fatal cases extremely lurid and the dingy, dusky appearance of the skin about the neck and breast was almost a constant attendant, cold clammy sweats and the pulse not perceivable at the wrist, with great restlessness and in many a general convulsion tormented the sufferings of the patient.

During the commencement of the epidemic bloodletting was had recourse to very copiously but during the latter period of the epidemic it was not found advantageous as in some instances the fatal event appeared to be hastened by it. Purgatives of different kinds were employed to a very great extent and appeared to have been beneficial in most cases. Ptyalism[25] was endeavoured to be brought on in general and where it was obtained freely about the third day it was successful, the mode in which I attempted to do it was by giving Calomel and Blue Pill combined in moderate doses at very short intervals.

The warm bath appeared to have been of service in some cases, but in others, it was of no benefit. Blisters on the head and nape of the neck were beneficial in relieving the headache and delirium in the earlier stages and useful on the pit of the stomach in checking the disposition to vomiting, but this last symptom was most effectually relieved by small doses of lime water and milk. Strangury[26] was a common effect of the blistering but easily relieved in a short time.

When the violence of the fever had subsided bark and other tonics were administered with advantage. The patients all expressed a great desire for Port and water as a drink, and it seems to have been of much benefit. The relapses have been numerous, and in many proved fatal as the constitutions of the fevered were greatly reduced by long services and the abuse of spirituous liquors.

Every measure of precaution to arrest the progress of the epidemic was adopted. The garrison was removed from Morne Bruce to a healthy village about two miles to the south of Roseau on the sea coast. The woollen clothing and the blankets and rags of the deceased were burnt, and the linen well scoured with lime and water. The barracks were repeatedly fumigated and whitewashed, the floors were taken up and ventilation allowed for several weeks.

The epidemic, however, did not cease till every one (with a very few exceptions) had been attacked with it, after which the troops were removed back to their quarters on Morne Bruce.

Signed
Edward Dow
Surgeon to the Forces

Extract of Observations on the Diseases That Occurred in the Detachment of Royal Artillery 35th Regiment Stationed in Dominica for the Period from 21 December 1825 to 20 December 1826 by N. Birrell, MD, Assistant Staff Surgeon

The 35th Detachment maintained good health for three or four months after their arrival here, during all which period the weather was generally dry and the temperature pretty uniform. About the beginning of July, there were frequent heavy showers, alternated with hot sultry intervals; it was perfectly calm.

The consequences of such weather must therefore be obvious. Its effects were first felt in the town of Roseau which from its situation was naturally to be expected. Several of the civilians (*the character of the civilians is not intemperate which proves that excess in drinking was not the exciting cause of the disease – the great proportion of soldiers subsequently seized with the above evidence shows how much more bodies, [debilitated to exhausted by intemperance] are susceptible of morbid impressions*) of Roseau were attacked with a severe form of remittent fever, in some of whom it proved fatal and death was generally preceded by yellow suffusion of the body and by something like black vomit. It soon afterwards appeared among the military stationed in or near Roseau. Ordinance Storekeeper Drake died of this disease in June and Ordinance Storekeeper Sevaine in July. It appeared in the detachment of artillery consisting of fourteen men (these all stationed at Fort Young close to Roseau) on the 6 July and very soon, one-half of this small detachment was attacked, of whom two died. The remainder at the recommendation of Staff Surgeon Lyons[27] were then removed to Melville Battery. But this change did not arrest the progress of the disease – the remaining half of the detachment, one man excepted, were attacked with the same fever of whom also two died. Thus, in a short period, four deaths happened in a detachment of fourteen men. Of three women and six children belonging to this detachment, all were attacked with fever, but only one, that of a girl, proved fatal. The surviving ten men were then ordered to Scotts Head and thereafter a residence of nearly two months, the only man who had previously escaped the fever at Roseau was in that healthy place attacked with fever of which he died. The total number of fever cases admitted from the 35th Detachment was 146, but generally speaking, the cases were mild until the beginning of August when it assumed the same type as it had done among the artillery that is that of the endemial remittent of the country. The deaths, however, in the 35th were proportionally few, six only having proved fatal being at the rate of 4 per cent. The question may naturally occur why the disease first appeared amongst the Artillery and why that small detachment suffered so much more than that of the 35th. That question is very easily answered, and has been stated in previous reports – that is the locality of Fort Young, from its low situation and from its being entirely enclosed, the heat of the sun is reflected and a [direct] current of the air is prevented, from which circumstances the temperature is frequently four degrees higher than it is at Morne Bruce.

The contiguity of Fort Young to Roseau must not be forgotten, by which there is every facility of procuring new rum and other spirits of bad quality. The men who composed the detachment of artillery had not been quite twelve months in the West Indies; they were young, robust and apparently healthy, [having] all the sanguineous temperament and of plethoric[28] habits of body. It must, therefore, be evident that such excitable constitution in such a place, during the existence of such variable weather as has been briefly mentioned, must have been very liable to morbid impressions. How much, therefore, this liability to disease must have been increased when the above unavoidable general and local causes was added that of the usual imprudence of soldiers – the indulging in ardent spirits.

The 35th Detachment on the contrary, are elevated more than four hundred feet above the situation of Fort Young. The temperature of Morne Bruce is in general some degrees less than that of Fort Young and scarcely a day passes without its inhabitants being in some degree renovated by the cool refreshing breezes from the mountains. There is not the same facility of procuring new rum on the Morne, as at Fort Young and finally from the greater number of the men of the 35th having been nearly six years in the West Indies, they were less liable to the impression of the morbid causes, which it has been attempted to be shown there existed.

The symptoms of the fever for the reasons just stated, amongst the artillery were much more ardent and speedier in their course, than in the 35th although the type in both were essentially the same. The symptoms were such as generally occur, when such endemics make their appearance in tropical climates – that is severe pain of forehead, painfulness and sense of stiffness in moving the eyeballs, great sense of tightness or of oppression in the epigastric regions and frequently tenderness there on the slightest pressure, constant irritability of stomach, urgent thirst, restlessness, and so on. The pulse varied according to the constitution and habits of the patient. The symptoms and the sensation which the surface produced also varied.

In the robust patients at the commencement of the disease, it was pungently hot and dry. In worn out constitutions and in the advanced stages of the disease there were frequent cold clammy perspirations. The tongue seldom presented anything remarkable, except in the protracted cases when it generally put on the appearance of the tongue in typhoid fever. It became brown, dry, incrusted and black and the teeth were covered with black and brown incrustations. The more severe forms of fever were always ushered in by universal rigours (such as I have also always observed in other islands), and which were generally mistaken by the patient for a fit of ague. These symptoms were, therefore, frequently no more attended to than by the patient drinking some warm punch which had the effect of producing perspiration and thus for a time suspending the symptoms at least, so far as the patient's sensations went. In twelve and sometimes not until twenty-four hours the patient had a similar attack then succeeded by severe pain of head and so on which *forced* the patient to report himself sick.

It has been ascertained, and the patients themselves have confessed, that they have contrived to conceal their complaint and to do their duty for two or three days after the first attack of rigours. The chances of recovering these patients must, therefore, it is obvious, have been very small. The most difficult symptom to contend with was the gastric irritability when this sign occurred in exhausted, dissipated constitutions, accompanied with tenderness of the stomach on pressure with an acrid or burning sensation of that organ. A small feeble pulse shrunk and anxious features and the prognosis always unfavourable. When the head was principally affected and the patient had strength to bear venesection[29] and other powerful evacuates, the disease if taken in time was easily overcome. According to the register, the *four first* fatal cases [within the] artillery had the usual black vomit immediately preceding death and that one man recovered after having had that usually fatal symptom (Register No. 11 Folio 117).

In no case did that symptom appear after my taking charge of the hospital. The fatal cases that came under my observation had generally more or less a yellow appearance of skin and irritability of stomach continued to the last, but the matter ejected was merely the food taken in, or the medicine, mixed with mucous and dark-coloured bile.

From the post-mortem examinations, the principal morbid appearances were in the liver and stomach. In the majority, the liver was of a pale yellowish colour, in some it was dark red with congestion, the gall bladder sometimes empty, or nearly so, and in a few containing a substance of the colour and consistence of tar. In the four first Artillery, cases that proved fatal, the stomach contained about a pint of a dark fluid resembling coffee grounds. In some there were dark patches about the *cardia* and pylorics[30] resembling effused blood into the substance of the coats – as was seen in the case of Sweeney, McGuinness's case differed by having its mucous coat vascular throughout. In Corporal Smith also, the internal coat was vascular and covered with a thick layer of brownish coloured matter. In some, the mucous coat was only at different places vascular, principally about the two orifices. In a few, the mucous coat of the duodenum had several florid red patches and in Private Hutchins's was covered with matter resembling pus, and this appearance in this patient was observed in a less degree throughout the small intestines. In Bell's case, the duodenum was vascular. In all, the coats of the stomach were more or less thickened. Seldom any morbid appearance was observed in the thoracic cavity – the lungs, indeed, were in general quite healthy and even free from adhesions. In a few, there was a slight vascularity of the *pleura costalis*[31] and a slight effusion of the serum.

Signed:
Birrell,[32] MD
Assistant Staff Surgeon
Prince Ruperts
Dominica, 24 February 1827

Extract of Yearly Report of Disease and Medical Occurrences at Dominica Ending 20 December 1826, by John Glasco,[33] Surgeon to the Forces

Remittent Fevers

These take a lead in all parts of the West Indies and lay the foundation for others; they are to be met with at all seasons and in all classes, though rarely in the Negro; but they are most prevalent in or after moist, variable weather, when there have been alternate calms and gusts of wind and a great range of thermometer.

Such has been the case during part of the first and all the third quarters, and the results have been proportionate. From the middle of January to the end of February, the rains were incessant with calms and gusts of wind. For six weeks, the Morne was in a constantly miry state. The huts in which the married people resided were almost inaccessible, and it was from among these the first cases of severe fever were admitted.

In the third quarter, it was stated that from the latter end of June to September, there was scarcely a dry interval; and these were remarkably calm, close and sultry. The intermediate quarters were generally dry and accompanied by a refreshing breeze.

The state of disease seemed to follow the weather, and the remittent fevers abounded during the period of rains – in the dry quarters of the year, the garrison was tolerably healthy.

In the first quarter, the symptoms are stated to have been great prostration of strength, and languid pulse, cold surface and rather moist eyes, dull little thirst, tongue tremulous and covered with white sores, stomach irritable. In the second quarter, the attacks were ephemeral, brought on by intemperance and exposure to the cold. The disease partook of the contained more than the remittent form, and the treatment was without embarrassment and was removed by a brisk cathartic of Calomel and Jalap with saline purgatives.

In June, cases of fever in the severe form took place among the inhabitants, while the military were exempt. Early in July, it first made its appearance among the artillery. Many circumstances tended to give it force among these troops. First the robust habits of the men, the unfavourable situation of their barracks, and their easy means of indulging in ardent spirits from the living in town. In this detachment, there were eleven admissions, one a relapse form of which proved fatal. At the same time, three women out of four, and five children were seized with fever, all belonging to the same detachment. One of the children died with black vomit. The detachment was removed to a neighbouring battery up an adjoining eminence (Melville Battery), but this did not arrest the progress of disease as one-half the admissions were from this place. After their removal to Scotts Head, the detachment remained free from disease, and during the whole year, not one admission with fever took place from that post.

The Artillery consisted of fourteen robust young men. On 6 July, these were all healthy. On the morning of the 7th, three were attacked with fever, without any evident cause, and on the same day, a Sergeant, 35th, doing duty in town, and Assistant Staff Surgeon Birrell were also taken ill. Thus, in one day, five out of fifteen individuals living within a short distance of each other were attacked with fever, all of whom were in apparent health the day previously. Of these five, three died. After passing through nearly all the artillery, it assumed the severe form among the 35th Detachment, which was in the beginning of August; several of the women and children of the 35th Detachment were also affected, but with two exceptions, they were all slight and no mortality occurred.

Of six officers stationed at Morne Bruce, four had severe attacks of fever and three have been sent home – one in an extreme state of debility and subject to frequent spasms of fever. He had remained a long time in hopes of doing duty with his regiment, but could not gain strength, tending to prove that this situation is ill-calculated for convalescing.

The officers serving in the town suffered more severely than those at the Morne. The fort adjutant, his wife, servant and two children were all at the same time confined to bed. The lieutenant of artillery also suffered, although he had been several years in the command. The ordinance storekeeper both in Roseau and from Prince Rupert's fell victims, as also the engineer officer and the son of the major general commander. The majority of the cases were marked *Febris Contenna Com*, but the type generally speaking was remittent. The characteristic signs of all the cases of artillery on admission were languor and great debility, pain of forehead and eyes, with a sense of fullness in the hypochondriac and hypogastric regions, irritability of stomach and dark foetid alvine dejections, skin hot and dry, and as the disease advanced, alternating with cold perspirations, thirst extremely urgent, the state of the tongue varied in appearance, sometimes white and loaded at others brown and in some of the mouth it had a fiery but clean appearance. In the fatal cases, it became dry and incrusted as in the last stage of typhus fever. All the fatal cases had the usual appearance of black vomit, as also had one child. One man recovered after having had that symptom.

The disease appears to be the severe form of the bilious remittent and in the 35th, although there was constant irritability of stomach, the matter ejected bore no resemblance to the coffee-ground vomit. In the post-mortem examinations, the external surface of the body was yellowish and ecchymosed.[34] Thorax – both cavities contained a large quantity of fluid blood; the heart was large and firm and had many small dark points upon it.

Abdomen – the intestines were healthy. The liver of a pale or straw colour, the gall bladder contained a substance like tar; the stomach was thickened and contained from one to two pints of a dark coloured fluid, owing to flocculent matter described as resembling coffee grounds. There were several dark red patches about the cardiac and pyloric orifice resembling effused blood into the substance of its coats. In one, the stomach contained one-third pint of black grumous matter; its mucous coat was vascular throughout and not in patches as in the former case. In another, the inflammation extended to the duodenum. Such were the appearances in the Artillery cases. In the fatal cases, the stomach and liver had similar appearances except in the absence of the black matter above described. In the brain, there were diseased opacities of its membranes, turgescence of all the vessels, and effusion of serum in all the ventricles and spinal canal.

Of the three officers who died at this station, the first District Ordinance Storekeeper Drake was attacked on 11 June with rigours; skin hot but moist face flushed, headache excessive; pains in his loins and limbs; great thirst, tongue whitish and moist, pulse full and quick. He took fifteen grams of Calomel with the same quantity of Jalap and was put into the warm bath. By these means, it was hoped the paroxysm would assume the intermittent form, but failing in this, active depletion was used. He sunk on the fourth day, having black vomit for ten to twelve hours.

The second case was that of Deputy Ordinance Storekeeper Serayne. He was first taken ill at Prince Rupert's, and the time lost in his removal allowed the disease to make such progress that he gradually sunk after his arrival in Roseau. The third was lieutenant of the engineers, a young man of delicate frame, who seemed to suffer from visceral disease, was seized on 27 September with chilliness and constriction of skin, followed in the evening by headache, pains of the limbs and other febrile symptoms. From his habit of body and time of residence in the West Indies, it was not considered advisable to try the Lancet but twelve grams of Calomel were given and salts which freely acted on his bowels. The following day, he appeared very free from fever. On the third, day he was very restless and there were great jactitations.[35] In this stage, an endeavour was made to bring the system under the mercurial action for which purpose small doses of Calomel were given at intervals. On the fourth day, strong hopes were entertained. He was cool and more tranquil than on the preceding – pulse 84; tongue moist. But in that night, he became restless and feverish. [His] tongue furred, and the next morning things appeared very unfavourable which gradually advanced, and he died on the evening of the fifth day. He had black vomit for three or four hours previously. Sulphate of Quinine with Opium seemed to have a temporary effect in suspending a little the vomiting. In this case, the first, third and fifth days were marked by stronger fever than the second and fourth.

Signed
John Glasco
Surgeon to the Forces
P.M.O.

Extract of Annual Medical Report of the Garrison of Dominica, 31 March 1839, by F. Macaw[36] MD, Staff Surgeon

Prevailing Diseases:

Fevers were, therefore, during the past year not only the most prevalent class of disease in the garrison but the most fatal also, circumstances which are to be attributed to the existence of a severe epidemic, to be more particularly noticed in the succeeding paragraph.

About the middle of May 1838, some cases of the fever made their appearance in the garrison of a form different in many respects from any which had been seen here for many years. And this form of fever continued to prevail here to the exclusion of almost every other amongst the white troops from that time until the latter end of September, when it may be said to have entirely ceased as an epidemic. When the disease first appeared the garrison of the island consisted of 144 white men and 125 black, not including officers. Amongst the blacks throughout the whole course of the epidemic, not a single case of the disease appeared nor did the cases of continued or remittent fever which really occurred amongst them during that period (fourteen in number) exhibit any of the peculiar symptoms of the epidemic or terminate fatally in any instance.

The disease there may be considered as confined exclusively to the white or European part of the garrison amongst the commissioned officers and privates of which 101 cases of fever of the continued or remittent form appeared during the months of May, June, July, August and September, of which number 35 died. Amongst the officers of the garrison also (white Europeans) the fever prevailed to a considerable extent and with great severity. Seven cases, three of which proved fatal, having occurred in that body. As these facts and others connected with them will admit of being exhibited more clearly in a tabular form than by words alone, the annexed table has been prepared in which however no attempt is made at minute accuracy in the proportions, the nearest whole number being sufficient for our present purpose.

Table 6.4: Strength, Cases, and Mortality Report, May–September 1838

	Original Strength	No. of Cases	No. of Deaths	Proportions		
				Cases to Strength	Deaths to Cases	Deaths to Strength
Men	144	101	35	2 in 3	3 in 9	1 in 4
Officers	17	7	3	2 in 5	3 in 7	1 in 6

With respect to the history of the disease or of the symptoms and so on which appeared in the course of its progress during the five months it prevailed in this garrison, it would be impossible to enter here into any minute details, these symptoms, having undergone during that time various changes, both with respect to intensity and form. The peculiar or characteristic symptoms, therefore, will alone require to be noticed here, and with respect to these, it will be sufficient at present to observe first that the fever presented no distinct *remissions* in any part of its course and that it was essentially of the *continued type*. Second: that yellowness of the surface was uniformly present in every fatal case and in almost all the others to a greater or less degree. Third: that a dark turbid fluid usually denominated black vomit was in a great majority of the cases ejected from the stomach during life and that traces of such fluid or a quantity of it were invariably found in the stomach after death in all the fatal cases examined. Fourth: that in the fatal cases life was seldom protracted beyond the seventh day and that death sometimes took place so early as the third. Fifth: that in all the bodies examined after death, the internal surface of the stomach presented appearances of morbid vascularity varying from a slight but distinct degree of redness to the most intense appearance which recent inflammatory action might be supposed capable of producing.

Signed
F. Macaw, MD
Staff Surgeon P.M.O.

Extract of Annual Medical Report of the Garrison of Dominica from 1 April 1841 to 31 March 1842 by James Connell,[37] 2nd Staff Surgeon

Two companies of the 92nd Highlanders relieved two of the 89th in the beginning of April 1841: at the time of their arrival, the garrison was in perfect health, there being only five or six men in the hospital. The 92nd also continued pretty free from severe disease, although the numbers treated were numerous up to 12 August when yellow fever appeared among the white troops quartered on the Hill. A brief account of which will be given in the body of this report. The 92nd continued in the island until 27 November when they embarked for Barbados, and the island remained without white troops, except a few sick and hospital servants left by the 92nd until the arrival of two companies of the 33rd Regiment on 12 January 1842.

The endemic of the island is dysentery which generally prevails during the autumnal months at times as an epidemic. During the past year, although numerous cases have occurred, some of which proved very protracted and troublesome, it has not been very fatal; yet it has, in many instances, laid the seeds of organic disease.

Having but lately arrived in the island, I can only speak of the epidemic fever which raged with so much severity from August to the end of November, when the troops were removed; from the report of Assistant Surgeon Millingen[38] of the 92nd Highlanders, who has given an account of it, and who was in charge at the time, and from that of Staff Surgeon Dr Birrell, who was sent from Barbados in September. It appears from the reports of these officers that the fever first made its appearance in the town of Roseau towards the end of July, when it attacked Lieutenant Reilly, 1st West India Regiment, Fort Adjutant who expired on the 28th of that month, as also the colonial secretary who died on 1 August, and on the 12th, it appeared among the troops on Morne Bruce. It would appear from Assistant Surgeon Millingen's report that a brig – the *Tunchall* – arrived here in the beginning of July from Martinique and that she discharged a cargo of salt fish, and in the space of a few days, twelve of her crew were attacked with fever and three died.

The disease seems not to have been confined to any class of soldiers as the temperate were not more spared than those of dissolute habits; indeed, the former seems to have suffered in a greater degree. One of the great sources of mortality was owing to the delay which many allowed to take place before applying for medical aid, and the serjeants are particularized as being those amongst whom this practice was most usual. The table of deaths among the different ranks will clearly show those amongst whom it proved most fatal.

I shall now proceed to mention a few of the leading features and characteristic symptoms of the disease as described in the reports before alluded to. On the invasion of the disease, the patient complained of headache, confined principally to the frontal region; severe pain in the eyes (which were suffused) and intolerance of light; a foul furred tongue of a bright red at the edges, which were clean in the most severe cases. [The patient also complained of] intense thirst, pain in the back, sometimes extending over the abdominal surface, sense of weight at the epigastrium accompanied by tenderness, *dyspnoea*, and at times nausea; languor and pains of the extremities, heat of the skin and above all great prostration of strength with anxiety. The cold stage which precedes most febrile affections does not seem to have been well marked in this owing perhaps to the delay allowed to take place by the patients, and the discrepancies in their own accounts; it in all probability may have been overlooked by them and most likely had existed prior to their admission. In others again, the stage of excitement had gone by, prior to admission and reaction only took place after the use of the warm bath. Some, however, died without its coming on. Yellowness of the skin is stated to have occurred about the second day in those cases which proved fatal and was present in all those attacked, though in some to an almost imperceptible degree.

Black vomit was present in all the fatal cases, and only one patient, a child, recovered where this fluid was well marked in its character.

•••

Violent convulsions and delirium accompanied by tremor of the whole frame generally came on before death; bleeding from the gums, nose and from the rectum is also mentioned as having occurred in several cases.

•••

Post-mortem appearances do not seem to have thrown any light on the course of treatment best to be pursued. The head exhibited no abnormal appearances except effusion in the ventricles when delirium had been severe, the chest was also healthy; the stomach generally inflamed; its villous coat much thickened, corrugated and easily detached from the subjacent one; in the corrugations the flakes contained in the black vomit (which generally filled the cavity of this viscus) adhered strongly and could with difficulty be washed away. The liver is said to have presented a gamboge colour. It was generally found exsanguinous; the gall bladder usually nearly empty and containing some very dark and viscid bile. The small intestine [is] generally healthy but sometimes [contains] some of the dark fluid found in the stomach; the same remark applies to the large ones but in them the black vomit was seldom traced.

Signed
James Connell
2nd Staff Surgeon P.M.O.

Extract of Annual Medical Report of the Garrison of Dominica from 1 April 1845 to 31 March 1846, by Robert Smith[39] staff Surgeon, 2nd Class

Febris Remittens:
The prevailing disease has been remittent fever. It is stated that several of the admissions presented the form of yellow fever. It was ushered in

with the usual symptoms followed by heat of skin, lassitude and sense of extreme debility, headache, general pains over the body, feverish tongue, incessant and distressing thirst, increased frequency of pulse and what was not observed in former cases of this fever terminating in a copious warm perspiration, with so much relief to the individual that the most favourable prognosis was entertained of the case. This, however, proved fallacious. About twenty or thirty hours after admission, the patient began to complain of undesirable uneasiness of lower part of the chest and epigastrium, which was speedily followed by nausea and vomiting. The vomiting at first of bilious matter, ending in the usual black coffee ground-looking fluid, [was] attended with delirium, sinking of the vital powers, coma and the patient was cut off on the third or fourth day. Of twenty-five admissions of the disease, seven proved fatal. They presented bilious suffusion of the skin, but the black vomit was not to the same extent that it occurred in cases of the previous quarter. The treatment in the early stage consisted in the use of saline purgatives and effervescent draughts. [It was] the warm bath, Calomel with James's Powder, turpentine *sinapisus* and blistering the epigastrium. When there was any remission, however short, Quinine was freely given, with a moderate use of wine and light nourishment. The *Oleum Terebinth*[40] in combination with *sp. aeth. nitric* and *mistura camphorae*[41] was also given internally without any good effect. With a view to relieve delirium, one man was cupped in the nape of the neck and another muscular man was bled from the arm to sixteen oz. They both expressed themselves relieved for a short time, but the disease pursued its course to a fatal termination on the fourth day. The blood drawn presented the bright scarlet surface, was of the consistence of glue without a particle of serum so often seen in this form of fever.

The post-mortem appearances were more or less "black vomit" in the stomach and bowels, the mucous membrane vascular having clots or patches here and there of Ecchymosis without softening or any abrasion of the surface – nor was it corrugated into the large folds observed in fatal cases in February 1845.

Besides the death of Ensign Wood at Prince Rupert's there was one very severe cases of remittent fever which occurred in the person of Major Myers, 71st Regiment. On the twelfth and thirteenth day, the prostration of strength was very great. He had every appearance of sinking, and there is no doubt but his life was saved by the free use of champagne. He drank one bottle within half an hour, and he had a second bottle in the course of the same night. The stimulus was afterwards kept up by giving the wine in more moderate quantity. His bowels were particularly torpid. He had no "black vomit" nor sickness at stomach to any extent, nor was the febrile action high. Convalescence was very slow.

Signed
Robert Smith
Staff Surgeon 2nd Class /Dominica/18th April 1846

7. Reports from Grenada

Preview: The reports for Grenada, beginning with those for 1816 and ending in the 1840s, offer fairly detailed commentary on the health circumstances experienced in various named regiments. The observations on cases of yellow fever provide important insights into the medical philosophies that were held by the various medical practitioners over this period. The environmental factors which are often described in the reports fit well into the views of miasma as the principal cause of the disease, held by most doctors in the British military forces at this time.

Copy of Remarks Dated from 25 December 1815 to 24 June 1816 by F.A. Loinsworth,[1] Surgeon to the Forces at Grenada

At the close of last year, this garrison was suddenly augmented by the arrival of the Left Wing of the Royal York Rangers from Trinidad, where they had suffered much from sickness, particularly intermittent.

This regiment is composed principally of men who have commuted their punishment for West India service. Many of them have been years in the West Indies and are very intemperate in their mode of living. Their constitutions are much broken, and they are generally affected with chronic diseases of the abdominal viscera. The Left Wing of the York Chasseurs also composed part of the garrison till the early part of March when they were removed to Tobago. They are also men who have commuted their punishment but differ from the former corps in being mostly young, healthy men only a few months from England. The remainder of the garrison consisted of three and, for a very short period (the last month), five companies of the 4th

Battery 60th Regiment, all foreigners. They were removed to Barbados in April, leaving the York Rangers, the only corps in the garrison, with a few of the foreign artillery.

The 60th Regiment, while in garrison, was remarked for their orderly conduct and great sobriety. During the last twelve months, an unusual quantity of rain fell accompanied at the close of last year, and beginning of this with cold winds from the north and north-west and the great increase of troops to the garrison having occasioned the necessity of occupying the post, Hospital Hill (north barracks at a considerable elevation above the sea and to Leeward of a marsh) the bilious remittent fever[2] of the country very soon made its appearance amongst the troops, accompanied with great affection of the brain, general effusion of bile and that aggravated unmanageable symptom vomiting of black or dark-coloured bile. The mortality was consequently very great, but a marked distinction was to be observed between the York Rangers and Chasseurs, the former with constitutions broken down by intemperance and long residence in this climate, generally died from debility upon fever, the latter corps dying under the action of fever. The most powerful stimulants were used in the stage of debility but generally without success. Medicines seemed to do little good. With the Chasseurs bleeding largely in the commencement of the disease and keeping up a constant action of the bowels with mercurial purgatives appeared the most successful mode of treatment. With the York Rangers, bleeding in most cases was inadmissible. What effect cold effusion might have had could not be ascertained, the small quantity of water that could be procured for the use of the hospital being barely sufficient for drink for the patients and for the purpose of cooking. There is, unfortunately, no tank to the hospital. Sponging the body with vinegar and water was found beneficial, as were also spirits.

Towards the end, the 60th Regiment became sickly, which may be attributed to the influence of the marsh already mentioned and to the crowded state of the barrack rooms in Fort George where they were quartered, but the mortality was by no means so great nor the disease so aggravated in every case as in the former corps and would I think have been less, but for the impression of terror that was upon the minds of the foreigners at the idea of going into hospital. The appearances on dissection resembled each other: general inflammatory state of the brain, the blood vessels tinged with blood, especially those of dura and pia mater, inflammation of the coat of the stomach and intestines. In several of the men of the York Rangers, enlargement of the spleen and incipient disease of the lungs and liver were observed.

Towards March, the weather became more dry and settled, and the wind to its usual quarter in the east; the garrison became healthy and less crowded by the removal of part of the troops since when no sickness has occurred requiring a remark. At the present period the garrison may be considered healthy.

Signed
Frederick A. Loinsworth
Surgeon to the Forces

Half-Yearly Medical Report of Diseases from 25 June 1816 to 24 December 1816 by Frederick A. Loinsworth, Surgeon to the Forces

Grenada,
25 December 1816

When the last half-yearly return was made, the garrison was healthy and principally consisted of six companies of the Royal York Rangers, the greater part occupying the elevated military post, Richmond Heights. Three companies have since left this island for Tobago and been replaced by the 15th Regiment (about five hundred strong) from Martinique. Upon the arrival of the latter corps, the three companies of the Royal York Rangers and detachment of Royal Artillery (thirty strong) occupied Fort George the 15th Regiment Richmond Heights, giving a detachment of thirty men to the Sauteurs situated at the northeast extremity of the island, and one company at Hospital Hill. That company, upon the setting in of the north wind, having given some cases of remittent fever, were recalled to Richmond Heights and Hospital Hill occupied by the Black Invalid Garrison Company (hundred strong).

The 15th Regiment, while stationed at Martinique, was quartered at Fort Edward, nearly surrounded by marsh and the weather excessively hot and wet. They consequently suffered much from fever produced by marsh miasmata and, upon their arrival in this island, brought more than one hundred hospital cases and nearly the whole regiment suffering from intermittent fever, the latter and diarrhoea have been the principal diseases that have occurred since their arrival. The few cases of remittent fever being very slight, with the exception of three from Hospital Hill. This regiment has been twelve years in the country. A great many of the men several years have suffered much from fever and bowel complaints at different times and are generally speaking much broken down in their constitutions.

They may, however, be considered at this period healthy. Their disease being mostly of the chronic kind, and many of them recoverable if soon removed to a more temperate climate. The Royal York Rangers were very healthy till the beginning of November when a fever made its appearance in the town of St George's resembling in its malignant symptoms and consequent mortality that destructive disease known in this part of the world under the name of yellow fever. In this return I have distinguished it under the head of Bilious continued fever, the liver being the part principally affected if not the seat of the disease.

It first made its appearance in that part of the town known by the name of The Bay and where the fish market is situated, a close dirty place badly or not at all ventilated, having the sea in its front and a high ridge extending itself in the rear upon which part of the town is built intercepting the breeze and exposed to the whole of the afternoon sun. The contractor for supplying the troops with fresh beef occupied a house and large yard in this place, and where, for some time, the cattle were killed, occasioning a most offensive stench to arise from the half-putrid hides that were left to dry in the yard.

In the commencement of the fever, it was confined to plethoric young persons lately arrived from Europe and residing in that part of the town, but it soon extended its baneful influence to the other part and to the troops quartered in Fort George situated on elevated rocky ground at the south-west angle of the town and finally to the shipping moored in the careenage, a most dangerous unwholesome anchorage in point of health, partly surrounded by marsh and brushwood, joining the south-east boundary of the town of Saint George's, Fort George being placed at the north-west side of the entrance to the careenage.

A few cases also made their appearance in the neighbourhood but at no great distance from the town. That portion of the garrison of Fort George quartered in the Citadel and exposed to the northerly wind, at first suffered so considerably as to render their removal expedient, which had the desired effect as they sent fewer cases to hospital when placed in a more sheltered situation, one company quartered in that part of the fort but sheltered from the north wind sent the fewest cases to hospital until the fever became general thro' the fort.

The symptoms which marked the first stage of the disease were giddiness, pain of the head as if arising from the pressure of a tight hat, eyes dull and watery and suffused with a yellow tinge. Tongue foul and dry, skin hot and dry, pulse full, quick and strong, loss of appetite (though in a few cases, it was much increased a few hours previous to the patient being attacked), languor and debility with great restlessness and tossing about in the bed, great anxiety of the countenance, pain along the spine extending over the lumbar region through the groins down the inside of the thighs and legs to the feet, accompanied with chill, nausea, great thirst and difficulty of respiration, the secretion of urine greatly diminished and sometimes stopped altogether. What little was passed of a deep saffron colour, the bowels obstinately costive and torpid evacuations being procured very scantily and with great difficulty. Though, in some instances the reverse was the case, when they proved obstinate and mostly fatal cases. The faeces passed were of a deep brownish-black or grass-green colour and extremely fetid. The skin was slightly discoloured but in the early state, not sufficiently so to strike the eye unless closely examined. When uncured by medicine, the symptoms in the second seemed completely relieved, leaving the patient labouring under a slight debility as if arising from fatigue attended with a drowsy disinclination to any exertion and a careless indifference to what was passing, never asking or wishing for anything, and requiring to be spoken to several times before an answer could be obtained, as if unconscious that he was spoken to. Such was the second stage so mild in all its symptoms as to induce the patient's belief of having obtained complete relief from which he fancied to be a cold either by the medicines given or by some remedy of his own. A few hours fatally convinced him of his error by the return of all the symptoms of the first stage considerably aggravated, accompanied with violent vomiting of dark-coloured fluid like coffee grounds. Low muttering delirium, bowels again obstinately torpid, the skin now becoming of a deep dirty yellow colour rapidly changing to a dark brown. The limbs cold, stomach towards the end torpid, retaining everything even in the largest quantity. Coma, accompanied with *Singultus*,[3] the only active symptom that never left the patient till death, generally without a struggle, put an end to his sufferings.

Upon examination – post-mortem – the brain, from its very healthy appearance, did not seem to be the seat of disease. The only trace of inflammation that could be observed showed itself about the optic nerve.

The thoracic viscera was even unusually healthy except when the patient laboured under a pulmonic affection previous to the attack of the fever.

Upon examining the abdominal viscera, the liver exhibited one mass of vitiated bile or was in a general state of putrescence, its internal substance being always in a state of abscess or decay. The gall bladder unusually empty and distended with air. In two instances, it had burst, and in one, it was filled with vitiated bile. The stomach filled with the last substance swallowed mixed with the black flakes like coffee grounds and, similar to what the patient had vomited. The pyloric orifice and large curvature were much inflamed, as was the internal surface, which was always covered with mucous slime and full of small pustules filled with the same. The small intestines seldom appeared much deranged except when the tendency to putrefaction was very great, and then they had numerous livid spots.

When the fever first made its appearance, recourse was had to the usual remedy of depletion by copious bleedings, baths and purgatives, a mode of treatment attended with the greatest success in the remittent fever of the West Indies, but the loss of five men who were bled out of seven admitted made a change of treatment necessary at first from the mitigation of the symptoms. The greatest hopes were entertained of its success, but the rapidity with which the patient sank after bleeding soon frustrated those hopes, notwithstanding the most powerful stimulants were used internally and externally. Of the other two cases out of the seven, one (Private Bradd of the Royal York Rangers), was admitted whose debilitated state rendered Venesection inadmissible. He, after a strong purgative of *Hydrarg: submuria: g^r x Pulv Jalapi ʒj* was given, took *Hydrarg: sub:* every two hours. As the only thing his stomach would retain, it relieved the sickness immediately. In three days, copious Ptyalism commenced when he was again freely evacuated with Calomel and Jalap, in the same quantity as the first dose aided by *Sulpha Magneesia ʒi* and a strong purgative enema. His recovery was rapid when intemperance at the time he was to be discharged from hospital to his duty brought on a relapse, which, from its violence and his debilitated constitution, broken down by habitual drunkenness, soon proved fatal. Several trials more were made to bleed strong, robust habits – where the arterial action was great – but repeated failures prevented repetition. The plan then adopted and which appears to have succeeded best is on the first admission to give a strong purgative of *Hydrarg Submuria g^R x Pulv: Jalapi ʒjs*. Soon after (six or eight hours), the exhibition of *Infusi Semor ʒjy Magnesive bitartrate ʒi*, aided by a purgative enema, generally had the desired effect of freely evacuating the bowels. When this was accomplished, *Hydrarg submurias ʒfs* was given every two hours, and *Ung^t Hydrarg fort ʒi* rubbed in as often till copious Ptyalism came on, which was usually in forty or fifty hours when saline purgatives greatly diminished the irritability occasioned by the mercurial action when salivation was complete, bark Gentian or Quassia with liberal use of Madeira Wine.

Porter and a nourishing, stimulating diet soon recovered the patient. The sickness and irritability of the stomach were generally overcome by blisters to the part, as was the pain in the head by the application of a blister to it or between the shoulders assisted by the warm bath. The heat of the skin was relieved by frequently washing the patient with highly rectified spirits of Ether, dissolving the muriate of quicksilver. The spirit used as a wash was found very useful in producing Ptyalism speedily. In low delirium coma and *Singultus,* much benefit was derived from the application of Mustard Poultices to the feet, legs, on stomach, aided by the free internal use of brandy and capsicum.

Reports from Grenada

The diet in the first stage consisted of nutritive acidulated drink, such as barley or rice water and lime juice, when Ptyalism was complete, as was observed before the most nourishing stimulating diet became necessary.

Most of the cases terminated favourably where complete and copious salivation was brought on. The calomel, when given in the large doses of thirty or forty grains had rather a constipating than an aperient effect and in no one instance produced griping or any dangerous symptom. In the distressing case of sickness and vomiting, it never in any one instance failed to relieve it, more especially if given in the form of powder rather than pill. In the numerous cases admitted into hospital, little or no variation was observed in the symptoms more than the malignity of the disease was increased or diminished by the constitutional habit of the patient.

This fever does not appear to be an endemic disease produced by some peculiar cause in the atmosphere as is frequently the case in the West Indies from its being confined to the town and not in any one instance extending its influence to Richmond Heights situated in a direct line not more than three-quarters of a mile from the town. But rather, it may be supposed to have had its origin in the filth and dirt of the fish market bog where the first made its appearance and to have increased in malignity. The disease kept up by the excessive rains and very great heat of the weather acting upon the exuberant as well as decayed vegetation that surrounds the town in every direction. The fever is, by most persons, supposed to be not contagious, but all the hospital attendants being attacked. However, every precaution used to prevent them induces me to believe it to be a contagious fever.[4] I am greatly confirmed in that belief by the circumstance of the Royal Artillery occupying a barrack joining to a room that was occupied by an officer with the fever and where the symptoms were of the most malignant nature, having been suddenly attacked, they were immediately removed to another part of the fort apparently more unhealthy, when the disease disappeared amongst them altogether.

Signed
Frederick A. Loinsworth
Surgeon to the Forces

Extract from Half-Yearly Report to 20 December 1817 in Grenada by Alexander J. Ralph,[5] Assistant Surgeon, Queens Regiment

The left wing of the regiment occupied the barracks on Richmond Heights on its arrival in the island of Grenada, a few days after one company with an officer was ordered to garrison Fort George. Our men were not many weeks in Fort George when Lieutenant Hill, the officer commanding, was seized with smart symptoms of fever, evidently of the remittent form when remedies were used successfully. In a few days, he recovered. Shortly after, Mr Powell, an officer of the commissariat, who resided in a house lately purchased by the department (which stands on the Leeward side of the careenage nigh to the fort, was taken ill and died on the fifth day of the disease. I did not see Mr Powell, but I have been informed by Dr McEwen, who attended Mr Powell and who is the most esteemed of the civil practitioners of this island, that he died of malignant yellow fever. Two days after this gentleman's funeral, Private William Bayendale of the Queens Regiment (who was doing duty in Fort George) was sent to the hospital on Cardigan Heights as a patient who had been ailing for some days. I visited him on his arriving there and saw clearly that he was labouring under alarming symptoms of yellow fever, which had made such progress as to threaten his speedy destruction. Twelve hours after his admission into the hospital, black vomit and hiccough (hiccup) made their appearance. In forty-eight hours, he died. The nature of this man's disease cannot be questioned. He was placed among many surgical patients but did not communicate fever.

On 18 September, Private William Mills, servant to Lieutenant Girdlestone who relieved Lieutenant Hill at Fort George, was seized with severe symptoms of yellow fever. I treated him on his becoming indisposed; he recovered, notwithstanding that the gastric affection was alarmingly severe. On 19 September, Lieutenant Girdlestone was taken ill and conveyed to the hill with fever. He recovered. Alarmed by these occurrences, which declared that there existed in and about Fort George a cause which produced the most malignant form of yellow fever. I waited upon the commanding officer of the wing and urged the necessity which existed of removing without delay the whole of the detachment from Fort George. I acquainted him with the whole of the facts and begged him to represent these to General Riall. I did not fail to appeal to our past melancholy experiences, which had so decisively convinced me of the local nature of the cause of yellow fever. General Riall immediately directed the whole of the detachment to be removed to Richmond Heights and thus relieved our apprehensions.

Previously to the detachment marching from the fort I minutely inspected it and was gratified to observe that the men appeared to be healthy. I watched them narrowly, fearing that the morbid cause imbibed at the fort would affect them on the hill. I was correct in my conjecture. On the 20 September, I admitted three patients: on the 21st, two; on the 22nd, one; on the 23rd, four; on the 24th, two; on the 26th, one; on the 27th, one; on the 28th, two and on 29th, one patient, making a total of seventeen fever patients, every one of whom had been quartered in Fort George. The fever distinctly evinced a tendency to remit; three assumed a continued type and had serious gastric affection. The whole seventeen happily recovered. As yet, no case of fever had originated on the hill.

On 7 October seven patients were admitted into the hospital with remittent fever. They had been living in the West Spur Barrack, and since that period, eleven cases have been received into the hospital and twelve women from the same barrack treated with fever. No death has occurred.

The number of attacks in the lower apartments of the barracks was far more numerous than the upper, being 18, although the inhabitants of these apartments were fewer. Mr Harrison, deputy assistant commissary general, died on 8 October of malignant yellow fever. He had resided in the same house in which Mr Powell died. Not a single instance of fever attacking either officer or soldier living in Fort Matthew has occurred. I have not heard of a single case of yellow fever occurring among the civil inhabitants of Saint George's. That Mr Powell, Private William, Baxindale and Deputy Assistant Commissary General Harrison died of malignant yellow fever is certain. Surely, we have reason to presume that the fever affecting the soldiers in the fort was the same in kind in all, as they were living under precisely similar circumstances and as in five examples it showed the same symptoms precisely. In all, it manifested a disposition to remit. In the slighter cases, it remitted obviously, which is precisely what I observed in the epidemic fever which raged in 1816 at Barbados.

On Richmond Heights we observed a mild form of remittent fever attacking a few individuals living in the West Spur Barracks and selecting particularly such as resided on the basement floor of the building. It did not spread generally, nor did it affect any individual living in Fort Matthew. The removal of the detachment from Fort George caused a cessation of the malady and, I believe, sincerely saved many lives. That the fever in question did not originate in infection must be admitted as the disease did not previously exist in the island and that it was not propagated by infection is moreover to be inferred. Fever was not communicated to any of the many individuals who held communication with the sick.

I shall not make any further comments, and as I consider the cause of fever to be Malaria, I shall proceed to notice the local peculiarities of the places in which it appeared.

Fort George stands upon a hill elevated about 140 feet above the level of the sea. It is situated in the Leeward side of the careenage, exposed to the easterly winds which eddy around Cardigan Heights and blow through the valleys which open at their feet. These winds move over the marshy and pestiferous land which skirts the lagoon, and passing this stagnant sheet of water, charged with noxious emanations, they play upon the fort. The military post of Fort George has always been extremely unhealthy, and when fully garrisoned yellow fever has repeatedly reigned there epidemically.

West Spur Barrack stands on a height at an elevation of about six hundred feet above the level of the sea and is completely exposed to winds which move over a swampy valley below. Fort Matthew is placed adjoining it on a rising ground, twenty feet higher than the West Spur Barrack and is completely protected by the fortifications which encircle it to windward. I believe it owed its salubrity to this protection. During the period in which the fever prevailed, heavy rains occasionally fell. The atmosphere was excessively sultry and calm. The winds, for the most part, southerly. The thermometer was repeatedly observed to rise to 90° and 93° in the shade in the fort. When on Richmond Heights, the mercury stood at 86° and 87°.

Tropical miasmata give rise to the following forms of fever in subjects susceptible of their influence.

- 1st – aggravated form of remittent fever with obscure tendency to remit, frequently consisting of a single paroxysm: malignant yellow fever (originated at Fort George)
- 2nd – aggravated form of remittent fever with obvious tendency to remit: malignant yellow fever (originated at Fort George)
- 3rd – severe and remittent fever exhibiting distinct febrile paroxysms and remissions (Fort George and the lower apartments of West Spur Barracks)
- 4th – mild remittent fever (upper and lower apartments of West Spur Barracks)
- 5th – intermittent fever (two cases of quarter ague have recurred. Individuals residing in Forth Matthew).

The several varieties are occasioned by:

a. depends upon the condition of soil, heat, weather.
b. causes which may influence the concentration of miasms such as winds and substances which may attract them.
c. distance from place of generation of miasmata – they become weaker as they are more distant.

Circumstances of the constitution of the individual affected:

a. having passed the severer forms of the disease impairs the susceptibility to the influence of marsh poison.
b. debility lower induced favours its operation.
c. habit renders marsh poison comparatively innoxious and vice versa

Period after attack at which disease is treated

a. the earlier it is treated, the more obvious the remission
b. it may be remarked that the fever, when neglected, often destroyed life in a single paroxysm.

The above table was constructed from observations made in Barbados when the fever raged epidemically in the Queens Regiment. It is here applied in illustration of the cause of the several forms of fever which have appeared in the left wing of the regiment since their arrival in Grenada.

Fever produced by drunkenness – During the epidemic reign of yellow fever, many examples of a species of fever or rather of febrile irritation, came under observation, which appeared to have their origin in drunkenness and which not uncommonly terminates in mania or even death when improperly treated. Its existence was marked by an extreme degree of sensibility in the nervous system – a disordered function of the stomach. Cold, partial and clammy sweats, tremors, sleeplessness and extreme debility in the muscles usually attack the habitual drunk, especially such as drank rum.

The disease alluded to is one of frequent occurrences and certainly demands attention as it is often confounded with and treated as yellow fever when that disease prevails generally. It requires a diametrically opposite treatment – liberal administration of stimulants and cordials – opiates sufficiently powerful to procure sound sleep, partial application of cold to the head and a particular attention paid to the regulating the excretions, was found invariably successful.

Two cases of the fever briefly described above have been treated in Grenada. The patients were both delirious during three days; excessive and continued intemperance was the cause of the disease. The shower bath was used with the most decided benefit, although the skin was bedewed with perspiration, which ran off from the surface in drops. In other respects, the treatment was precisely that mentioned in the above remarks.

Signed
Alexander J. Ralph
Assistant Surgeon
Queens Regiment

Extract of Annual Report of the Diseases of the Troops Serving at Grenada from 21 December 1827 to 20 December 1828 by John Glasco,[6] Surgeon to the Forces and P.M.O.

The artillery is generally placed in some fort at a distance from the main body of the troops, with only one officer to superintend them and their duties are of a laborious nature. They indulge more freely and are less under restraint. They will be found to produce more serious cases than the Line Regiments throughout his command, and this year has given Grenada an example of my position. The disease first showed itself among them and has only been prevented, making further devastation by their removal to Richmond Hill, where I am in hopes they will remain. At Dominica in 1826, the same remarks will be found to have applied. Disease of a serious character first manifested itself among the artillery in the beginning of July and found its way among the troops occupying Morne Bruce not till the interval of one month.

In the first quarter of the present period, the weather was cold, accompanied with strong breezes from the north. The only prevailing disease was the epidemic, which had run its course from the northern islands visiting each in succession and from its regularity in the time of travelling. I cannot imagine it originated from the weather at any particular island. I saw it at Dominica in December and January, and it appears to correspond with the description given by Dr Simpson of the disease which took place in Grenada in March. Dr Simpson has, in the spirit of the times, endeavoured to divide the disease into three species, but which amount to nothing more than some trifling difference in the mode of attack. He says it began at once with *Synocha*, or second the pain of the joints accompanied the fever or third febrile symptoms were preceded by languor. However, by whatever mode it commenced, there is a striking similitude in the disease as it appeared here and in Dominica. In both places, the attack commenced in a similar manner. The duration of the 1st stage was the same that is from thirty-six to forty-eight hours, followed usually by pains in the joints, knuckles, elbow, and shoulder and about the third or fourth day, there was frequently an eruption not unlike the measles. The pains continued more obstinate in the aged and delicate, and after subsiding they were frequently brought back by a fit of intemperance or any debilitating causes. The artillery in both places, as usual, came in for a greater share than the troops occupying the elevated situations.

June and July give little increase to our sick, but towards the latter part or beginning of August, we may expect a succession of cases of well-marked remittent, and these continue till the latter part of October. This, I think is the usual period for the prevalence of remittent fever but let us take the facts as they occurred during the present year. In giving the state of the weather, Assistant Surgeon O'Callaghan[7] says, "Towards the middle of August, the wind became very variable, shifting frequently towards the north. The weather now became intolerably oppressive, insomuch that the oldest practitioners of the island could not remember anything like it since the memorable year 1817; their apprehensions were naturally excited, and the accompanying return verifies but too truly their well-founded alarm".

Now, before I quote more of this passage, I will just put in a remark: the same oppressive weather prevailed at Dominica, and strong suspicions were entertained, yet remittent fever was not more than usual, but in the garrison, bowel complaints took its place. He then goes on to state, "that remittent fever of the worst form suddenly made its appearance in the unhealthy position of Fort George, at that time occupied by a detachment of artillery, and the first cases proved fatal almost immediately. He suggested to the major general commanding that the immediate removal of these troops was the only measure likely to save the remaining few with constitutions already shattered by their intemperate habits". We here see it flatly stated that I have all along witnessed that the artillery are the first to suffer. They are under less restraint and have more pay.

After their removal to Richmond Hill, the sick report is very much diminished. Still, we have one death terminating in black vomit. The 27th Regiment began to suffer at the commencement of September. Three cases terminated fatally, exhibiting the same character throughout their progress as the artillery cases. The symptoms were lassitude and general debility for some days preceding a severe rigour, in which the patient always supposed he was dying. The reaction was not attended with any high vascular excitement. There was usually a haggard countenance with a frightful expression of anxiety. The breathing was quick and laborious. The stomach always irritable, the skin dry, the pulse sometimes not quicker than natural; at other times, it would rise to ninety-six but uniformly tremulous and compressible. The eyes were muddy and glazed, and the man looked as if he had been debauching all night. The bowels were generally open. The patient complained of distressing pain in the back and lower extremities.

The fatal cases that were noticed in the quarter were marked by symptoms of high congestion, eyes suffused, red and muddy, tottering as if drunk, and sometimes convulsions which recurred at intervals. Others remained in a state of coma from which they were reluctantly roused and expressed a wish to remain quiet when, by degrees, the strength failed, and they sunk between the 3rd and 5th days towards the termination. The skin became yellow.

The post-mortem examination gave the following appearances:

The surface of the body yellowish; vessels of the dura mater and the brain, as also the sinuses gorged with blood. The liver and spleen enlarged, the latter sometimes resembling a mass of putrid blood. The lining membrane of the stomach was vascular, with patches of spots resembling extravasation into the capillaries. The stomach often contained a dark-coloured fluid like the sediment of Port Wine floating in a transparent mucus. The duodenum was dark and gorged with blood. Its texture destroyed and yielded to the slightest force. The gall bladder was distended with tar-like bile. The omentum[8] was shrivelled, the colon remarkably contracted.

With regard to the treatment, Mr O'Callaghan, 27th Regiment, who had charge of these cases, states that the *Plumb: Superac:* given in grain doses in solution every hour, was successful in allaying the irritability of the stomach and enabling him to exhibit a strong purgative of Calomel and Jalap. By this treatment, the secretion of the liver was generally directed to its proper channel, and the recovery was as rapid as the attack. But it sometimes happened that the stomach could not be tranquillized by any means, and in these cases, it always terminated in black vomit. Still, it was not a hopeless case, and the records of the hospital, attested by the evidence of his brother's medical officers and an old civil practitioner of the first repute, exhibit several interesting cases to prove that this formidable symptom is not a harbinger of death. He has been induced to try the internal exhibition of lead in extraordinary doses in these desperate cases. In four or five instances, the quantity was four and even six grains and he has never seen any of the dangerous effects usually attributed to it. Such is the statement of Mr O'Callaghan, and I think the inference is that the sugar of lead has been successful in several cases of black vomit, attested by an old and well-informed civil practitioner and by his brother medical officers.

Now, upon these two assertions, I must pause. Mr McEvan, the gentleman alluded to, is unquestionable evidence both from his experience and intelligence. But what says Mr McEvan? That he only saw one case, that of Gillespie, who decidedly laboured under the symptom. He used the lead and recovered. Assistant Staff Surgeon Cuddy,[9] the other gentleman, is himself ready to allow that his opinions as to the appearance of black vomit were not sufficiently formed at the period, for he had never witnessed the symptom previous to his coming to this island. But let us advert to the cases themselves as given in the register. I examined twenty-one of them stated to have had this symptom, and I find ten recoveries, which indeed might be considered as an extraordinary proportion. Every author mentions recoveries, but they are only points here and there. I find the cases differing from the description given by Jackson, Moseley and others. In their writings, the black vomit is given as a symptom of the last stage of the disease. In the cases before us, it occurs in every stage on the second and again on the sixth day in the same patient. It is frequently succeeded by high action. In my quarterly report, I have given the pages in the register from which I have made my statements, and it would be a useless repetition to introduce them here, but I cannot help inferring that some other description of vomiting which took place in the early stage of the disease was mistaken for the usual fatal symptom of black vomit.

Signed
John Glasco
Surgeon to the Forces, P.M.O.

Extract of Annual Report on the Diseases at the Garrison at Grenada from 21 December 1827 to 20 December 1828 by P. O'Callaghan, Assistant Surgeon, 27th Regiment

Towards the middle of August, the wind became very variable, shifting frequently to the north. The weather was then intolerably oppressive insomuch that the oldest medical practitioners of the island could not remember anything like it since the memorable year 1817. Then apprehensions were naturally excited, and events verified but too truly their well-founded alarms. Remittent fever of the worst form suddenly broke out in the unhealthy position of Fort George at the time occupied by a detachment of the Royal Artillery. Three of the first cases proved fatal almost immediately. Dr Simpson, in his annual report of the last year states that:

> the circumstances of Fort George not being esteemed healthy are difficult to account for. I should, on the contrary, suppose that its locality alone would afford prima facie evidence to make out a charge of insalubrity against it. It is situated on the extreme point of the tongue of land (as the sailors term it), which forms one arm of the harbour and upon which a great portion of the town of St George's is built. It is elevated about 160 feet above the sea and placed upon a loose calcareous stone, broken up into fissures and caverns by a very irregular stratification. These interstices are filled with a rank and noxious vegetation in the wet season, which undergoes the various processes of dry decomposition during the summer.

Stoney Hill itself does not exhibit a more complete model of a new-fashioned laboratory of this disease, [operating] upon the improved principle. But independent of the conjectural cause, there is one the opposite side an extensive lagoon separated from the careenage by a shallow flash over a coral reef. This deep lake of almost stagnant sea water is surrounded by a dismal mangrove swamp the exhalation from which is constantly wafted by a steady breeze in the direct line of the fort. The estate has been always reckoned unhealthy, and several houses occupied by white people have been actually abandoned from the same cause.

As senior medical officer at the time I suggested to the major general commanding that the immediate removal of these troops was the only means likely to save the remaining few with constitutions already shattered by their intemperate habits. This measure was promptly carried into effect, and it was very gratifying to observe the sudden decrease of our sick list.

Shortly after the removal of the artillery to Richmond Hill, the disease made its appearance in the detachment of the 27th Regiment, first commencing with a corporal of that corps sent in command of a guard to Fort George. One or two of the men of this guard were admitted into hospital immediately after and this duty was given up to the 1st West India Regiment in consequence. It then made its appearance in the detachment hospital by attacking several of the patients admitted for slight surgical diseases with its usual fatality, and here it resumed a character very much resembling contagion. Not one of the servants of the house escaped and its awfully sudden termination in the cases of four orderlies alarmed the detachment so much that I found considerable difficulty in supplying their places. It was remarkable that all these cases which broke out in the hospital were confined to the patients or attendants in the surgical or lower ward. The immediate evacuation of this ward, and shortly after the abandonment of the hospital altogether, for the purpose of it undergoing a thorough lime washing and fumigation.

The insulating the disease by opening a detachment ward for these cases, the establishment [of] a separate mess and quarter for the convalescents, and the placing the whole of the white troops on an extra allowance of fresh meat once more restored the garrison to its usual state of efficiency and the disease disappeared for a time altogether.

The premature re-occupation of Fort George by a new detachment of artillery is a circumstance much to be regretted, for the sudden reappearance of this horrible fever, the alarming extent of its progress, the fatal rapidity of its career together with the perfect regeneration of the detachment by its removal to Richmond Hill, will stand forever as recorded proofs of the unhealthiness of this position. Since this period, the disease has continued to hover over us, marking by the irregular disproportion in our casualties the capricious uncertainty of its visits.

In my September report, I have given the following general description of the disease:

> The symptoms were lassitude and general debility with listlessness and disinclination to any exertion of the mind or body for some hours preceding a severe rigour in which the patient thought he was dying. The reaction was not usually attended with high vascular excitement. There was a haggard countenance with a frightful expression of anxiety and distrust; the breathing was irregular and apparently laborious. The stomach commonly irritable, the skin dry and harsh, the pulse was sometimes not quicker than natural, occasionally running to ninety-six, but it was uniformly compressible. The eyes were muddy and glazed, and the man looked as if he had been debauching all night. The patient generally complained of "a load and oppression at his heart" with distressing pains in his limbs and "lightness" of the head at this period of the disease. The solution of the super acetate of lead was commonly successful in tranquillizing the stomach and enabling it to retain a strong purgative of calomel and compound powder of jalap, by which treatment the secretion of the liver was generally directed into its proper channel. The recovery was as rapid as the attack. But it sometimes happened (particularly in those cases where the disease had been making an insidious progress in a latent form for some days before the patient complained) that the irritability of the stomach could not be allayed by any means in our power. These cases invariably terminated in black vomit.

I cannot avoid remarking in this place the common error into which most writers have fallen in likening the matter to "coffee grounds". I have never seen it granular or in solution in the fluid with which it was ejected. I should rather be induced to compare it to a quantity of the surface of rotten mushrooms suspended in a clear viscid fluid.

The usual post-mortem appearances were an enlarged liver looking externally as if it had been boiled but when cut into highly vascular. The spleen generally resembled a mass of putrid blood. On cutting into the stomach, it was found to contain more or less of the black matter ejected before death. Its mucous membrane was mottled with vascular patches. The duodenum appeared to have been actually disorganized, its coat commonly giving way under the fingers even when separating it cautiously with the hands or the scalpel from its cellular attachments.

This livid and vascular state of the mucous membrane might be traced throughout the entire canal. The secretion of the kidneys was usually suspended and in these cases, their pelvises were found full of mucus and the bladder thickening and shrunk. There was more or less venous congestion in the head with engorgement of the lungs and generally a quantity of yellow serum in the pericardium.

I have stated that I was induced to try the internal exhibition of superacetate of lead in these cases with the happiest results even after black vomit made its appearance. How far I have been borne out in this assertion, I shall endeavour to show, and as I am satisfied that the fearless exhibition of this medicine, to an extent[1] unheard of before, will introduce an important improvement in the treatment of this formidable disease. I have ventured to make it exclusively the subject matter of this report.

Case 1st taken from the notes of Hospital Assistant Robertson[10] in the Medical Register up to 17 September. The latter part of the case was treated and recorded by myself. Private Anthony Gillespie, 27th Regiment, aged twenty-two years, was admitted on 14 September 1828.

Signed
P. O'Callaghan
Assistant Surgeon 27th Regiment
In charge of the Garrison Hospital

Extract of Annual Report of the Diseases and Medical Occurrences of the Troops at Grenada from 21 December 1828 to 20 December 1829 by John Glasco, Surgeon to the Forces

Comparing the period embraced at the commencement of this report with that of its termination, there may be found a wide field for medical investigation, one that has hitherto eluded its researchers and has baffled its best efforts. The question is simply this: what are the internal causes which acting on the human body excite fever? This question, though old and often asked, is again forced on my attention by what took place during the present year. Let us compare the close of

1828 and that of 1829. We shall find that neither the quantity of rain which fell nor the range of the thermometer will present any material difference and that during both periods, the winds were pretty regular, usually east or somewhat to the north. Such being the case, we would naturally have expected a similar influence on the human frame, but in the former year, a fever of a malignant concentrated type prevailed and continued its ravages from August 1828 to April 1829, picking off from time to time some of our youngest and best soldiers, which during the corresponding period, as far as it has gone that is from August to December, not one case of a similar description was to be met with. The only solution which I can offer is wide indeed from anything like accuracy, that a hot close state of the atmosphere, as was the case in 1828, gives rise to the fever in question and that this cause, once produced, is capable of being continued during a state of weather which would not have excited the miasma or whatever name one may choose to give it.

It may be useful in order to explain what I have above stated, to give a short review by which it will appear how close an affinity existed between the early and latter months of the present year, and how little there is to be found which could throw any light upon the subject now before us. From December to March, the whole has been, with the exception of a few showers, remarkably dry. The soil has assumed a parched surface and the wind which strikes upon it was returned hot and scorching. In these hilly islands, we usually experience either puffs or calms, but during the present season, the wind had been pretty steady from the eastward, sometimes a little to the northward or southward of east. It will evidently appear from this that we cannot bring the effect of moisture to explain the existence of disease. The decomposition of vegetable matter totally fails us. Where we have had much moisture with luxuriant vegetation, we often betook ourselves to it as a ready solution for any prevailing sickness.

The theometrical heat will also give us little assistance. The maximum was eighty-three; the minimum was seventy-six. Nor was there any inordinate range at any time. The second quarter, from March to June, was remarkable for its dryness, having only a few days of showers, but towards its termination, there was some lightning and thunder, which is considered the precursor of the rainy season. The prevailing wind was easterly and southerly. The thermometer ranged during the period from 78° to 85°.

We have now a statement of weather for the time when severe and malignant cases were too frequently encountered. From this to the termination of the year, there was not among the troops a single case presenting even ordinary difficulties, although it was reasonable to have expected such an occurrence in as much as the rainy season set in and from July to September, the weather was close, sultry and oppressive with a higher range of thermometer and the year as usual terminated with cool, pleasant weather. Its vicissitudes gave rise only to catarrhal affections.

Fever must form the principal disease in this island as well as in most West India possessions. In some years dysentery will prevail in some of our settlements [such] as Dominica and will, in the long run, prove more destructive, but in the drier islands, this will not be the case. We have also to remark that diseases will be found to have a variety according to the place of residence in these islands. The inhabitants of the dry elevated situations at the leeward side are seldom attacked with intermittents, but at the windward, where this is a low marshy soil. Intermittents and remittents of a bad type are common visitors at the latter part of the year. Among the troops not a single case of the former was treated; two are marked as such, but they consisted of a single paroxysm, which not infrequently takes place after some irregularity. It requires but little curative means. Clearing out the punitive vice will always be the answer, and I may add that the administration of bark is useless. We have had remittent of the most violent form terminating in black vomit. We have called the disease by this name because, in the majority of cases, there was a remission with a subsequent accession of heat of skin, but in other respects, it bore a strong analogy to the endemial causes of writers on tropical fevers. It presented the high arterial action at its commencement; the yellowness of the skin ended after the second or third day and terminated by black vomit. It attacked the young and robust, and the newcomers of the inhabitants and sailors were particularly its prey. The seasoned residents were wholly exempt. It has almost been a settled opinion that this fever is excited by violent exercise and by too free an indulgence in the luxuries of the table. Newcomers are peculiarly exposed to temptations of the kind. Novelty of scenery and the attention of friends to strangers have often been adduced as causes.

That these have their influence no person will deny, but it must also be confessed that the most guarded in their conduct and the most temperate in their habits have also shared the same fate as the others. I knew two young gentlemen remarkable for their guarded and steady conduct who fell victim to the disease. The scene which I am now recording occupied four months of the former year and the same space in the present one. The number of sick at any time did not exceed the ordinary proportion. Often for days, not one case of an unfavourable aspect, then an admission and shortly afterwards a death. In this manner, we were frequently deceived in supposing the fever had ceased and as often were disappointed.

The fever of which I am now speaking is not a common occurrence in this island. It made great ravages in 1816 and 1817 and from 1820 to 1828, not a case of black vomit was known. The troops occupying Richmond Hill enjoyed complete immunity in 1816 and 1817. The disease was confined to that part of the garrison stationed at Fort George, and I regret to say that owing to some opinions of its contagious character. The sick and well were strictly confined to the scene of disease, thereby augmenting its evil four-fold. The sick, in my opinion, should have had a separate ward in our excellent hospital. The others should have had the benefit of an elevated situation, even at the expense of hiring detached buildings, as has been the case more than once in the Guiana district of the command when a change of situation was deemed advisable. Last year, when the few artillery quartered at Fort George were suffering severely, Assistant Surgeon O'Callaghan, then P.M.O., recommended with great propriety and succeeded in removing them to the forts on the heights. The result was that from that time, their sickness was terminated.

The fever which has done much mischief, differs in no respect from what we have recorded in the preceding year and was solely confined to the 27th Regiment among the troops. The sailors on board the merchant shipping lying in the harbour suffered severely, and the mode of attack and the duration of the disease was precisely similar to that of the 27th Regiment. Whenever black vomit made its appearance in the hospital, and it was observable in all the fatal cases with one exception, death invariably took place. Nor have I witnessed any remedy capable of controlling this symptom.

The disease commenced usually with a very slight rigour or a sense of chilliness which came on during the night or evening. There is much reason for supposing the soldier is not sufficiently on his guard during this stage of his illness, and some cases are well ascertained to have been concealed for more than forty-eight hours. I can only account for this on the supposition that men cannot be brought to believe that the attack is anything more than a severe cold or indisposition, and they will not take that view of their situation, which may admonish them of a speedy termination to existence after the cold stage, which is generally short. The reaction succeeds with heat of skin, headache and thirst, eyes red and suffused with a glassy appearance and muddy. The patient tottered as if drunk and after a time, his manner was heedless and indifferent as to surrounding objects. He became altogether listless, scarcely giving an answer to the questions which might be put to him. In the early part of this stage, the patient complained of pains down his back and in the calves of his legs. The tongue was usually moist and with a very slight coating of white sores. The pulse was often full and quick, in some cases only ninety beats. The irritability of the stomach, which afterwards becomes so distressing, is now frequently absent. The respiration was usually oppressed from the commencement. After forty-eight hours, there was almost invariably a remission in the morning, and this was succeeded by an evening accession, which was attended with delirium. About the third morning, the state of collapse began to manifest itself. The heat of skin was found to be below par. It was cool with a greasy, unwholesome feel. The respiration became very laborious, the vomiting distressing and there was a burning sensation at the *scrobiculus cordis*. The contents of the stomach which were ejected at the commencement were clear and looked as if they contained particles of boiled rice; after a time, sediment was observed not unlike jalap in its colour and this, if suspended in water, was found to have a fibrous texture and a stringy adhesiveness. When this was the case, black vomit shortly succeeded. We have witnessed cases where the patient did not throw the black matter, but it was found in his stomach after his death. There was a combination of appearances where the termination was about to be fatal, that it was impossible to mistake. However imperfect we may be in communicating it in writing, if [in addition] to the listless manner, we had the hurried respiration and at the same time a tossing about in the bed as if the person were overheated and gasping for fresh air. I have invariably witnessed a fatal termination. He will scarcely answer the question you put to him. At the next visit, within a few hours, the change of countenance is quite striking. His face exhibits a leaden mottled hue with a strong expression of anxiety. The neck and shoulders have also a yellowish tinge mixed with brown. This is not uniform but in patches. The pulse is seldom under 120 weak, and each beat running into the succeeding one. The vomit is now fully developed. It is either like coffee grounds or sediment in Port Wine or of a deeper colour as if soot had been mixed up with gruel. The patient is now in the very last stage. He becomes completely comatose, and a convulsive fit closes the scene. The duration of the disease was between three and six days.

The post-mortem appearances in the thirteen fatal cases gave very constantly the following results. The vessels of the pericranium were loaded with blood. Sometimes, the quantity was such as to inundate the table on which the body was placed. The membranes of the brain were also gorged, and its substance, when cut into, presented a number of red dots. The lungs were found congested. The stomach when opened, contained a quantity of the same fluid as was vomited. When removed and mucus cleared away, it presented large patches of red points, almost coalescing and resembling an efflorescence, especially towards the cardiac orifice. On attempting to remove the stomach by passing the finger under the duodenum that part gave way upon the slightest force and poured out the same fluid as the stomach. Its texture was quite rotten and gangrenous. This was not always the case, but it was so in the majority. The gall bladder was distended with dark-coloured inspissated bile. There was one exception to this, where the bile was now fluid and of a light gas colour. The colon was found always contracted much within its natural dimensions but without any other diseased appearance. The urinary bladder was contracted also.

I have often reflected on what information was to be derived from the inspection of the dead body, and my mind is strongly impressed with an opinion that the liver secretes bile of a poisonous quality and that, as yet, we have not discovered any means of correcting this secretion. Other gentlemen with whom I have spoken on this subject have expressed to me similar sentiments. They have not the same facilities as army surgeons for post-mortem examinations, and it is only now and then that they can make them, which we invariably do. The poison which I suppose to be secreted will, by coming in contact with the duodenum and stomach, explain the appearance of gangrene in the one and high vascular action in the other, and the turgescence of the vessels of the brain may be accounted for as produced by the state of the stomach. If simple congestion was alone to be encountered, one might expect that the lancet would have been found eminently successful, but we have to record the failure of this as well as every other practice and the relief from *venae sectire*[11] was found to be only momentary. I do not mean to infer (sic) by what I have put forward that the lancet is not be used. I only mean to assert that there are cases where it is totally useless.

The cases of the severe form of fever which terminated favourably were also marked by high action and continued to the eighth or ninth day, but in these, the countenance was good, the manner was steady, the ideas not confused, and there was more alarm and apprehension of danger than where it really existed. As the season advanced, no case, whatever may have been its early appearance, gave any cause of alarm. They frequently commenced with symptoms of high arterial action, but they were mild in their progress and no doubt essentially differed from the preceding. The skin, though hot, was not harsh to the feel; the countenance, though flushed, had no expression of anxiety and above all, there was no hurried respiration. A profuse perspiration came on in about thirty-six hours and forty-eight hours. The patient was often convalescent.

It commenced with a chill or rigour which was followed by heat of skin, headache, thirst, and pains in the lumbar regions and down the extremities. The pulse was often quick and soft and sometimes full and bounding. In other cases, there was a succession of chills and flushings and one case in July would have been at a former period looked upon with great suspicion. The man appeared oppressed, stupid and sleepy with suffused eyes as if recovering from a debauch. Another point of difference in these mild cases arose from the patient's habits and mode of life previously to the attack. The stomach evinced a greater degree of irritability with a white tongue, and the skin more easily became relaxed, but when it owed its origin to exposure to cold, the skin was hotter and drier. The pains in the back were more severe. At the close of the year, we had one case of the genuine mild remittent fever when the evening accession was regular, and the remission was very decided. On the fourth evening, delirium came on, which was checked by a dose of opium and Ether, and on the subsequent day, quinine was given, which stopped a recurrence of fever.

The ephemeral fever was commonly met with at every season and as frequently during the period of severe sickness as at the latter part of the year. They were the most commonly the result of a debauch and commenced with a trifling chill followed by heat of skin for which a purgative was admitted. The following day the patient expressed himself much relieved, all the symptoms of the disease having gone and on the third day, he was well. Towards the close of the year, a good number of cases turned up which were blooded with a catarrhal affection. They were accompanied with an excitement of the living membrane of the fauces, *nares* and bronchia, sometimes with muscular pains of the thorax. The early cases more resembled the common continued fever, except that their duration was shorter.

I have now summed up my view of the fevers as they were observed by us during the year at this station. They exhibit the complaint in its extremes from the most active and virulent, evincing from their onset the concentrated type and terminating with that worst symptom, black vomit, to the mildest forms of sanguineous excitement with which the human frame can be pervaded. The bilious remittent was but obscurely defined in any of the cases and I have noticed only one case of the simple remittent. These are the fevers which commonly terminate in intermittent in either the quotidian or tertian shape, but of these we had not a single case. They are the inhabitants of low and marshy situations. The ground upon which the barracks are built is a species of sand rock. The rainwater can make no lodgement upon it and to this, I attribute exemption from this class of fever.

Before concluding any remarks on fevers, I wish to make a few observations on this disease as far as regards the other classes of this community. The officers differ essentially from the soldiers in their habits and [in] a great measure from the civilians. Generally speaking, their mode of life is more temperate than the latter, and they also enjoy the advantage of a cooler residence. They have experienced immunity from sickness with the exception of one or two attacks of mild fever. One young gentleman, the son of an officer, aged seventeen, fell victim to the severe concentrated type. The seasoned inhabitants were at this time totally exempt, but as the year advanced, the middle-aged and elderly, in some few instances, were obnoxious the last stage of it in a gentleman of active pursuits whose mind had been overstrained by a complexity of engagements. He had fever for four or five days previously. During the day, the remission was well-marked. At night, his mind usually became disturbed. He was then restless, slept very little and his pulse was quick. On the day on which he died, he attended the courts of justice and transacted business, but at 5:00 p.m., he complained of his head. When I saw him at 9:00 p.m. his pulse was 120, small and soft, his breathing laborious, his manner quick and irritable. He asked questions with a sharp, suspicious aspect and muttered a good deal to himself, respecting his affairs and also on light, passing subjects. But by degrees, he became totally insensible and expired. This case appears to me to have been remittent fever in which the brain was much engaged and that the disease had supervened on a state of much excitement of that organ in consequence of inordinate anxiety and worldly affairs.

Signed
John Glasco
Surgeon to the Forces, P.M.O.

8. Reports from Montserrat

Preview: There are only two reports listed for Montserrat, and these are for the 1820s. In the earlier report, for 1820–21, there seems to be some adherence to a theory of miasma. The doctor who reports here informs his superiors that "When any marsh exhalations do arise from this swamp,[1] fever usually prevails among the Negroes on the estate in its immediate vicinity." However, in the second report, there is a denial that any such issue exists in Montserrat. There are not many references that identify specific cases and any medical treatment administered, unlike the case in many of the reports for the other Caribbean territories.

Extract of Half-Yearly Report 21 December 1820 to 20 June 1821 from Montserrat by William Parry,[2] Hospital Assistant

The present quarter has been remarkably dry, sultry and oppressive, the thermometer in the shade ranging from 87 to 89. The wind has been extremely variable, hanging in the early part to the north-west and latterly ranging from East to South. This very unusual weather moved the prognostic of much sickness in the island. I regret to say that the concentrated endemic has been raging with uncommon severity in the town during the last two months and continues its ravages with unabated violence.

It made its appearance on 5 May in a European family residing in Parliament Street. The symptoms were decidedly those of yellow fever. The black vomit was thrown up on the third day, and the disease terminated fatally on the fifth with hiccough, *subsultus tendinum*,[3] *vibices*[4] and intestinal haemorrhage. Immediately on the death of this and in the same family, another case occurred, which pursued a similar fatal course. The next case was a soldier of the detachment. He was attacked on the 7th and died with the same symptoms on the 13th. The disease was for some days confined to Parliament Street and the lanes and alleys in its immediate vicinity, but towards the latter end of May it appeared in other parts and soon after spread generally through the town. Neither sex nor colour enjoyed exemption from it. Males and females were indiscriminately and nearly equally attacked, but in the different classes, it assumed various modifications of form, according to the various degrees of susceptibility, from a slight ephemeral attack in the negro to the highest degree of concentration in the European. A considerable proportion of the former were attacked, but all terminated favourably, the disease in most instances subsiding within twenty-four hours. The coloured inhabitants suffered more severely. The form here, as well as the white creole, was that of the remittent, and the remittent were, in general, very distinct, but there were four fatal cases in Parliament Street where they were by no means evident. The final terminations in these were characterized by black vomit and haemorrhage from different parts of the body. The Europeans, whether long resident or newly arrived, presented all the symptoms of the highest grade of yellow fever, and the disease proved almost uniformly fatal. Fortunately, there were not above three European families residing in the town or the mortality would have been incalculably great. Assistant Commissary General France and his daughter with six children and the two soldiers whose cases are detailed in the *Quarterly Report* have been the victims.

This formidable endemic is generally supposed to be produced from the exhalations of an extensive swamp called Bransby's Pond, situated about two miles to the North-West of the town, and that these exhalations were in the present instances conveyed into the town by the North-West winds which prevailed for some days previous to the appearance of the disease. This swamp appears to me, however, to be wholly incapable of affecting the town, for there is a very elevated hill or ridge running from east to west and interposed so as to intercept all communication between them. When any marsh exhalations do arise from this swamp,[5] fever usually prevails among the negroes on the estate in its immediate vicinity. They frequently suffer from fever when the town is perfectly healthy, but they are entirely free from any at present and have been for a long period.

There is another swamp less extensive called the Wash Pond, lying in the same direction and within half a mile of the town, which may possibly affect it, but I think that the principal source of this fever will be found to arise from the filthy state of the town. There are no established police regulations, animal and vegetable substances in a state of putrefaction and, therefore, allowed to accumulate in large masses in every street. There are also several ruinous buildings in different parts of the town, which are receptacles of similar substances. All these, when acted upon by an unusual degree of atmospheric heat, will be found sufficient to generate effluvia capable of producing the very worst forms of tropical fevers.

These morbid effluvia appeared to be much more powerful and concentrated about Parliament Street than other parts, for the mortality was mostly confined to this quarter. All the deaths among the coloured inhabitants occurred here. Assistant Commissary General France, most imprudently and regardless of every advice, removed into this street from a healthy situation to Windward of the town soon after the endemic made its appearance. The daughter was attacked with the disease on the 5th and died with black vomit on the 9th. Conceiving this melancholy event might now induce him to remove into the country. I renewed my advice. I represented to him the dangerous and fatal consequences that would inevitably ensue by his remaining in the town but all had no effect. He was attacked on the 18th and fell a victim to the disease last night. The disease in Miss France was ushered in with a violent headache, inflamed watery eyes, pungent heat, anxiety, apprehension and burning sensation in the stomach with excessive thirst, incessant vomiting and uncommon vascular excitement, the pulse beating at the rate of 175 in the minute. The febrile heat abated on the 2nd day. The pulse fell to 120 but intermitted, and the gastric irritability was almost unconquerable. On the third day, dark brown glaring matter were (sic) vomited and continued at intervals to be thrown up in large quantities.

She died on the fifth day, having retained her intellect perfectly clear to the last moment. She was free from yellowness and had no livid discolorations, the body preserving its natural colour for several hours after dissolution.

• • •

Having been particularly called upon to investigate the subject of contagion in yellow fever, I can, without the least hesitation, declare that the present endemic did not in any instance manifest such properties. If such could have existed, its operation would not have been so exclusively confined to the town but would also have extended to the country for many families among whom the disease appeared removed from the town, but they never communicated the disease to others in the country. The detachment presents also the strongest evidence of the contrary. Here is a company of strong, robust soldiers only four months in the climate, quartered within three hundred yards of the range of the disease, but enjoying almost a total exemption from it, while every class suffers more or less in the town. These men have frequently exposed themselves to any infection, if such existed, by frequently visiting the town during the day and often committing great irregularities, but every exertion was made to prevent their leaving the barracks at night, to which circumstance may be attributed their exemption. The two men that were attacked were the most intemperate characters,[6] and I have no doubt they exposed themselves to the noxious exhalations of the town at night, for men of such description will sometimes find means of cheating the greatest vigilance. No precautionary measures were adopted to interdict the general intercourse. The sick of every class were invariably attended by their relatives. No one apprehended or even believed in the existence of contagion. In short, no circumstance occurred either among the inhabitants or the troops that could afford the slightest grounds for believing in the existence of such properties.

Signed
William Parry

Extract of Annual Summary Report of Diseases Treated in the Detachment Hospital and Prevailing on the Island of Montserrat from 21 December 1826 to 20 December 1827 by A. Tonnere,[7] Assistant Staff Surgeon

Notwithstanding that, towards the end of the year, bilious remittent fever in an epidemic form spread widely through the island for eight or ten weeks, attacking indiscriminately every class of inhabitants without distinction of constitution, age, colour or sex. The troops, on the whole, may be said to have enjoyed a state of tolerable good health as only two of the officers and five of the soldiers suffered from this disease in one of whom it proved fatal on the 9th day, and only twenty-three cases admitted into hospital during the season.

The epidemic to which I have just alluded so extensive and fatal in Antigua and many of the surrounding islands as well as in Montserrat, did not show itself until after a long continuance of wet, usually boisterous weather, unprecedented in the recollection of the oldest inhabitant; nor even then till after the prevalence for some time of [an] oppressively hot, calm, cloudy, sultry state of the atmosphere, with light rains, thunder and lightning and frequent sudden squalls at night from the south and south-west, lasting from ten to fifteen minutes before leaving the atmosphere as still and motionless as if they had never taken place with a range of temperature in the shade from 88 to 96 Fahrenheit thermometer by day and seldom lower than 84 or 83 during the night. And as this form of bilious remittent fever disappeared, with as great rapidity on the approach of the cold weather, when the northerly winds set in. The atmosphere became dry and clear with a range of temperature from 81 to 82 Fahrenheit thermometer without remaining in any part of the island. It will be necessary to take a view of the state of the weather and atmospherical phenomena during the year 1827 in order, if possible, to ascertain its source or from what cause it originated.

By medical writers of the first character, the remote cause of remittent and intermittent fevers is solely attributed to the miasma of marshes or marshy ground; Dr Cullen[8] strongly held this opinion and all those who since followed his general theory. Dr Mason Good (sic)[9,] in his elaborate treatise, says that these disease[s] unquestionably originated only from this cause, and I could quote a hundred others who make the same assertion, according to this doctrine, wherever marshes or marshy land exist these fevers must ever be present both in Europe and this country, but this is not the case in either for at this post, (English Harbour), although it is almost surrounded by marshes there is not a single case of fever of any description at the present moment in the neighbourhood – although no individual either white or black or coloured escaped and no less than forty-five of the inhabitants of this small community died of remittent fever in November and December last when it prevailed generally in this island. Again, here, will this doctrine hold good, or what arguments will its supporters adduce as to the origin of intermittent and remittent fevers of every type and character existing and daily taking place? Here, there is neither marshes nor marshy ground to produce this contagion nor what you please to call it, for search the whole island of Montserrat, and there is not a foot of land to be found in it deserving the name. Yet, it is not only subject in common with the other West India islands to the above diseases but occasionally visited by the very worst species of yellow fever, and everyday experience proves that the same diseases are met with in all inter tropical climates perfectly free from the above-supposed cause. Therefore, we must look for some other than marsh miasma for their production as it would be absurd to suppose an effect could be produced by a cause which did not exist.

We find that up to the latter end of September or beginning of October, no fever generally took place in the island. I am speaking of that so long as the temperature of the atmosphere did not exceed 86 or 87 and continued clear and dry with a fresh current of air, it continued healthy, and that it remained equally so during the heavy rains when the temperature became reduced to 81 or 82. But as soon as it became close and sultry with slight showers, the temperature advanced above this range, causes which acted powerfully in suppressing both animal and vital energy and producing an unequal or partial distribution of blood to the *sensorium*, liver, stomach and other viscera, thereby exciting a greater degree of irritation in these organs, than essential for their salutary functions. A change which could not long exist without producing derangement in the entire system and, therefore, a fever as the immediate result, differing in character and duration in a ratio with the injury these organs had already sustained and as the cause was general, its results became endemic or epidemic in proportion to the extent and influence of the predisposing cause. That this was the case has been demonstrated to a certainty by the following facts. During the last and present year, while remittent fever raged in every other part of the island of Antigua, not a single case of the kind occurred amongst the men of the 93rd regiment, or Highlanders quartered in the Ridge Barracks, which is situated on a dry rock eminence, on the South-East part of the island about two hundred feet above the sea which washes its base and exposed to the direct current of the trades as they traverse the ocean without crossing over any portion of the island and what helps to move more fully the superior advantage of such situations. In point of health, an object that ought to be impressed on the minds of those who occasionally are employed in selecting situations for military posts and which I regret to say from the local position of many at present in this country display to the world a most profound ignorance or total carelessness regarding this most important of all considerations.

While remittent fever prevailed in all its various forms and was so general in Montserrat, not a single case of fever occurred at the estate of Roaches, situated on the south extremity of the island on a rocky soil and elevated about five hundred feet above the level of the sea which also washes its base and like the ridge exposed to the sea breeze, although the population consisted of 230 whites, blacks and coloureds.

It also may be necessary to add that the islands that suffered most from the hurricane of August and the subsequent changeable state of the weather suffered also much more from remittent fever and other diseases than those where its effects were less severe or escaped it altogether. After what has been stated, I shall conclude this subject by asserting that both intermittent and remittent fevers of every type and variety will take place in any situation, especially in intertropical climates. Subjected any time to the combined influence of heat and moisture with a calm, close, sultry atmosphere, they only acquire an endemic or epidemic character, and their continuance or existence altogether depends as well as their mildness or malignancy solely on the force, extent, duration of the above-combined causes and effects produced on the constitution, with only any aid from marsh miasma or any other source whatever. The disease which occurred amongst the men of the detachment during the year was as follows:

Feb: Remt: six, *Feb: Con.* one, *Phlegmon*[10] one, *Paryrrchia* 1; *Rheumatis Acut.* one; *Hepatitis Chron* one, *Phthisis Pulmon*[11] one; *Catarrhus Chron*[12] one; *Dysenteria* acute three; Delirium tremens one; *Bubo Simplex*[13] one; *Flaus* five; total, twenty-three; and two cases of remittent fever amongst the officers making a total of twenty-five altogether.

Febris Remittens – seven cases. The first stage of this disease was generally ushered in with a sensation of chilliness (seldom going to rigour), vertigo, sickness of stomach, succeeded by vomiting, coldness of the lower extremities, a nervous agitation of the upper and lower limbs, fullness increases in the head, face becomes collapsed, and pale, and generally covered with a dense cold perspiration, which falls from the forehead, temples and neck in large drops; eyes glassy and suffused with tears, great prostration of strength with a sense of soreness and weariness, in the muscles of the back, loins and extremities, great anxiety and uneasiness, deep respiration often with a sense of fullness and oppression in the chest.

The second stage rapidly succeeds the first. Pain increases in the head, especially over the eyebrows and anterior portion, seldom passing a line drawn across the centre or forepart of each ear. The temperature of the body becomes much increased; vomiting more frequent, throwing up large quantities of yellow or dark coloured bilious fluid fullness and pain in the *praecordia*[14]; obstructed respiration, face flushed and dry, eyes suffused and heavy, pulse rapid, sometimes full, both generally small and easily compressed, increased pain in the loins and muscles, inability to stand any time in an erect posture with obstinate constipation, increased restlessness, want of sleep, coma, delirium, impaired articulation, urine scanty and high-coloured, etc.

Signed
Andrew Tonnere
Assistant Staff Surgeon

9. Reports from St Christopher (St Kitts)

Preview: As in the majority of reports hitherto transcribed, those that follow for St Kitts follow a fairly typical pattern. Doctors are writing detailed descriptions of post-mortem examinations, all in an attempt to ascertain the cause of the yellow fever epidemic. Additionally, special attention is paid to environmental conditions. Of particular issue here is the view that emerges that yellow fever attacks may at times be class-specific. Thus, in one case, it is observed that the attacks are more severe on the rank-and-file troops, while the officer class might be spared on some occasions. Again, these reports offer us first-hand commentary on the prevailing medical and other philosophies held by these doctors.

Extract of Observations on the Yearly Return of Diseases That Were Treated in Her Majesty's Military Hospital at St Christopher from 21 December 1826 to 20 December 1827 by J.B. Patterson,[1] *a Staff Surgeon and Medical Officer*

The remittent fevers amounted for the year to twenty-five. In these, the most striking circumstances were noticed in my September report viz the severe headache with the general derangement of the portal system, the epigastrium being greatly distended, the fullness there was often the first symptom complained of; the bowels were obstinately confined at the commencement, and after the action of medicine the faeces were dark green and which could not have been occasioned by the use of Calomel as asserted by the island practitioners and for the reasons given in my last quarterly summary. Croton Oil, infusion of senna with a small proportion of Tartar Emetic, Alvetic medicines,

Calomel, and saline purges were all on different occasions. When any of them failed, the Croton Oil soon caused the peristaltic motion to be excited.

These greenish dejections[2] continued for about seventy-two hours, but where Calomel was administered, the evacuations were not so long of that appearance, and in two patients where salivation was induced from the taking of mercury twenty-four hours after admission, the croton oil injections being given at the same time, the stools assumed on ptyalism[3] supervening, the natural colour altho' the previous evacuation was a complete spinach one.

The history given by the patients themselves, together with the uneasiness felt in the right hypochondrium[4] days before they were obliged to report themselves, evinced that the headache was sympathetic, nothing being more likely to produce excitement of the brain sooner than a morbid state of the liver, cold applications to the head. Blisters to the *nucha*; mercurial purgatives were now persevered in. Afterwards, this medicine was combined with sudorifics to equalize the circulating fluid. In most of the cases, blisters were early applied to the epigastrium, which, with warm baths, procured ease from, I apprehend then resolvent or relaxant powers.

The exacerbations began generally at half past 10:00 or 11:00 a.m. The deviation being seldom more than seven hours and, in a few, nine hours. As the remissions after the second paroxysm were inclined to this regularity, Sulphate of Quinine, with a few grains of Calomel, was ordered every second hour and with marked benefit. This fever in the June quarter had a *synochus*[5] form, but in the two last quarters, it put on more of the garb of *synocha*. It may be thought that I have carried the purgative plan rather far and probably that bleeding was not sufficiently often called to our assistance in fevers. Upon this, I have only to say that the latter resource could only be used in particular cases and under certain conditions of the atmosphere to have a beneficial consequence. With purgatives, it was otherwise, and nearly a similar answer may be given as the advocates of bleeding have offered in support of their system, that is that one ounce of vitiated secretion on the body may cause death, but that no immediate fatal effect can take place for want of eight or twelve ounces of even healthy secretion brought away by purgatives.

Reports from St Christopher (St Kitts)

The bleeding practitioners will perceive by the above remark that the alteration of the sentence which they frequently quote is the word *secretion* being substituted for *blood,* but the most triumphant reply is that the success of the discriminating practice is superior to the bleeding plan in a ratio of five to one.

In support of this, I shall merely mention one case in point: the returns of this island for 1825, *the year before my taking charge*, includes 401 patients treated in hospital, of which number 18 died. In the September return alone, seven men died of continued fever, the duration in the longest case being only nine days. Here, bleeding was extensively tried, and at the very onset, the period being also a healthy one through the West Indies in the present year, 578 admissions are recorded, and the deaths, including John McRays's, not of this post amount to four, none being really from fever notwithstanding Corporal Melville's complaint was at the first termed so. Words may gloss over and hide errors, but there are facts that speak at once to the heart and conviction of more than fifty theoretical essays and, besides, 117 patients above the numerical strength of 1825. It is true that the garrison is much stronger now than it was then, but this is likewise in favour of my argument.

The returns of both years are officially registered and the director general will draw his conclusions.

The diet, I may say, was antiphlogistic,[6] but not such as to torment or fret patients by denying them many little things which they anxiously craved; upon a change of type or conversion into a milder form, a change of diet also took place narrowly watching the results which entirely guided me in the administration of wine, as well as food. These results were my only instructor.

It may not be considered extraneous in this place to state, as the question of contagion and non-contagion of the malignant remittent fever seems not yet hard at rest, nor is it likely soon to be, that the remittent malignant itself can engender its resemblance from whatever cause it may have originated, is a truth as well established as that death will happen to us all; without referring to the well-authenticated facts witnessed at Middleton North Amboy New York, and Ascension Island within the last twenty years, I beg leave to observe that the malignant remittent fever which occurred in St Kitts in 1818 was introduced by a man of colour of the name of Waller Fernando, who arrived from the island of St Thomas which he left on account of the pestilence then raging.

Being at the time, Health Officer to the Port of Sandy Point in this colony and acting under instructions from Governor Probyn, I visited the man who is still alive and residing with his family here; he was landed in the night to evade quarantine regulations, the company who were visitors at his mother's were the first that took the malady then the neighbours. The fever spread from this spot in all directions – from a centre to a circumference. By gradual degrees affecting all, as it proceeded in less than five weeks, it reached the garrison of Brimstone Hill, a distance of two miles to the southward, and the mortality that there took place is too well known to be here recapitulated. In short, the fever soon became prevalent throughout the island, and the treatment for a time was chiefly venesection; this error in which the late principal medical officer himself caught the fever from a disregard to precautionary measures, and to which I at an early period, called the public attention.

This advice altho' offensive at first, was in the end pursued and with favourable consequences. It is necessary to remark that the island was seldom healthier than before the arrival of Fernando and that for eight or ten days the sickness was confined to his friends and neighbours.

I have barely alluded to this endemic at present as I do not find any observations on it in the books of my predecessor, but as I intend that the medical world shall one day be acquainted with the fever as it appeared and was treated here, it would almost be superfluous to dwell longer on the subject in this summary. Two cases were all that were put under mercurial fumigation as noticed in former reports, the other remedies being found sufficient.

Signed
J.B. Patterson
A. Staff Surgeon and Senior Medical Officer
St Christopher
29 December 1827

Extract of Annual Report of Medical Transactions and Prevailing Diseases at St Christophers, Nevis and Tortola from 1 January 1836 to 28 February 1837 by Staff Surgeon W. Munro[7]

I believed with too much confidence that if in times past there existed any causes favourable to the development of epidemic disease, these now were either exhausted or had become wholly innoxious. But the melancholy experience of nine months has dispelled this illusion, showing me that no circumstances of locality in the climate, however unfavourable in appearance to the development of fever, can be trusted. This island, as I have had occasion to notice in former reports, exhibits a form of surface and a soil little favourable to the collection and stagnation of moisture declining continuously on every side from a high central range of mountains to the sea. Its soil is sandy and gravelly to a great depth insomuch that wherever wells are dug, their bottoms must descend to the level of the sea before water appears.

The weather during the past year differed in nothing appreciable from that of preceding years. The drought and heavy rains which characterize the different periods of the year were neither irregular nor excessive. These phenomena, therefore had no obvious influence either in originating this epidemic or modifying its several varieties. In proof of which I here subjoin a table of the admissions of fever cases at Brimstone Hill and of the weather in each month from 1 May to 18 December.

Table 9.1: Admissions of Cases at Brimstone Hill, Each Month, Noting Weather Conditions

Month	Cases	Weather
May	25	Clear and cloudy; frequent slight showers
June	36	Similar to that in May
July	47	Clear and cloudy; frequent rains and thunder one day
August	61	Similar: thunder two days
September	90	Similar: thunder one day
October	53	Similarly, the rains heavy
November	22	Similar (drier) thunder one day
December	13	Clear and generally dry

The above table shows the infrequency of thunder and lightning. To what physical agency this fever may have been owing appears to me to be inscrutable. Its octeology[8] may have had reference to the less frequently visible activity of the electric fluid, but that may be, that it originated in some specific agent altogether independent of local causes is, I think, sufficiently probable.

The 67th Regiment occupied this station and the detached posts of Basseterre, Nevis and Tortola until the end of April and though several cases of remittent fever and a good many severe cases of dysentery came under treatment up to that date, that corps was relieved here and at Nevis and Tortola on the 1 and 15 May by the 14th Regiment and was removed in a tolerably healthy state to Demerara, leaving behind several cases of dysentery. The removal of the detachment from Basseterre where the epidemic first appeared, seemed to suspend its progress in the relieving detachment of the 14th Regiment. As no case appeared in the latter for seventeen days, but on 17 May, it broke out suddenly and continued to prevail with great severity until the detachment was removed from the town to a small house in a ruinous colonial fort at one extremity of the Bay on which the town is situated. There, though the accommodation was so limited as to render it necessary to place a part of the detachment under canvas, the epidemic entirely ceased in a few days. Thus, showing the utility of moving men under such circumstances, though to an inconsiderable distance, for the temporary barrack provided by the colony in the town, though not unexceptionable in site and construction, had moved for the two preceding years remarkably healthful. Epidemic fever visits this island at very distant periods. The last that appeared here was, I believe, in 1819. Though an isolated and fatal case of bilious remittent does occasionally present itself, none of these islands is less obnoxious to febrile disease.

The epidemic constitution of the atmosphere would seem to have extended to Tortola, which is a hundred miles directly to Leeward of St Christopher, for between 9 and 30 May, forty-one cases of fever appeared in the detachment of the 14th Regiment then recently stationed there. On the other hand, Nevis is not more than one or two miles directly from Windward to St Kitts. St Kitts was at this time very healthy. However, that island is annually visited by remittent fever, which is generally malignant, whilst in the Dutch island of St Eustatius, seven miles directly to Leeward, fever was fatal. The number of sick having rapidly increased at Brimstone Hill and the hospital being consequently full on 27 July, I recommended to the officer commanding that a house should be hired at the foot of the hill for the reception of convalescents, whom it became necessary to discharge from hospital sooner than under ordinary circumstances would be necessary. This unavoidable haste rendered the direct return of those men to barracks ineligible, and I feared to recommend the inefficient shelter of tents, particularly during the rainy season.

I also submitted for the consideration of that officer that as it became necessary to discharge men from hospital at an early stage of their convalescence, the daily allowance of fresh meat for a certain period thereafter would be beneficial. A brief pause in the increase of fresh cases took place at the end of August, but about 8 September, the number again began to increase rapidly. I now suggested to Colonel Everard the possible advantage of placing a portion of the men in barracks under canvas, but as I could not strongly recommend such a measure, the suggestion was not attended to. A few days thereafter, I represented what I conceived to be the absolute necessity of reducing the number in barracks by procuring detached accommodation for at least a company, for though circumstances did not warrant the inference that this fever was essentially infectious, yet in the somewhat crowded state of the barracks such a contingency did not appear to me to be impossible. Whilst a reduction of the number gave an opportunity of more thoroughly ventilating and of again white-washing the barrack rooms in succession, a house for that purpose could not be procured at a less distance than the village a mile and a half distant. Thither a company was removed, and the convalescents from the other temporary quarter were successively transferred to it, preparatory to their return to duty. Yet the adoption of these measures had no marked effect in checking the epidemic in the frequency and malignancy of which no decided abatement took place before the end of October. Indeed, though more admissions took place in

September, the disease was most fatal in October in proportion to the number treated. About the end of that month, it began to decline and continued slowly abating throughout November until about the middle of December, when it may be said to have ceased, though severe and even fatal cases continued to appear at intervals until the middle of January.

The company of the 14th Regiment stationed at Tortola was removed to Brimstone Hill on 9 July. This change was intended to precede the removal of the right wing of that corps to Antigua, but unfortunately, the arrangement was not completed, and the barracks were somewhat crowded at a most inopportune time. If the whole Regiment had been removed at that time it would probably have been one of the most effectual means of putting a stop to the ravages of this fatal fever. The detachment was withdrawn from Basseterre on 30 November, and the improved health of the garrison permitted the return of the company, which had been removed to the village on 12 December. These changes were also in anticipation of the long-expected transport, which should take away part of the garrison. The transport did at length appear on 28 January and transferred the Right Wing of the 14th Regiment in a healthy state to Antigua.

To the fact of the detachment of artillery being here for five years and quartered in a spacious and detached barrack may probably be ascribed its immunity from this fever to so late a period as the 12 July. Though one man died, the cases were comparatively much less severe than those in the 14th Regiment, recently from Europe.

The cases of remittent fever which appeared in the 67th Regiment previously to April were of men who had been ill at Tortola and removed from thence in an early stage of their convalescence along with the detachment. One of these men was in an extreme state of exhaustion on his arrival here, and with symptoms of dysentery supervening, he died two months thereafter.

About the beginning of April fever first appeared amongst the natives in the town of Basseterre, the mortality amongst whom was considerable. I understood from the civil practitioners that the accession was generally very sudden. Headache, quick pulse and heat of surface were preceded by rigours so slight as to be little noticed, neither vomiting nor pain at the epigastrium were frequent. Those gentlemen invariably placed their chief reliance on the speedy introduction of mercury into the system after clearing out the *primae vire*.[9] They also used blisters to the epigastrium, warm baths, cold applications to the head – general or local. Bleeding was rarely resorted to. This practice was exclusive. It was, however, better suited to the constitution of the native and of the European long accustomed to the climate than to that of the soldier recently arrived, but I was unable to collect any data respecting the proportion of deaths to the number treated, the practitioners being too much occupied to assist me on this point.

At the end of April, two men of the detachment of the 67th Regiment, then stationed at Basseterre, were the first soldiers affected. They both died on the fifth and sixth days of the disease. In one of those cases, the urinary secretion ceased on the second day, as was distinctly ascertained by the repeated introduction of the catheter, and the civil practitioner attending the detachment informed me that that was a common and a fatal sign in the epidemic fever of 1819. The 14th having replaced the 67th Regiment at that post on 30 April, the further progress of the epidemic seemed to be suspended (at least no case appeared) until 17 May when, as already observed, it broke out with great violence and continued with little abatement until the detachment was withdrawn from the town.

The rather low though quick pulse and the moderate heat which the civil practitioner usually noticed did not, in his opinion, warrant the frequent abstraction of blood. He chiefly adhered to the mercurial plan of treatment and endeavoured to obviate gastric congestion by blisters. On the fitness of this practice with reference to the constitutions of Europeans recently arrived I was not then nor am I prepared to give an opinion. In this as in most other epidemics, the moral agency of fear had the most powerfully depressing effect at its first invasion. The first case of fever appeared at Brimstone Hill on 1 May, from which date till the end of September, the disease spread with alarming but unequal rapidity. Its progress and decline were marked by frequent and sudden pauses. We have repeatedly been deceived by a decrease in the number of fresh cases and a universal improvement of those under treatment occurring simultaneously and continuing for two or three days when an unfavourable change would as suddenly return for which we could assign no satisfactory cause. The atmosphere at such times indicating no remarkable vicissitude, though it probably was the vehicle of the occult miasma.

The mode of propagation of this epidemic was erratic and anomalous, somewhat resembling the progress of spasmodic Cholera passing localities which in ordinary times are not considered the healthiest to locate itself in places more remote. In the village of Old Road, which is halfway between Basseterre and Brimstone Hill no case occurred for many days after the disease had appeared at the latter. In this way, it made the circuit of the island, remaining for an indefinite time in each parish, but it had ceased long before this in the place where it first appeared (Basseterre). As it is now pretty generally believed that constitutional immunity from disease in tropical climates depends much on the age of the soldier, I here subjoin a table of the number of cases of fever treated here from the first appearance of the epidemic until it ceased.

Table 9.2: Number Treated between 1 May and 18 December, Exclusive of Blacks

21	Age not above 20 years	Of whom died	1 in 7
220	Age not above 25 years	Of whom died	1 in 5 ½
81	Age not above 30 years	Of whom died	1 in 8
41	Upwards of 30 yrs	Of whom died	1 in 10

From this it would seem that the age best fitted to withstand the influence of tropical climates is that of thirty and upwards, and the least favourable age between twenty and twenty-five. This epidemic was fatal to those negroes (military labourers) attacked, with three dying out of four cases treated, but it must be observed that those men are generally old and worn out in the service.

Symptoms

At the first appearance of fever on Brimstone Hill in May, the symptoms remitted obscurely and irregularly, but no long time elapsed before it began to assume the character of *Typhus Icterodes*,[10] though yellowness of the tissues was not invariably observed. Its invasion was generally sudden. Rigours were more or less severe and were quickly followed by a dull headache of the forehead, attended with great mental depression, which was probably aggravated by fear. The skin became hot and dry, but the pulse, except in sanguine temperaments, was seldom excited in a corresponding degree, particularly in force. Generally, there was tenderness at the epigastrium accompanied with nausea; the eyes and face became somewhat flushed, and the tongue furred, though often moist.

On the second day, prostration of strength was usually great. The heat of the surface decreased, the tongue became drier, frequently showing a defined red streak in its centre, and the pulse became less frequent and full. On the third day, if no favourable change took place, vomiting came on, the fluids ejected at first tinged with yellow bile, subsequently became of a dark colour, low delirium supervened and frequent deep sighing was observed. The pulse became weak, the skin clammy. The thirst was rarely urgent except after vomiting. The bowels were sometimes confined, the dejections always dark, frequently black. Suppression of urine and oozing of blood from the gums were usually observed in fatal cases. The first especially was a sure sign of approaching death, but many individuals recovered in whom oozing of blood from the gums took place. The duration of the attack extended to the third and seventh days. If the symptoms continued unabated beyond the third or fourth day, an unfavourable termination was to be expected. A sudden cessation of all the symptoms was noticed in a few cases, but in an hour or two, delirium, vomiting, a quick and feeble pulse suddenly returned, followed by coldness of the extremities and death. The continued type prevailed with little modification until July, when it was characterized by higher vascular action, greater heat of surface, a stronger and quicker pulse, more intense headache and acute pains of the back and limbs. About the end of July remissions began to take place, which gradually became more distinct and frequent in August, but without regularity in the periods of remissions. Frequent alternate chills and flushing, attended with diarrhoea and profuse perspirations, were often premonitory symptoms of the remittent type. The attack usually began with vomiting and painful tenderness at the epigastrium, a quick, small pulse, and great prostration of strength. There was often a tendency to syncope[11] on the erect posture being assumed. The stage of excitement usually lasted forty-eight hours when collapse was to be anticipated.

In some cases, this type first manifested itself by a state of collapse followed by little reaction. In such of these as recovered, the progress of convalescence was very protracted. In the majority of cases, a deep yellow tinge of the tissues took place as early as the third day but this appearance at so early a period was not unfavourable. In fatal cases, a less intense yellowness appeared at a later period. When vomiting of black matter occurred, it usually appeared as in the continued type on the third day, but it was not always a fatal sign. Mr Dowse,[12] surgeon of the 14th Regiment, has recorded haemorrhage from the stomach and urethra in one or two cases. Haemorrhage from the gums was a very common symptom. It was considered for some time to be symptomatic in some degree of the action of mercury, but it took place in several cases in October in which the exhibition of that medicine was from the extreme prostration of strength deemed unsafe.

Vascular excitement gradually became less remarkable throughout September from the commencement of October, assumed more of a low typhoid character, and the disease was in this month most fatal in proportion to the number treated. Relapses were also very frequent in October, particularly in convalescents who had not yet been sent out of hospital. In these, the relapse generally took place at such times as all the fever cases in hospital suddenly and simultaneously became worse, and such changes were repeatedly noticed. In this month, prostration of strength and a tendency to collapse, with irritability of the stomach, were frequently so severe from the first accession as to take away all hope of recovery. In such cases, the pulse was generally frequent but feeble, the heat of the surface little above the healthy standard, skin dry, the tongue rather clean and of a dull red, sometimes moist but more frequently dry and shining. The thirst was usually urgent. The bowels were either torpid or disturbed – no great pain was complained of either in the head or at the epigastrium, but a heaviness was felt in the former. Haemorrhage from the gums was, as in all the types and varieties of this epidemic, very common. In a few of the more protracted cases in the same month, abscesses and sloughing bed sores supervened, rendering the free administration of wine and a nutritious diet indispensable.

Erysipelas[13] supervened in four cases, in one of which it appeared on the head and face and proved fatal. In the others, suppuration took place. The symptoms observed in those negroes who died were of that low typhoid character which I have now been describing, but as I have already observed, those men are generally enfeebled by age and length of service.

The stomach was never free from marks of inflammation either in numerous distinct patches chiefly between and around the orifices or the greater part of its internal surface appeared of a uniformly deep red colour. It generally contained a viscid dark matter mixed with the fluid *ingesta*.[14] Inflammation resembling that observed in the stomach often pervaded the duodenum and was sometimes observed in the lower portion of the ileum and *caput caecum*.[15]

The officers and women of the garrison were equally with the soldiers [suffering] from this fever. On 30 April, Assistant Commissary General Hare, aged upwards of sixty years, living at the foot of Brimstone Hill on the road leading from the town where the epidemic was then raging, was the first person of the garrison seized with fever. He died on the fourth day. The officers living in the garrison enjoyed the immunity of a month thereafter whilst fever was making progress amongst the men.

On 5 June, the surgeon and Mrs Dowse (14th Regiment) were attacked at the same time. The latter died on the 10th. The Fort Adjutant was taken ill on the 12th, besides several women (one of whom died) and children. After the lapse of another month, Captain and Mrs N 14th Regiment were attacked on 4 and 5 July. The former was dangerously ill. He had incessant hiccoughs and profuse bleeding from the gums. In both, fever was succeeded by jaundice.

The adjutant of the same corps was taken ill on 8 July. Another officer and his wife on the 14th, the Paymaster on the 22nd, and Assistant Surgeon Telfer[16] on the 30th. The adjutant had a very severe and protracted attack followed by symptoms of chronic hepatic disease from which he became so feeble and emaciated that his only chance of recovering appeared to be an immediate removal to England. (*That unfortunate officer and his whole family of five persons perished in a dreadful gale off the coast of the Isle of Wight.*) Two officers and two ladies were seized on 9, 14 and 28 September. One of the ladies (Mrs Hazlewood) died, and in her husband, fever was followed by jaundice and dysentery, whereby he was obliged to return to Europe. Surgeon Dowse and Assistant Surgeon Telfer had a second attack in September. The convalescence of the latter was very protracted, and he did not recover his health until he moved to Nevis. Many natives and Europeans long resident in the island died. I had flattered myself that an irksome sojourn of many years in this climate would have secured me from the widespread infection, but in that, I was mistaken, though it may be observed that my constitution resisted the malarious influence for nearly six months, and I was less severely affected than many others, yet the fever left me in a state of great and long-continued debility.

In concluding this imperfect sketch of this malignant epidemic, I am conscious that my description conveys no new information on West India fever, but I have aimed at avoiding prolixity, and I am sure that I have not used the language of exaggeration.

Signed
Mr Munro
Staff Surgeon
28 February 1837

Extract of Annual Report of the Prevailing Diseases among the Troops at St Christophers from 1 April 1839 to 31 March 1840, Staff Surgeon, D. Scott[17]

Since 18 March, we have had a most destructive fever prevalent here, which carries off the patients rapidly by "black vomit". It appeared unexpectedly after a lapse of two months of unusual absence of severe disease of any kind while the white native population had suffered considerably from fevers, many of which proved fatal, but the disease had for three or four weeks disappeared, when on 18 March the first case showed itself on this hill and in less than ten days, five soldiers died out of ten admissions of fever, all of them with yellowness of skin and black vomit. Some of them [had] high febrile excitement the first two days, and others [had] a low type from the beginning. Pain of forehead and back, loins and limbs, with much heat of skin in some and none in others, and a rigour or a shiver in all, are the first symptoms. Great weakness, a low, slow pulse, heavy and sighing respiration and irritability of stomach quickly followed, and the fluid brought up from glary mucus, or the ingesta, by degrees became greenish and dirty rusty here and then brown and of coffee ground appearance characteristic of black vomit.

The first cases admitted were of a most aggravated form. They all died and seemed to have all been attacked about the same day, though some of them delayed reporting their illness more than others. The first fatal cases went in on 18 March, the next on the 22nd, the two next on the 23rd and the last with five slight cases on the 25th. There was an intermission of a week from more attacks till the 31st, since which there are numerous cases, some mild, some severe. There is no accounting for this visitation.

The weather was dry and windy, hot by day and chilly by night, but the same kind of weather frequently prevails here without producing any unusual sickness. The disease reappeared among the civil inhabitants simultaneously with our first attacks.

As to treatment, various means were tried, but as usual, they all failed. Nothing can be done in those fevers but keep the bowels clear, and combat symptoms. Bleeding was tried when the state of pulse and apparent determination to particular organs would reasonably suggest its adoption, but with no success in any case. Cold effusions, when there was heat of the skin, appeared to moderate the force of circulation and reduce the pulse but had no influence in averting the course of the disease. Blisters to the head, epigastrium, legs and thighs, sinapisms to the same, stimulants medicinal and dietetic, wine brandy and porter were administered with good effect when the stomach retained them, but this was rarely the case.

The post-mortem appearances were not different from what is generally found after these fevers, with the exception of the uniformity of the small size and firm texture of the spleen, which organ is commonly rather large and very generally soft and friable. In one case where there had been no urine passed for twenty-four hours before death and it was supposed there was none secreted, the bladder was found distended beyond the brim of the pelvis by urine of a natural appearance.

Extract of Annual Report on the prevailing diseases among the troops stationed at St Christopher from 1 April 1840 to 31 March 1841 by D. Scott, Staff Surgeon

Table 9.3: Monthly Admissions and Mortality from This Disease Category among White Troops

April	Admitted	28	Died	5
May	Admitted	50	Died	8
June	Admitted	23	Died	11
July	Admitted	12	Died	3
August	Admitted	18	Died	10
September	Admitted	5	Died	1
October	Admitted	12	Died	4
November	Admitted	10	Died	3
December	Admitted	12	Died	3
January	Admitted	1	Died	1
February	Admitted	1	Died	1
March	Admitted	1	Died	1
	Admitted	173	Died	51

The above statement shows an awful amount of mortality from this disease, with nearly one-third of the garrison having perished in nine months. The fever commenced suddenly in March last year in a most virulent form after some months of unusual healthiness. From that time till the end of December, the disease remained unmitigated with occasional intermissions of a week or ten days, attacking chiefly the young, the robust and the least acclimatized, as shown in the following table, compiled at the end of the first quarter, when the entire force exposed to the influence was present.

Table 9.4: Mortality by Age, Strength and Service Duration

Ages	Strength	Of Which Died	Of Which Deaths under 2 Years in the Command	Deaths under 3 Years	Deaths under 4 Years	Deaths under 5 Years
Under 21	11	1	1	2	"	"
Under 22	113	12	7	4	3	"
Under 23	50	7	3	"	"	"
Under 24	28	1	"	"	"	1
Under 25	13	3	"	"	3	"

As to acclimatization, see the following table.

Table 9.5: Acclimatization to Disease

Periods	Strength	Of Which Died
Under 2 Years Residence	94	11
Under 3 Years Residence	34	3
Under 4 Years Residence	29	6
Under 5 Years Residence	58	4

At first, the disease showed a partiality for particular localities in preference to others. It began in the Citadel among the men of the 89th lodged in the *case-males* or Bomb-proofs, and for some time was confined to one room occupied by ten men, five of whom died. By degrees, it spread to all the other *case males* and soon appeared in the Bedlam barracks also in No. 5 house, where it committed its ravages for more than four months before a man was attacked in No. 4 house;

though the distance between the two is not more than a few yards and in the interim had visited most of the detached quarters all over the hill of different elevations and every kind of aspect viz the officers' barracks. The artillery officers' quarters the fort adjutants, the barrack serjeants, the artillery serjeants and the artillery barracks from the latter, which is considered the best barrack on the hill for roominess and airiness as well as for being sheltered from the chilly blasts, which often blow off Mount Misery, the worst cases that occurred during the season were admitted. Two only of the whole detachment escaped fever, six out of eighteen admissions died, and several of those that recovered had been despaired of. Subsequently the regimental medical officers' quarter, the engineers, and ordnance clerks' quarters were visited. It was long a question wither (sic) the removal of the troops to an encampment in some other parts of the island was feasible or likely to be useful, but there were many obstacles and objections to it. In the first place the fever was prevalent all over the island where it could meet proper subjects. Secondly, a limited number only could leave the garrison to any distance because the powder magazines and stores must have guards. Thirdly, there was a difficulty in getting a place where water could easily be procured, besides some minor objections. These considerations conjoined with now and then a lively hope (from occasional relaxations in the severity of the attacks) that the disease was on the move, prevented the measure from being carried into effect for some time after it was agitated. At last, it was resolved owing to several very virulent cases having been sent to hospital on 24 August just as we were sanguine in our hopes, from the milder type of the cases admitted for some time previously, that the enemy was about to decamp. The next day (25 August), all the men of the 89th that could be spared were put under canvas on a dry, airy situation near the sea on government ground at the foot of the hill so that they were able to furnish the requisite guards from the camp. There they remained until 6 October when it became necessary to break up the encampment on account of boisterous wet weather having set in which upset the tents and rendered the men uncomfortable as well as produced some bad cases of dysentery that terminated in fever.

Contrary to the expectation and prognostications of some of the garrison, the change from barracks to canvas proved extremely beneficial for a time, notwithstanding the distance was not above a mile and a quarter. Six cases of fever were sent from the camp in five weeks, of which only one proved fatal. A relapse while in hospital, so I think there can be little doubt, considering the virulence of those admitted on 24 August, that the excitement of a move saved many, that had they remained in the monotony of the usual routine, would have been seized.

With regard to the phenomena of the disease, I can add little to my account of it [in] my hemestral[18] report for June, in which the symptoms were detailed as correctly as I could describe them and close observation in the subsequent months merely tended to confirm my previous experience. The disease was usually ushered in by chills, headache, pains of back and limbs, in some very severe, in others moderate, nausea, vomiting, heat of skin, flushed countenance, dull, heavy looks, great despondency, high arterial action, the pulse being quick full and firm, tongue white, with great thirst with strong disposition to sleep in the intervals of vomiting, the attacks coming on generally in the night, the patient awaking with headache and pains "all over" him, some with "cramps" in the legs.

But although this was the most common mode of attack; there were a great many exceptions. In some of the very worst description of cases, the invasion was so insidious that the patients were in imminent danger before they were aware of being ill almost, complaining merely of a little heaviness, want of usual appetite with a slight frontal pain or some thirst, which were disregarded till sudden debility supervened. On the second or third day, sometimes earlier, sometimes later, the pains, vomiting and high excitement disappeared, and a different train of symptoms ensued. The pulse fell (generally below the natural standard), the skin became cool, the pains abated, or at most, a slight uneasiness remained in place of the intolerable ache. The patient expressed great relief, fancying himself quite recovered. But want of sleep, a heavy and sighy respiration, a dull yellowish injected eye, dirty, dingy hue of skin, a sallow and haggard countenance, a whitish dirty, slimy tongue and much thirst with vertigo on getting out of bed or sitting up, excited much apprehension as to the issue of the disease. This state lasted generally for a day or two without any apparent decided change, when the patient slowly improved, or more dangerous or fatal symptoms followed about the fourth or fifth day, such as restlessness, drowsiness, *subsultus tendinum*,[19] picking of the bedclothes, vomiting of dark fluids, cold clammy perspirations, feeble faltering pulse, bleeding from the gums and nose, *singultus*[20] and stupor which soon ended in death. The alvine discharges[21] all the time very variable both in different individuals as well as in the same person at different periods at one time of a dark or dark grey colour, at another nearly natural (even within a few hours of death) sometimes mixed with dark blood and sometimes white with all the intermediate shades, but always offensive. The urine is generally high and scanty; sometimes limpid and abundant.

Although the above is as correct an outline of the general symptoms as I can give, it cannot be denied that almost every case presented peculiar features. In some, there were severe "cramps" of the legs instead of acute muscular pains. Others had violent pain of the back and body without headache and vice versa. Some were despondent and prostrated from the first, while others made light of their complaint, saying they had only a little cold. In some, there was great gastric irritability at first, which soon left them and never returned. While others had no vomiting till the black vomit came on near the close, and a few never vomited from first to last. In some the pulse continued quickly and full nearly to the last hour, though this was rare. In the majority, the intellects were sound within a few hours of death except in some cases in which coma appeared earlier. *Epistaxis*[22] at the commencement occurred in a few but it was more common along with bleeding from the bowels, mouth and bladder in the last stages, and usually a bad sign. One died in universal convulsions, and several others had partial fits of them a little before death. One case had the appearance of spasmodic Cholera from the first day. Cramps of the legs, surface bedewed with icy cold perspiration, face livid, fingers sodden and corrugated, breath and tongue cold, no pulse perceptible, constant vomiting of mucus and *ingesta*,[23] intellects clear, but the excretions were dark. One man on admission had pain in and discharge from the left ear. After death, an immense abscess was found in the corresponding side of the cerebrum without having excited any symptoms different from those common to fever, not even delirium till towards the last stage.

With regard to the predisposing or exciting cause of the epidemic (if it may be so-called), little is known. The only thing remarkable in the meteorological phenomena was the long continuance of southerly winds, which had blown almost without intermission for nearly two years (certainly for twenty months at least) while the usual trade wind is from the north of east, and that appears from the records of the office to have been always the prevailing wind here. An unusual absence of thunder and lightning was remarked in the commencement of the disease. For some months afterwards, but subsequently a good deal of both occurred without altering the nature of the complaint. About the new year, we had cold, northerly winds which have been dominant ever since, and with the appearance of this wind, the fever left us, whether from that cause it is impossible for me to say.

Most of the men were impressed with the idea that wind blowing upon them from open doors and windows gave them the disease, from finding themselves often stiff and chilly with the bedclothes off on awaking; others again attributed the attack to exposure to the sun or having "got wet" or taken a "glass too much" and having slept in the open air in consequence. There can be little doubt that all these may have been the exciting cause where the seeds of the disorder were already sown in the constitution. When the disease first showed itself and for some months before and after, the weather was rather dry and occasionally very chilly and squally at night, but the same kind of variations of temperature are frequently met with, and no bad effects result from them. Indeed, the last three months have been remarkable for sudden changes of this kind, yet there have been but few cases of acute disease admitted during that period. Relapses were frequent (about a third of the whole) and nearly as fatal as original attacks. Yet with common prudence in avoiding excess in eating and especially in drinking, a person having had an attack was considered pretty safe from a second, for most of the relapses could be traced to intemperance and inconsiderate exposure to the sun or cold and wet when heated, and some to being out at night in bad weather. The prognostics were extremely difficult in most cases. For the mildest symptoms at first, frequently after a few days, assumed a most dangerous and fatal character, and many, on the other hand, recovered who were considered hopeless. When the disease appeared to be stationary for a day or two, and a little sound sleep came on after extreme vigilance, when the skin from a harsh, dry feel became softer and when the urine began to flow after being scanty or altogether suppressed there was a hope that a favourable crisis would follow. In bad cases a free discharge of urine was a most favourable symptom, but there were some exceptions even to that. A sound sleep after long watchfulness was also a happy event, but in one or two cases, even this disappointed our hopes, particularly in one instance. A steady, good soldier whose case was considered dangerous, though not hopeless, after taking plenty of wine and nourishment, fell into a sound sleep which lasted for six or seven hours and was still fast asleep when the morning medical visit was made. He then appeared in a placid, sound sleep, breathing quite easy and countenance apparently good. About half an hour afterwards, he awoke, retched and vomited a large quantity of dark slough and died the next day.

The most fatal symptoms were the black vomit and coma. None in hospital recovered after these symptoms appeared. An officer recovered after having rejected some "black slough", but as the medical attendant did not see it, there was some doubt as to the nature of it, though an intelligent orderly and another officer who paid a good deal of attention to cases and took interest in them were quite sure it was black vomit. An accident prevented my seeing the matter. It is curious that the patient was most anxious that I should not see the basin, fearing I presume that I should declare it to be the much-dreaded black vomit, which all were perfectly aware to be a fatal sign. *Subsultus tendinum*[24] and picking the bed and trying to get up without any object were bad signs, but not always fatal.

It is surprising how little the tongue and pulse [varied] in this disease. The former was frequently found clean, moist and pliable to the last, and a slow, steady, full pulse was rather an unfavourable sign than otherwise. The heat of skin, too, was seldom above the natural standard in fatal cases after the first excitement subsided. In fact, in the absence of the above fatal appearances, the danger was judged chiefly by the looks of the patient. A dirty, darkish line of skin and a muddy eye generally indicated a severe disease. Heavy, slow breathing and sighing accompanying such appearances were almost sure to predict a fatal termination.

Post-Mortem Appearances
These were pretty uniform. All the tissues were of a yellow tinge, great congestion of the venous system especially of the membranes of the brain. The pia mater and arachnoids were frequently so thickened and injected that they appeared as a thick layer of coagulated dark blood. This extreme congestion offered in those cases which had [come before death] and [had presented with a] fiery injected eye. Seldom much serum in the ventricles, and the plexus was usually pale; the cerebral substance generally firm and oozing out dark, bloody clots when cut, sometimes rather soft; the thoracic viscera were usually loaded with dark blood; the lungs inflated, often infiltrated with bloody mucus; the heart large and flabby in some, small and firm in others – the right side full of blood, very little in the left or the arteries; the latter empty and in about one-third of the subjects internally tinged of a deep red colour, which could not be removed without peeling a pellicle of the membrane with it. There is seldom much *liquor pericardia* present. *Abdomen*: Liver generally large substance, often the reverse; the hepatic and portal veins full of dark blood; a small quantity of dark tarry bile in the gall bladder. The stomach contained more or less dark fluid (with very few exceptions), which smeared the mucous membrane; large patches of this membrane of various shades of red colour, from a bright cherry to a dark purple, sometimes uniform at other times arborescent, or dotted.
In most cases, this coat was soft and pulpy and easily scraped off. The small intestines were dark and distended, but no lesion was found; the colour being caused by a lining of dark mucus. The colon at one

time inflated with gas, at another much contracted; spleen smaller than is usually the case after fever, and very firm in several, but soft and brittle or "rotten" in others; kidneys large and congested, probably from the same cause which produced Strangury,[25] which seldom failed to be distressing after blisters to the head; bladder contained a small quantity of urine, dark in some, clear tho' high-coloured in others; in some cases full of clear fluid.

The fever fell with considerable weight upon the officers, six out of ten Europeans had smart attacks, one died, the latter (Captain Poppleton of 89th) a young man who had been about a year from Europe. He was taken ill on the 12th May and died on 19th. He was of a desponding disposition and despaired from the first. Lieutenant McDonald of the same corps was the only instance of recovery after black vomit. The women contrary to their usual fate suffered far less than other classes, owing, I suppose, to their having had less fatigue here than usual, all their washing having been done by black women with three or four exceptions, and all these had the fever in a severe form, two of them artillery women both young, one a year in the West Indies, the other about two years. One staff serjeant's wife had an attack though she had been ten years in the command (at Barbados, St Lucia, Antigua and St Kitts) without ever having been the subject of the disease before. The total strength of women was fifteen Europeans. One child died out of twelve seized, out of [a] strength of forty-nine; five of those attacked belonged to the artillery, but neither they nor the women were lodged in the artillery barracks in which the men suffered so much. Nearly all the women and children had the disease in the first quarter of the epidemic as well as the officers.

Among the blacks, three cases of fever occurred. They all belonged to the 1st West India. One was rather severe and of the same character as that among the white troops. He had dangerous symptoms for some days. The other two were mild cases.

Signed
D. Scott
Staff Surgeon

Extract of Annual Report on the Prevailing Diseases among the Troops Stationed at St Christopher from 1 April 1842 to 31 March 1843 by Staff Surgeon D. Scott

Febris Remitt

This disease has been a severe scourge to the troops of this garrison for the last two months. The previous months had been tolerably healthy with the exception of a short outbreak of fever in October and November. When the attacks were mostly of a mild character. In December and the remainder of January, the troops were remarkably exempt from acute disease. The 47th during the first month after their arrival had scarcely a case admitted of this class of disease, and they were rejoicing in the change from Barbados, where they had a good deal of sickness, and where they were quartered for a year and nine months since their arrival from Malta.

But about the middle of January, a case of rather a severe character was admitted in about a fortnight, after another which soon terminated fatally. After this, there was an admission every two or three days till the middle of February, when a sudden increase took place in the numbers attacked, and the disease put on a more formidable aspect, every case almost being of a most virulent form. From 12 February till the end of March, there were eighty admissions, twenty-five of which proved fatal. The acme of its virulence was about 9 and 10 March. Of nine admissions in those two days, seven died on the fourth and fifth day. On the 13th, there were seven dead bodies in the dead-house which, of course, created great alarm among all classes. Three of the officers quartered on the hill were seized on the 10th – all very severe attacks. One of them, the Commandant Major Gordon of the 47th Regiment died on the 16th. The detachment of artillery which remained on the hill when the 47th went under canvass – though mostly young men lately landed from England, with two exceptions – escaped the disease till the 23rd. On that day, two were seized and the next day as soon as these were reported, the men were sent to the camp and several were seized that night or rather reported themselves for they were ailing the day before. Two or three more were taken ill next day and slighter cases [in the] subsequent day or two, and there is little doubt that had they remained in their barracks, the greater number of them would have suffered, for the venom of the disease seems to attach itself by turns to a particular locality, and after a while, leave it for another. Very few of those who remained on the hill have escaped.

Three old gunners, married men who have had West India service in Jamaica but not lately, have hitherto escaped, although all their wives have been laid up. They did not remove to camp with the others and were quartered in separate houses from the barracks.

This is the severest visitation of yellow fever that is on record in this (P.M.O.'s) office, extending to 1819. I have examined all the returns, and there is none which showed so many deaths in so short a period out of so few admissions, although in 1840 more deaths in proportion to the strength of the garrison occurred. In the quarter ending 30 June of that year, there were 24 deaths out of 90 admissions of a strength of 139, while this season there are 27 deaths in 95 admissions in a strength of 194 whites. All I can say of the probable origin of this epidemic is that the weather was remarkably dry, hot by day and cool, even cold to the feelings by night. After the earthquake of 8 February, the weather became still more scorching; and bleak north winds set in. Vegetation was entirely checked, but this same state of weather held all over the island without having produced among the civil population any of the sickness that we had on this hill, to which it may be said it has been chiefly confined hitherto, for although many sick came from the camp, it was but in a few cases, it had a fair trial. The men were frequently on night duty on the hill attending the sick in hospital unavoidably, for every patient that was seriously ill was so helpless that he required an attendant to himself. Some of them, even two and as many of the men, had great aversion to the smell, filth and other unpleasantness, inseparable from such duties and many too impressed with the idea that the disease was "catching", as they term it, it is likely that they contracted it while on those duties. None of the officers who never slept on the hill has had even a slight attack. It was, however, very evident that those who were most exposed to hard work in the sun or exhausting fatigues, in any cases, were peculiarly liable to severe attacks. To this cause,

I attribute the extreme sickness and mortality among the hospital attendants. Three of whom besides the hospital serjeant died. They were harassed day and night, frequently much heated over vapour and hot baths administered to the sick, which produced perspiration and thirst; and they called for an unusual supply of liquid and excellent excuse for quaffing spirits, which with the soldier have the effect of keeping off the fever in spite of daily evidence to the contrary. Although occasionally there were coincidences which confirm their notions and favour their propensities, for instance. The only two perfectly sober men of the artillery were for some time the only victims of the disease. The drunkards ultimately came in for a heavy share of its fury. There was nothing in the nature of the disease different from what is usually met with in fatal cases of this fever – pain of the head, back and limbs, chills, nausea and vomiting, thirst and weakness were the most common symptoms at the onset, most commonly felt toward morning or in the night after the first sleep. The patient awaking with the bed clothes thrown off to which he attributes his illness, feeling chills at the time, but which is probably merely the accident of his feverish restlessness, during which the clothes fell from him. In some, a want of appetite or sleeplessness for some days preceded the full development of the disease, and if they had the sense to apply for aid in that stage, there is little doubt that many a severe attack would be rendered comparatively mild. But instead of that they have recourse to what is more agreeable and which sometimes proves effectual viz a good dose of hot punch, going to bed. [This], of course, adds fuel to the flame if it does not by perspiration carry off the complaint, which it seldom does. In nine cases out of ten, a clearance of the bowels is required, together with repose, to give the system time to return to its natural equilibrium instead of being excited still further by the usual stimuli of food and exercise, while weakened by the combined influence of the disease and the remedy.

I am convinced that by far the greater number of intractable cases are the consequences of neglect of applying for aid in time while there is a chance of cutting off or rather preventing the disease. There are instances, of course, where the invasion is so sudden and severe that this reasoning cannot apply. But in such cases, I apprehend that some violent exciting cause has been in operation, such as happened to five or six convalescents here during the present season, through the thoughtless ignorance of a non-commissioned officer. These men, although ordered to remain convalescent in camp until further orders were sent to the citadel in the heat of the day, a distance of a mile and a half and a height of seven hundred feet to take down their knapsacks, arms and accoutrements, the consequences were every one of them relapsed. In less than a week, three of them were dead, and a fourth was all but dead. It was when he imagined himself dying that he told me of the horrid outrage (though perpetrated in stupid ignorance of the consequences) and no doubt many similar excesses are committed, though never known. It was by mere chance that this instance came to my knowledge, for the informer was almost *in articulo mortis*[26] when he told me of it, and if he had not expected to die, in all probability, I should not have heard it, although of such serious consequences these premonitory symptoms were soon followed by a high state of fever. In most cases, that is much disturbance of the circulation evinced by a quick, high pulse, generally full and firm for a short time, but quickly becoming feeble. [There is] vomiting of greenish or darkish fluids; yellowness of eyes and skin; excessive debility; the patient being unable to stand without staggering or even fainting; excessive thirst; foul or slimy tongue or parched and black; drowsiness with flushed face and glistening eye or paleness approaching to ghastliness with a dead muddy look. In the former, skin very hot, in the latter, cold, except about the pericardia or head. Urine generally high-coloured and scanty, though sometimes the reverse, abundant and clear faeces usually dark and offensive but much variety existed in this also, being quite natural in appearance often, and other times almost white. There was but one symptom which was almost never absent – that is an urgent desire for drink even when there was a tolerably clean tongue and little heat of skin or vomiting. This last was the most distressing of all, however, when urgent, nothing would stay a moment on the stomach; and there was a most painful craving for liquids which were no sooner swallowed than rejected with distressing retching. These soon brought on prostration and cold clammy sweats and sinking of pulse, which soon stopped altogether. In these cases, the intellect were quite sound till the very close of the scene. The patient sensible to all around him when not a beat of the artery could be perceived in the extremities. Some cases had no disturbance of the stomach but had the head more affected, and these generally ended comatose, several of both had *epistaxis* and bleeding from the gums; and I believe from the lungs and stomach unless it was the blood from the former viz mouth and nose that was swallowed and inhaled. Some vomited as much as two quarts of dark, really black blood in the twenty-four hours besides constant oozing from the gums and dribbling from the mouth. Most of these recovered, contrary to every appearance. They were excessively yellow and had languid feeble circulation. The pain of head, back and limbs generally disappeared on the second or third day except in a very few instances. Cramp of the legs, which often accompanied those pains, seldom departed with them, but teased many patients for several days and was considered rather unfavourable prognostics. The most fatal symptoms were a fiery red and yellow eye accompanied by drowsiness; stupor with tossing in bed, cold, clammy perspiration with faltering pulse, no secretion of urine *subsultus tendinum*[27] and vomiting of dark fluids. This last one, when very dark, invariably pointed out a fatal issue. Patients recover occasionally from all the other symptoms, but I never saw any recovery from black vomit of any extent. The clerk of works, Mr Callender, recovered after having had a slight degree of it. That is, he brought up about a mouthful, which left a stain on his linen that could not be mistaken; yet he had a rapid convalescence. As to treatment, I have little faith in any remedy, active purgatives at the commencement, Croton Oil, Senna and Salts, Jalap and Calomel and so on. And afterwards, Seidlitz Powders were the chief remedies used. Cupping was tried, at first, in those whose heads were much affected and of full habits, but it proved of so little value that the practice was given up. In favourable cases, the spirit ammonia aromatic was thought to be useful in preventing a fatal depression of pulse, when the stage of excitement was over, at least latterly when it was more used than at first it got credit for cures, which probably had their cause in the diminished force of the venom of the disease. [There were] blisters to back of head which usually produced strangury and to the epigastrium when the stomach was unquiet, sinapisms[28] to the same in the same cases. Cold lotions to head and sponging, when the heat of skin required it, and vapour and warm water baths [were used as treatments]. *Pediluvia*[29] and hot bricks to the painful parts were frequently used. But stimulants in the shape of wine and brandy with frequent supplies of light farinaceous food; chicken or beef tea were the remedies mostly relied on when the stage of debility supervened, which it frequently did in a sudden way often within the first twenty-four hours. Yet I cannot say that much advantage was derived from their most liberal use in the generality of cases. But when the vital powers are rapidly failing and medicine evidently of no avail, the universal call is: support the patient. And what will do this, but wine and nourishment, when probably not an atom of them is assimilated or carried to the blood for the purposes of life.

The post-mortem appearances were pretty uniform: most of the viscera in the large cavities, head, chest and abdomen were usually much congested, particularly the brain and its appendages and the lungs. The heart commonly flabby but different in size and thickness of walls in different bodies seldom any blood found except in the auricles. The large veins were generally loaded, and the congestion of the viscera was of course chiefly venous. The liver of very variable appearance and consistence though mostly indurated. The stomach always contained black "coffee grounds"-looking fluids and the mucous membrane pulpy, thickened dotted more or less with ecchy spots, sometimes crowded and coalescing, forming nearly continuous redness; sometimes in separate small patches, invariably smeared with the dark contents which was easily washed off, leaving the membrane of a clayish darkish lime where the above redness did not occupy it. The spleen was rather small, often very much so, seldom larger than natural size, but always soft and friable, breaking down into a rotten mass when the envelope was destroyed by cutting or tearing. The *vesica fellea*[30] is usually small with a little thickish tarry bile in it. Kidneys are large and congested, their pelves yellow and sometimes containing a yellow thickish fluid-like thin pus. These appearances throw little light upon the pathology of the disease. They would indicate the free use of depletion if the experience of all practitioners that I have met with of any standing did not condemn it. The continued fevers occurred chiefly in October and November and were, in fact, milder forms of remittent fever. I could never make out a distinction between them, and when I meet fever of any kind, I am always unsatisfied till a decided change for the better appeared, whether there is a remission or not.

Supposed* to be D. Scott
Staff Surgeon

(*The term "Supposed" is in the original document.)

Extract of Annual Report on the Prevailing Diseases among the Troops Stationed at St Christophers from 1 April 1843 to 31 March 1844 by Staff Surgeon D. Scott

Strength Alterations

The average strength during the year had been 205 white and 55 black. On 11 June, the 47th detachment was strengthened by one captain, one serjeant and fifty-three rank-and-file from Antigua, part of the annual draft from Europe. On 12 December, the detachment of the 47th was relieved by 6 officers, 8 serjeants and 186 rank-and-file of the 85th Light Infantry from Canada via Barbados. The 47th embarked in the same transport for England after a sojourn here of twelve months to three days. In last year's annual report, we left this corps and the detachment of artillery under canvas where they remained till 25 May (from 20 February) rainy and squally weather having then set in and bowel complaints having appeared among the men, probably from damp and wet tents. It was presumed though there was no proof of it that the abundant rains had washed away the miasma of fever from the hill.

The men were very healthy after their return to barracks for two or three months. The 85th detachment became very sickly almost immediately after landing. Fever appeared among them which by degrees increased in virulence till they were removed from barracks and encamped below the hill where the 47th had been last year.

The change had the most beneficial effect on the health of the men.

The admissions to hospital in the period were 437 whites and 42 blacks exclusive of 33 whites remaining last year, which gives two admissions and about one-eights to each of the white troops in the year.

The admissions of the black were at the rate of about one to each man in fifteen months being forty-two to fifty-five in strength.

The deaths of whites were 34 being about 1 to 6 of strength or upwards of 165 per thousand. There were no deaths among the black troops.

Remarks on the principal classes of diseases: the following were the diseases treated during the year.

Table 9.6: Diseases Treated during the Year

	Whites	Of Which Died	Blacks	Of Which Died
Fevers	241	30	16	None
Diseases of Lungs	12	None	"	"
Stomach [or] Bowels	79	4	6	"
Diseases of Brain	6	None		
Dropsies	3	None	"	"
Rheumatism	5	None	4	"
Veneral (sic)	8	None	3	"
Ulcers and Abscesses	57	None	6	"
Wounds and Injuries	13	None	4	"
Punished	3	None	1	"
Diseases of Eyes	32	None	1	"
Diseases of Skin	1	None	"	"
Other Diseases	10	None	1	"
Total	470	34	42	0

It will be seen from these statements that fevers have been the most numerous classes of diseases exceeding by twelve all the others collectively. And the mortality was chiefly confined to them. There were thirty deaths or one to nine of treated, while there were but four deaths to all other diseases; and those in complaints of the stomach and bowels being four in seventy-nine or one in twenty nearly.

The fevers which prevailed were:
Febris Remittens – 85 white; 3 black
Febris Con: Com: 138 white; 13 black
Febris Ebriasitatis: 18 white; 0 black

So they were classed in the returns although it is very probable that there was no other difference between them than in the degree of severity; the cases being put down *Febris Con Com* when the symptoms promised a slight attack and the frequency of mistaking for a mild disease, that which eventually and speedily too turned out the worst species of remittent fever is proof either of there being no difference or the impossibility of diagnosing between them which comes to the same thing in practice at least.

Fevers have not been so rife in this garrison for many years (not since 1836) as they have been for the last twelve months, though the mortality has often been greater in proportion to the strength and the numbers treated.

The following are the monthly admissions and deaths from fever among black and whites from which it will be seen that when the white troops suffered most, the black were free from the disease.

Table 9.7: Deaths of Races by Month

	Whites	Of Which Died	Blacks	Of Which Died
April	20	3	4	None
May	6	"	"	"
June	9	"	2	"
July	11	1	"	"
August	15	1	4	"
September	3	"	1	"
October	16	1	"	"
November	26	1	3	"
December	18	4	"	"

	Whites	Of Which Died	Blacks	Of Which Died
January	26	6	1	"
February	42	10	1	"
March	17	3	"	"

In last year's annual report, mention was made of the white troops being under canvas from 20 February and [they] were obliged to adopt the same measure this season about the same time.

Last year, the sickness began to diminish in the end of April. May was tolerably free from it, the few cases which offered being of a mild character.

The troops returned to barracks in the end of that month and they continued tolerably healthy during summer and autumn. In November, there was considerable effect in warding off disease although there was evidently miasmal tendency in the atmosphere of the Hill, and three or four lives were lost in consequence of the delay of the vessel which had been looked for most anxiously for nearly a month. The newcomers were disgusted with their change of quarters from Canada to the West Indies and the report of the sickness of St Kitts having been much exaggerated; they landed impressed with considerable apprehension of yellow fever.

Under these circumstances and the predisposition of subjects fresh from a cold climate, it was but what might be expected that they would soon suffer from the prevalent miasma. Accordingly, they had landed but a few days, when some cases of fever of a very virulent character appeared amongst them. Before the end of December, they buried four men and a woman. Through January, the disease kept increasing in the number of attacks and not abating in severity.

In February, things became worse, the cases still more numerous and more fatal. Great alarm spread among all classes; though the disease was confined to the 85th, it was at first supposed that giving the men more room in barracks would tend to diminish the sickness. Thirty men were ordered to the artillery barracks on the Lee side of the Hill. This having no effect, No. 5 Bedlam Barrack, which was the sickliest and to which, for more than a month the disease was entirely confined, was vacated and the men put under canvass, on the low ground off the Hill. The sickness rather advancing than decreasing in No. 4 room, the men from it were in a few days removed to camp. There now remained on the hill of the 85th, the party in the artillery barrack and the married men in the Citadel, who had hitherto continued exempt from the disease and for nearly three weeks after the removal of the others, these kept free of attacks but at last two very severe cases came from one of the rooms which, of course, caused the immediate removal of all the other married men, as well as of the part in the artillery barracks, as a corporal, who was attending the "hard labour men", who slept in that barrack was attacked.

The camp had been quite free of anything but slight attacks, the consequence of ebriety, although the men have been exposed to all sorts of irregularities, from the difficulty of preventing them from escaping among the negro huts and getting drunk.

The artillery detachment all this time has not had a single case of fever, of any description. They landed here last year in the beginning of February from England, in the midst of the worst period of the fever and most of them had an attack of it; some slight, some severe. The detachment lost six out of eighteen, a mortality which might in all probability have been obviated had they been put under canvass at the same time as the 47th were, which was not done because it was supposed that the locality would continue free from the miasma.

Nature and Causes of the Disease

The character of the fever differed but little from that which usually prevails in the malignant fevers in the West Indies. There was perhaps a greater proportion of the low adynamic type than usual; where there was scarcely any arterial excitement or reaction from first to last no very evident disturbance of any function; a sort of narcosis pervading the whole frame; with the mind in many instances perfectly collected and calm till towards the close when mild delirium generally came on. To examine the skin, pulse and tongue, in some of these cases, one would imagine that the patient was in sound health, so deceptive were the symptoms that even an experienced medical attendant might very readily be led to an erroneous prognosis.

The unnatural, dingy, dirty appearance of the skin, the muddy injected or yellow eye, the great weakness, the viscid at first then dark, bloody saliva, and often the suppression of urine were the only guides for three or four days in these insidious attacks. If one of these patients were asked how he felt he replied, "quite well" or "I have no pain nor ache", "I hope you will let me up tomorrow", but he had no appetite, probably much thirst, and got no sleep – yet some cases were free from these symptoms, having no thirst, a good relish for food and slept tolerably. But with all these seemingly favourable symptoms, in a day or two, vomiting of dark fluids, an embarrassment of the circulation, *singultus*[31] and delirium came on, which soon terminated in death.

The same placidity of mind and body frequently (indeed, I may say in the majority of cases) succeeded in a day or two, to the severe pains of the head, back and limbs, to the violent retching and vomiting and high excitement of the circulation and the patients were more energetic in their expressions of comfort from their previous sufferings.

It has been observed in this island that fever is most intractable when cold north winds prevail, whether they have any share in the introduction of the poison into the system or not. During the last fifteen months or more, these winds sometimes changing to the west and north-west have been unusually prevalent and an increase in the number and severity of fever cases could always be predicted when a sudden change from an easterly breeze brought the chilly gusts from the north and north-west. To the feelings of newcomers, these winds are usually agreeable, as they reduce the temperature which so often oppressed the high fed and thirsty subjects fresh from a cold climate.

These subjects have [been] the only victims to the disease among the troops hitherto since it broke out violently in December. But in the previous months a good deal of fever was met with among the higher classes of civilians of long residence, some of whom died of it. The colonial secretary, Mr Harper, the Speaker of the House of Legislative Assembly, Mr Rawlins, and some others of less note were rapidly carried off.

The lieutenant governor (resident two years in the colony) had a narrow escape in November at the time that Mr Harper died. The disease has been very little under the control of medicine. As it has always been and probably ever will be, mercury is the principal remedy used by the civil practitioners, but with very little success.

Signed
D. Scott
Staff Surgeon

10. Reports from St Lucia

Preview: It is not clear why the filing listed under St Lucia only consists of two reports, the first dated in 1846 and the second, curiously, in 1839. In the first report, the reporting physician is clearly aware of a prevailing discussion on whether or not yellow fever could be transmitted by contagion. That possibility is dismissed, but there is some holding on to the view that it could be transmitted by miasma. Thus, the doctor declares, "It is certain that yellow fever of a malignant type may be produced in a previously healthy person by inhaling the air of a room [or] cabin of a sick [person] or other confined place where a number of fever patients have been for some time crowded together..." It is in that context that much of the report is devoted to identifying suitable locations for the housing of the troops. The second report has a similar focus.

Extract of Annual Report on Medicine Transactions and of the Diseases Prevailing among the Troops in St Lucia from 1 April 1846 to 31 March 1847 by J.P. Hawkey,[1] MD and Staff Surgeon 1st Class

In the detail of other subjects I treat, it may not be deemed irrelevant to terminate this report with a few remarks on the fatal scourge of the West Indies yellow fever, principally deduced from my own experience while stationed in Jamaica during the prevalence of the destructive epidemic of 1840 and 1841.

The conclusions to which I arrived from what I then observed are contained under the following heads.

    1. The numerous and diversified forms of intermittent, remittent and yellow fever are merely varieties of an identical disease

forming a complete chain, the extremities of which widely differ, but the adjacent links are harshly distinguishable from each other. All of these may be produced by the same morbific poison, and at the same time in different individuals, the varied effect on each arising from some natural peculiarity of constitution or some temporary state of [the body], at the moment of exposure.

2. The only original existing cause of this disease is a gaseous body, denominated malaria, usually emitted by the earth from the combined action of heat and moisture but which is capable of being produced under far different circumstances with the nature of which we are unacquainted.

3. Also, no variety of the above diseases can be communicated by contagion or defection properly so-called. It is certain that yellow fever of a malignant type may be produced in a previously healthy person by inhaling the air of a room cabin of a sick [person] or other confined place where a number of fever patients have been for some time crowded together. The concentrated miasma from the bodies of the infected [acts] in the same manner as the original malaria and in many instances [occur] in localities where the formation of the latter had never been known to occur. In this way, a pestilential atmosphere may be conveyed by a ship to distant countries, and there prove fatal to those respiring it, as was recently exemplified in the case of the *Belair* in England and in several others related to one when I visited New Orleans in the autumn of 1841.

4. The poison productive of the most virulent epidemic may be received into and remain dormant in the system for days, maybe even weeks, without exciting any appreciable morbid symptom whatever, and yet terminate life in a few hours after these had manifested themselves. It is consequently impossible in many cases to detect the existence of disease so as to make use of treatment till often too late to be of any avail. A remarkable and decisive proof of the truth of the remark occurred during the period I was in temporary charge of the medical department in Jamaica. One company of the 82nd Regiment was quartered in Kingston, another at Fort Augusta. The epidemic which then prevailed, having appeared among the former, attended with several fatal cases. I recommended their removal to Fort

Augusta, which was then and for a considerable time subsequent particularly healthy. That detachment was accordingly removed thither, but this measure, apparently so prudent, signally failed of success, then in question hardly one of whom exhibited a trace of disease when leaving Kingston continued for three weeks infected with a malady of unmitigated virulence losing a large proportion of their numbers, while the company of the same corps previously stationed at the fort remained perfectly healthy.

5. Malaria has the property of remaining suspended in the atmosphere without being dissipated through or diluted by it and so rendered innocuous. It can, therefore, be conveyed by the wind a considerable distance from where [it originates with no] material diminution of its intensity. The most delicate chemical tests have hitherto failed in elucidating its nature or even detecting its presence.

6. Yellow fever, never having been found to originate at the height of three thousand five hundred feet above the level of the sea, it is evident that malaria capable of producing that extreme form of disease can neither be generated at that elevation nor can ascend to it from inferior localities. If, therefore, we admit that malaria is a substance possessing the ordinary properties of bodies, we must conclude that in such a state of concentration, its specific gravity exceeds that of the atmosphere at the above altitude and cannot by any action of the wind be conveyed to it, without expanding and thus to a certain extent losing its virulence so as to be capable of producing the minor forms of the disease alone, such as intermittent and slight remittent fevers. We may also infer that in different states of density of the surrounding medium, it may rise to variable heights below the limit of three thousand five hundred feet before suffering the above loss of intensity, which will, in some degree, account for the variations in salubrity of those minor attitudes.

In selecting, therefore, localities for the permanent station or even temporary encampment of troops in those colonies, we should keep this important point continually in view and, whenever at all practicable, be exclusively guided by it. However, Jamaica, Dominica and St

Kitts alone, I believe, possess mountains of the required elevation. Our only other alternative in the case of an epidemic is to select for the encampment of the troops such site as has for a long series of years been found salubrious, leaving wholly out of consideration all local circumstances, however favourable in appearance, they being apt to lead us completely astray as is sufficiently exemplified throughout these colonies, where stations selected on such grounds have in numerous instances proved most unhealthy. On the contrary several that seemed to labour under every disadvantage have turned out eminently salubrious. In this case, therefore the experience of old residents must be our sole guide, no situation save at the altitude stated, affording any certainty of perfect immunity from a prevailing epidemic.

The military post of Newcastle in Jamaica was first inspected and reported on by myself under orders from Sir William Gounn. The successful issue of that selection has even surpassed expectations. The 2nd Battery 60th Rifles, on arriving in that island, occupied in the first instance Fort Augusta and other lowland stations and shortly after Stony Hill. In a very few weeks, they lost nearly a fourth of their entire number, including two Lieutenant Colonels. As I was myself resident in Kingston during the whole period that terrible epidemic prevailed, I feel convinced that the great majority of that ill-fated corps would have been swept away had they not been hastily removed to the still unfinished barrack at Newcastle. The mortality was instantly checked as if by magic, and in several months not more than half a dozen suspicious cases occurred, although fever still continued to devastate the plain of Liguanea. On each of those occasions I visited Newcastle and accurately examined the bodies of three of the above, which had terminated fatally. In all of these, I had the satisfaction to trace the disease, which in one instance only bore a similarity to yellow fever, to causes fully capable of accounting for its presence without impinging the character of the mountain station, which remains unsullied to the present day.

Signed
John P. Hawkey MD

Staff Surgeon 1st Class

Extract of Report (Annual) of Medical Transactions and Prevailing Diseases in the Island of St Lucia and Its Dependencies from 1 April 1839 to 31 March 1840 by Richard Dowse,[2] Surgeon 14th Foot

In the early part of the summer remittent fever of a malignant type began to make its appearance among the white population of the Town of Castries and other districts of the island. It quickly assumed the true Icteroid character and proved throughout its course much more severe and fatal than any other epidemic which prevailed here for many years; while it was thus committing its fearful ravages in almost every white family in the island, the white troops and population of Morne Fortune enjoyed a comparative immunity from fever, the black troops (strange to say) being the most obnoxious to disease; but short was the respite which the European troops were permitted to enjoy from the attack of this insidious enemy, about the second week in August the admissions of remittent fever of a more severe character began to be more numerous and quickly assumed a malignant and Icteroid type increasing in virulence and the number of its victims throughout September, so much so, as to render the Headquarters of the 14th Regiment unable longer to take the usual routine duty of the garrison.

It is worthy of remark that as the epidemic spread itself on the Morne, it subsided in the Town and entirely ceased there about the middle of September when the daily admissions at the Garrison Hospital were the most numerous. The medical history of St Lucia shows that although remittent fever is in general prevalent in the autumnal season yet that it seldom has prevailed as an epidemic of so malignant a character. The cause assigned by the resident medical practitioners for the severe visitation of the last year, and in which opinion I perfectly agree, was the unusually dry state of the weather for several months preceding the appearance of the fever, which caused the low marshy grounds which are partially inundated in general, to be in a comparatively dry state which together with the decayed vegetable and animal matter pent up in the deep and narrow ravines and accumulating for months for the want of the usual mountain torrents (the only effectual scavenger of such recesses) to sweep them away. Such, taken in conjunction with a high range of temperature and the long absence of brisk breezes, may reasonably and fully account for the acknowledged cause of such fevers (malaria) being generated more abundantly and in a more concentrated form than in ordinary seasons, perhaps some unknown and peculiar state of the constitution of the atmosphere may have assisted in developing or rendering the human system more susceptible to the influence of this marsh effluvia, for certainly the epidemic began to decline soon after a few days of boisterous weather amounting almost to a gale accompanied with thunder and heavy (tropical) rain took place.

Under such fertile causes of the fever long existing, it was not to be expected that the Europeans in garrison or Morne Fortune could escape [infection]. Its locality is but too well calculated to give full force to emanate from whatever causes it may emanate when we take such causes in connection with the then crowded state of the barracks with their dark walls from the bad state of the gutters of the roof. The *then* large open spaces between the top of the side walls and the roof through which the cold, damp wind rushed down at night to fill up the vacuum made by the more rarefied air in the lower portion of the over-crowded rooms, we cannot, I think, but be thankful that the scourge had not been even more severely felt.

During the time, this scourge of the tropics had been harassing us on the Morne and traversing the other districts of the island. Pigeon Island and the adjacent district enjoyed immunity from fever early in November; however, it was doomed to undergo the ordeal which the rest; suddenly, fever of a most malignant character appeared among the troops at that station and in a few days, ten cases were admitted into hospital of which I am sorry to say five proved fatal, nothing in the distribution or duties of the new, nor the locality of their barracks could be assigned as a cause for this sudden appearance of fever among them. We may, I think, in fairness, look for its etiomology[3] in the dry state of the marshes of the opposite Windward district of Gros

Islet, the population of which were at the same time suffering from fever varied in its type, according to the habits and constitutions of the subjects of its attack among the white, I am informed, it appeared in its more aggravated form, while with the black and coloured it assumed the remittent and quotidian intermittent character.

In this opinion as to the cause at Pigeon Island, I opine I am fully borne out as not a case occurred there after the wind veered so much to the north as to evade the noxious exhalations from that isolated spot.

Signed
Richard Dowse
Surgeon 14th Foot

11. Reports from St Vincent

Preview: The following reports from St Vincent follow a pattern that is very similar to those of other islands. The reports begin in 1819, and then there is a gap until other reports are presented in the late 1820s. The final reports cover periods in the 1840s. In all of the various periods, the reports offer commentaries on the fate of some victims and include, in some cases, a few remarks on the type of treatment followed and on the environmental conditions in the various localities. Unfortunately, the treatments tried by some doctors included administering Calomel and the use of venesection. In at least one case that [was] reported for 1829, the treatment tried illustrates that, perhaps, the patient might have been better off without the medical attention. In that case, the doctor reported: "I was induced (although I must candidly confess in opposition to my usual practice) to give the Acetate of Lead a fair trial; I must, however, say without any desirable advantage as my patient expired on the fifth day retaining to the last moment his intellectual faculties."

Extract from Remarks on the Half-Yearly Return of the Sick at St Vincent, in December 1819 by G.W. Cockell,[1] Surgeon to the Forces

The weather has been uncommonly hot and sultry and very oppressive so as to be almost stagnant, with little wind and much rain. During the time the above state of the atmosphere continued, the health of the troops was not at all affected by it, and a decrease of two has taken place in the last month.

The diseases have been very similar to the preceding month (with the exception of the persistent fever) and were mild and not of long duration. The case of persistent fever was violent in its attack, and the symptoms were of the aggravated kind and closed with black vomit. This case occurred during the oppressive state of the atmosphere.

Previous to this man being attacked, a disease of a similar kind had appeared at the upper part of the town. It carried off five or six of the white inhabitants, particularly those lately arrived in the island. The disease was attributed to the state of the atmosphere at the time, for it appeared to subside immediately on the change taking place; from that oppressed state to that of strong wind and rain.

The period at present is healthy – thermometer from 77 to 87.

Signed by
G.W. Cockell
Surgeon to the Forces

Extract of Report on the Diseases Treated in the Left Wing of the 27th Regiment St Vincent from 21 December 1828 to 20 December 1829, by Thomas Mostyn,[2] Surgeon, 27th Regiment

Febris Intermittens

Only six cases under this head were admitted and solely confined to a few of the old soldiers who had contracted the disease at Demerara and have occasionally had slight attacks since their arrival. The stages were well marked and soon yielded to the treatment employed; one case excepted, which I shall afterwards detail.

The treatment consisted of purgatives of Calomel followed up with a mixture of Senna and Salts in the first instance and, during the intermission the Sulphate of Quinine in doses of ten grains three times a day. The convalescent stage now followed when a generous diet with wine or Porter was given.

The fatal case was not strictly intermittent. The patient, a man of very dissipated habits, was admitted in March and for the first three days, he was evidently labouring under ague and on the fourth, the disease assumed the continued form. He complained of headaches and pain in his joints. The body was perfectly yellow, the stomach excessively irritable, the matter ejected of a dark colour resembling coffee grounds, stools of the same nature, pulse ninety, hard and irregular.

I was induced (although I must candidly confess in opposition to my usual practice) to give the Acetate of Lead a fair trial; I must, however, say without any desirable advantage as my patient expired on the fifth day, retaining to the last moment his intellectual faculties.

The post-mortem examination was not very satisfactory. The stomach contained fluid of the description already mentioned. The liver and intestines were highly tinged with bile but perfectly healthy in their structure. Nothing remarkable could be observed in the remaining viscera.

Febris Continuous

Seventy under this head were treated, and with the exception of thirteen cases of an obstinate and aggravated form, the remainder in three or four days yielded to the prescribed treatment – ten grains of Calomel followed up with an infusion of Senna and Salts and repeated if necessary until the bowels were freely evacuated, after which small doses of Calomel and Antinomial or James's Powder, of each three grains every second or third hour, invariably succeeded. The Sulphate of Quinine and a generous diet formed the latter treatment.

The aggravated cases required a more active treatment – three of the numbers were fatal. The symptoms from the commencement were most unfavourable – headache, very acute pain across the forehead, dryness and excessive heat of the body, tongue parched and dark in colour, pulse ninety, soft and intermitting occasional intellectual aberration. The body on the second and third days becomes perfectly yellow and notwithstanding the promptest measures of diligent attention, they expired; the first on the fifth day and the remaining two on the sixth and eighth days.

The stomach contained a quantity of dark, bilious matter which was frequently thrown up before death. The abdominal and thoracic viscera were perfectly healthy.

Ten cases were successfully treated. The Lancet was decidedly of use and blood to the extent of thirty-two ounces abstracted; an active purgative composed of Calomel and Croton Oil was then administered as the stomach was so irritable. The beneficial and almost immediate effect of this valuable medicine I experienced in the formidable fevers that were treated in the Regimental Hospital of the 27th Regiment when stationed at Demerara.

After the bowels were freely evacuated, a pill composed of equal parts of Calomel and James's Powder with a small quantity of Opium was given every second or third hour. On the sixth and seventh days, the disease disappeared, and scarcely any remission was observed from the commencement.

The convalescent stage was protracted; a generous diet with stimulating drinks together with a few doses of Sulphate of Quinine formed the remaining treatment.

Signed
Thomas Mostyn
Surgeon, 27th Regiment

Extract of Annual Report on the Prevailing Diseases in the Garrison of St Vincent from 21 December 1828 to 20 December 1829, by Alex Melville Jr,[3] Staff Surgeon P.M.O.

In the class of fevers, very few indeed of the intermittent type have been met with during the last year. Although they were by no means infrequent, for some time after the arrival of the 27th Regiment from Demerara to the station where, there is abundance of the putrid exhalations.

This immensity is caused no doubt by there being no ground of this nature in the vicinity of the garrison, but in some of the valleys, both to Windward and Leeward, where the Rivers communicate with the sea and the land low, the water frequently stagnates. The inhabitants in the city are at all times more or less subject to remittent and intermittent fevers, particularly after heavy rains and succeeding hot and dry weather.

For their removal, it is necessary to repair to other situations, not under such baneful influence. I have before remarked that harsh effluvia from whatever cause, as well as malaria, acts differently on subjects within its vortex.

In the newly arrived Europeans, an attack of continued fever may be fully expected. In those for some time resident, the remittent type and ultimately the intermittent fever, terminating in enlargement of some of the abdominal viscera, if a change is not embraced either that of a healthier situation in the island or a northern climate.

There has been a diminution of admissions generally throughout the year, those of fever of the continued form being the most numerous. The cases of which, with a few exceptions have been extremely mild, a few were severe and protracted.

In the beginning of the year, I, for the first time during the last three years, observed the black vomit in one patient only in the 27th Regiment hospital. During this period, as I mentioned in the quarterly Report, several cases occurred in Kingstown with this appearance together with the mottled yellowish colour of the surface of excessive irritability of the stomach, which designated the aggravated, continued or West India fever.

None of the type has been observed since the termination of the first quarter, and the instances being few compared with the majority of new arrivals about that period. The disease could not, therefore, be said to prevail epidemically or be called infectious.

Signed
Alex Melville MD
Staff Surgeon

Extract of Annual Report of the Prevailing Diseases in the Garrison of St Vincent from 1 January to 31 December 1835, by Alexander Stewart,[4] MD, Surgeon to the Forces

August, September and October – catarrhal influenza was general among the inhabitants, and in December several sharp attacks of remittent fever occurred in the families residing in the low, damp situations of Kingstown entirely from local causes.

Towards the close of November, I saw a severe case of bilious remittent fever with dark yellow suffusion of the skin, black vomiting to a great extent, several basins-full ejected in the course of a few hours resembling the very darkest coffee; the patient expired on the fourth day – he was a young, mercantile gentleman of most abstemious habits, on his passage from Glasgow to St Vincent the vessel called at Antigua. He went on shore for a few days to see his friends; this form of fever was then prevailing there and where he must have contracted his attack, it being the only instance here.

Signed
Alexander Stewart
Surgeon to the Forces

Extract of Annual Medical Report of the Garrison at St Vincent to 31 March 1840, by F. McCann,[5] MD, Staff Surgeon

Prevailing Diseases

Ample details on this subject are given in the Annual Returns of sick and of deaths which accompany this Report.

It is sufficient, therefore, to say here that fever was the most prevalent disease during the past year and that it existed for many months in the garrison as an epidemic.

State of the Epidemic

About the middle of March 1839, some cases of fever appeared in the garrison here, presenting the true characters of that form denominated yellow fever.

Of these cases, four proved fatal before the end of March … in one Officer and three men of the 70th Regiment, from which period no other death took place until 18 April from fever.

From 18 April, however, to the middle of September, no week elapsed without one or more deaths from fever. During that time, therefore, the disease may be said to have been epidemic in the garrison, or rather to have existed as an epidemic among the white troops in garrison, for amongst the black soldiers and labourers, not one case of the disease appeared nor any case of fever of a fatal character.

In the class of white troops, European officers of all corps are, of course, included amongst whom the disease mostly prevailed and even with greater severity in proportion to the numbers than amongst the men.

The annexed table will exhibit the principal facts connected with this subject in a clearer point of view than words alone can do.

Table 11.1: The Prevalence of a Fatality from Epidemic Fever in the Garrison of St Vincent from 1 April to 30 September 1839

White Troops	Strength – 1 April	No. of Cases	No. of Deaths
Officers	18	11	5
Men	334	370	75

Notes

It being impossible to say on what precise day the epidemic either began or ended, I have deemed it better to include in the foregoing table the whole of April to September and thus embrace probably every case of epidemic disease.

Signed
F. McCann MD, Staff Surgeon
St Vincent, 31 March 1840

Extract of Annual Report of Medical Transactions in the Garrison Hospital at St Vincent for the Period Ending 31 March 1842, by Staff Surgeon John Hall[6]

Bowel Complaints: One of the cases of spasmodic Cholera was attacked in December at the outbreak of the Yellow Fever epidemic and died in a few hours in the blue stage, having had vomiting, rice water purging and violent cramps.

The other was landed in a dying state from a small schooner in which he had come down from Barbados to join his regiment, the 33rd. He was taken ill on 13 March, the day he embarked at Barbados and died about six hours after his admission into hospital here on the night of the 15th. On examining his body after death, a quantity of dark fluid, resembling black vomit, was found in his stomach.

Fever

The class of diseases most dreaded and fatal to recently arrived Europeans in this climate comes next under consideration, and I could wish our list of casualties from that source was not quite so large as it unfortunately is; however, on a comparative, average of the ten preceding years, we have not much to complain of, and if we take the year ending 31 March 1840, when yellow fever raged epidemically in the 70th Regiment, there are even grounds, melancholy as they are, for congratulations.

Table 11.2: Attacks and Deaths, 1831–42

Years	Average strength of Garrison	No. of Attacks of Fever	Proportion of Attacks per cent to Thought	Number of Deaths	Proportion of Deaths Per cent to Attacks	Proportion of Deaths Per cent to Thought of Garrison	
1831	3310	123	39.68	3	2.4	.97	
1832	3344	22	6.4	2	9.1	.6	
1833	3379	20	5.27	2	10.0	.5	
1834	5567	17	3.0	0	"	"	
1835	5588	32	5.44	1	3.1	.17	
1836	4454	57	11.26	3	5.88	.66	
1838	2245	12	5.0	0	--	--	
1839	3376	131	34.84	3	2.2	.8	
1840	331	412	120.8	75	18.2	22.0	Yellow fever prevailed this year in the 70th Regiment
1841	3302	57	17.2	2	3.9	.66	
1842	3349	131	37.53	13	9.9	3.72	Yellow fever prevailed this year in 92nd Highlanders
	3337.6	198	57.61	26.67	8.1	7.82	Average of the three preceding years
	3390.5	87.1	24.88	9.1	4.89	3.14	Average of the ten preceding years

Yellow fever, which had been raging with fatal effect at Dominica for three or four months amongst the men of the detachment of the

92nd Highlanders in garrison there, made its appearance at Barbados about the middle of November in the artillery and 33rd Regiment quartered in the Stone barracks at St Ann's. On 11 December, it broke out with great violence in the bomb-proof barracks at Fort Charlotte in this island.

Some fatal cases of fever terminating in black vomit had appeared amongst the recently arrived Europeans in the town of Kingstown prior to the disease making its appearance in the garrison of Fort Charlotte. Amongst the rest, a young man named Weight died at a place in the mountains called the Whim.

This young man, son of a stipendiary magistrate of that name, was in delicate health, and had not visited Kingstown or its neighbourhood for some time previous.

The Whim where he resided is an open, dry, healthy situation, and his medical attendant, Dr Melville, an intelligent practitioner of the town, was at a loss to assign a satisfactory cause for his complaint in such a locality. The young man was fond of gardening and had been amusing and exercising himself by digging up the beds of his garden a few days before he was taken ill. This exercise he had been in the habit of taking on former occasions with impunity, and as the soil was dry, it can hardly be supposed to have generated the fatal disease of which he died.

When the disease was ascertained to exist in Kingstown, the men of the garrison were restricted as much as possible from going down into the town. Three men of the artillery, who were sent from Barbados to make room in the barracks there, were not permitted to communicate with the garrison but were sent off to Fort Duvernette. One of them was complaining when he arrived, and two days afterwards, it was found necessary to remove him to the hospital at Old Normans Point.

On the same day (26 November) that this man was admitted into hospital, a man of the 92nd, [by] the name of Fraser, was admitted from Fort Charlotte with severe fever. Fraser was a steady, well-conducted man belonging to the band. He had neither been down in Kingstown nor had he had any communication with the detachment of the artillery from Barbados so that his attack of fever, whatever it was owing to, could not be traced to any imprudence on his part.

The disease, however, was so decided and characteristic of what followed that I look upon his case as the commencement of the epidemic. Indeed, when the yellow suffusion and bleeding from the mucous and blistered surfaces took place, I communicated to Dr Bone,[7] the inspector general of hospitals.

Fraser's case was followed on 6 December by that of a lad of the name of Carrick, who had intense yellow suffusion and severe cramps in his legs but recovered. On the night of 11 December, four cases were admitted, when the disease may be said to have fairly developed itself, for within little more than a week, out of about 220 men of the 92nd in barracks, upwards of 50 were admitted into hospital and had not prompt measures been taken to remove them and place them under canvass at a distance from the fort, I am convinced the disease would have run through the whole of them in less than a month.

As it was, every soul that remained in the fort after the men were encamped on the 20th was attacked with fever, and even a man and his family (Elder, the Schoolmaster), which were removed into the Servants Rooms at the commandant's house, did not escape.

This epidemic visitation was not preceded by any remarkable atmospheric vicissitudes. Unless one takes refuge under Dr Parkins' theory of Volcanic Agency, as there was a small shock of an earthquake about the middle of August, I do not know what to ascribe to it (sic).

During the early part of October, a heavier fall of rain took place than had been witnessed for many years previous. It amounted to five and a half inches in twenty-four hours, but the sea breeze continued regular and strong during the whole month. In the beginning of November, the sea breeze was moderate, but towards its end and at the beginning of December, it blew with great force.

On 13, 14, 15 and 16 December, after the disease had manifested itself, the sea breeze was light and from the south-west during the day and chilly land winds at night, but these were immediately followed by wet and boisterous weather from the north-east, without any abatement of the disease. The mean average range of the thermometer for October, November and December was 81°, that of the barometer, 30.18. The quantity of rain which fell was 19.29 inches; the average dew point was 70.3, and the natural state of moisture in the atmosphere, saturation being 1,000.

The epidemic may be said to have fully developed itself on the night of 11 December. On the 17th, measures were taken for encamping the men on a dry knoll about a mile from the fort called Lowman's Ridge, and on the 20th, the whole of the 92nd was under canvass; and on the 24th, the detachment of the artillery was removed to Fort Duvernette.

The removal of the men from the focus of disease acted like a charm, and not a man except those who took the seeds of the disease along with them from barracks was admitted into hospital from camp. After two or three days, the disease entirely disappeared.

The 92nd continued to occupy the encampment until 6 January, when they were released by the 33rd from Barbados and embarked for that island in HMS *Cleopatra*, leaving all their sick and convalescents behind them, amounting to one officer, sixty-one men, seven women and eleven children.

But on 31 January, one officer, fifty-four men, seven women and eleven children of these were enabled to follow the headquarters to Barbados. Of the seven who remained, four died in the 33rd hospital, and three finally rejoined their regiments.

The following table will give the number of yellow fever cases treated by the surgeons of the 92nd and 33rd Regiments at different periods.

Table 11.3: Cases of Fever Treated by Two Doctors, 1841–42

	Number of Attacks	Those Terminating in Black Vomit	Died	Recovered	Relapsed	
Cases of Fever Treated by Surgeon Palmer,[8] 92nd from 26 November to 31 January 1842							
Officers	1	0	0	1	1	Dr Steven's saline mode of treatment adopted by Surgeon Palmer with moderate depletion at the commencement of the disease
Men	56	9	7	48	1	
Women	2	0	0	2	0	
Children	6	1	0	6	0	

	Number of Attacks	Those Terminating in Black Vomit	Died	Recovered	Relapsed	
Cases of Fever Treated by Surgeon Drysdale[9] of 33rd from 7 January to 31 March 1842							
Officers	0	0	0	0	0	Free venesection at the commencement. Calomel Colocis with purges with Saline remedies in the more advanced stages
Men	7	0	5	2	0	
Women	3	0	3	0	0	
Children	1	0	1	0	0	
Total	76	10	16	59	2	

The 33rd Regiment took up the encampment of the 92nd on their arrival at St Vincent. It remained there until 1 February when one hundred men and some recruits who had just arrived from England were marched into barracks, and on the 9th, the remainder followed, and the encampment was broken up.

The Royal Artillery remained at Fort Duvernette until the end of the month. On 8 January, a man of the artillery of the name of Bowden, who had been left behind in Fort Charlotte to take charge of the Engineer Yard when the rest of the detachment were removed to Fort Duvernette and who was noticed in my quarterly Report for December as being the only individual who had escaped an attack of fever, was admitted into hospital of the 33rd Regiment in the last stage of the disease and died the following day.

On the 17th, a man of the name of Gall, who had been left behind by the 92nd as a convalescent from fever, relapsed and died on 10 February on the same night that Gall relapsed. A man of the 92nd of the name of Russell who had been employed as an Orderly in the hospital during the whole of the epidemic and who lost his passage in Highland HMS *Cleopatra* on 6 January from having been employed and detained in giving over the hospital and stores to the 33rd was attacked with fever and died on this 18 February.

On 31 January, a man of the 33rd was admitted from the encampment with fever and sore throat. The fever assumed the character of the epidemic, and he died on 11 February.

When the 1st Division of the 33rd was moved into barracks from camp on 1 February, a man and his wife of the name of Holmes were put into the small house in the engineer's yard without my knowledge, out of which Bowden of the artillery was admitted into hospital on 8 January with fatal yellow fever and where his wife had previously had an attack of the same complaint.

This house, not being considered a quarter, had escaped the fumigation and purification which the barracks in the Citadel had undergone, and the consequence was that Holmes was attacked with Yellow Fever on 8 February and died on the 15th. His wife was taken ill with the same complaint on the 9th and died on the 14th. In the same way, the Servants Rooms in the commandant's yard, where Elder and his family of the 92nd were taken sick in December, were occupied by Corporal Fellow and his family when the 2nd Division of the 33rd marched into quarters from camp on 9 February. These rooms had been fumigated by my orders, but unfortunately the free exposure to fresh air which the barracks had undergone had not been so strictly observed.

On 26 February, Fellow was attacked with a fever and admitted to hospital. On 2 March, his wife was taken ill with Yellow Fever and died on the 11th, and on the night of the 4th, her son, aged eight years, was attacked with the same complaint and died on the 9th.

On 12 February, Mrs Bradshaw, the wife of a man who was employed in the barrack store in remaking the mattresses which had been used by the fever cases of the 92nd, was seized with fever and died on the 15th.

These sporadic cases of fever, which were admitted into the 33rd Hospital during January, February and March, were much more fatal than those of the 92nd, which occurred during the height of the epidemic in December, but as I have already entered so fully into the history and symptoms of the disease and the modes of treatment adopted by the surgeons of the 92nd and 33rd Regiments in my quarterly reports of sick for December and March, it is unnecessary to revert to them here, as these subjects will, I have no doubt, be fully detailed in the Annual Reports of those gentlemen although as yet

I have not been favoured with either of them, but I am unwilling to delay my Report any longer on that account.

Signed
John Hall
Staff Surgeon
St Vincent, April 1842

Extract of Annual Report of Medical Occurrences at St Vincent during the Year Ending 31 March 1843, by Staff Surgeon John Hall

Except for the case of yellow fever in the serjeant of artillery and the case of remittent fever in the corporal of the 46th, which came down from Barbados and proved fatal, all the cases of fever that have occurred here have been of a trifling nature.

Febrile Complaints: The serjeant of artillery had just arrived from England with his company, and while in Barbados, he, a corporal and a Bombardier were permitted on account of the crowded state of the artillery barracks to hire lodgings for themselves and families in one of the small houses near the Savannah. The corporal died of fever; the Bombardier was left in a dying state when the detachment embarked for St Vincent. The serjeant's wife was very ill, and the poor man, in his anxiety to get her away, must have embarked with the disease on him. After his arrival here, he neglected to report himself until those symptoms had set in, which rendered medical aid of little or no avail.

The corporal's case was aggravated by the exertion of marching up from the landing place to Fort Charlotte with his pack on. He lingered for some days, and at one time, I had hopes of his recovery, but he sank into the stage of passive haemorrhage from the mucous surfaces.

The serjeant had incessant vomiting after his admission, and as nothing had been done for him during the first stage of his complaint, his case was quite hopeless.

The corporal, on the contrary, was seen early, and perhaps too much was done for him, for I was induced from the violence of his symptoms to bleed him from the arm.

In the after stage of the disease, I regretted this, but the chances are if I had not done it, he would have died sooner, and I would have felt equal regret at having omitted it.

Signed
John Hall
Staff Surgeon
St Vincent
5 April 1843

12. Reports from Tobago

Preview: The reports for Tobago cover various years from the 1820s and then rather abruptly switch to the 1840s. Of particular interest throughout the various reports are the several case notes describing the course of the disease and even ending in death of the various patients. Such detailed case notes are instructive on the course of treatment employed and when death came and were followed, in many cases, by detailed post-mortem examinations. Apart from these general observations, we also note cases where there are discussions on the various theories concerning the cause of the yellow fever outbreaks. In one report, the reporting doctor appeared to be questioning the utility of miasmatic theories. In that case, he observes: "A medical gentleman walking near a cane field, on his observing the canes growing luxuriantly, though no weeds or moisture was to be seen on the ground, turned up his nose thinking that he perceived miasmata. Another looking at a field to windward of his quarters which was dry and cultivated and where even vegetation was scanty, asked me if it was not apprehended that deleterious miasma would arise from it. Such theorists by a little ingenuity of reasoning (and it certainly requires some) contrive to extract miasma to suit their purpose from the arid Rock of Gibraltar and even onboard English ships of war to form artificial swamps (very artificial ones indeed) by means of the solid timber cut down for fuel, so as to constitute (in their minds) hot-beds for the production of miasma, when necessary for the occasion of accounting for sickness…"

Special Report on Fever from Tobago by Dr John Arthur,[1] Physician to the Forces

Having again had to witness the melancholy destructive ravages committed by the malignant commonly, though I conceive improperly termed, yellow fever, during its late visitation at the island of Tobago, I beg to offer the following remarks on it, as it fell under my observation there. The first cases that attracted notice from their suddenly fatal termination and the severe symptoms they had been attended with, I was informed by Staff Surgeon Panting,[2] principal medical officer, occurred in the town, towards the latter end of November, all within the near neighbourhood of one another. Of the military, the first person affected was the ordnance serjeant armourer's wife, who happened to live then in town in that neighbourhood, and fell an early victim. It soon afterwards reached those in garrison on the summit of the hill, conically formed and about the base of which, on the leeward side, the town principally lies at least that part of it where the disease was first observed. The garrison consisted of two companies, Royal York Rangers, an old regiment in the command, and about two-thirds of those stationed I was informed by Commanding Officer Captain O'Keefe were the survivors of those that had been sent from Trinidad for change of air on account of the impaired state of their health, and who were then so far recovered as to be capable of doing duty. Fourteen artillery men and 153 young African negroes [are] employed as military labourers and pioneers.

It appears to have commenced among the white troops of the garrison early in December 1818, and spread so quickly through them that on the 18th or 19th of that month, within twenty-four hours, there were nine deaths. One officer was dead, another dying and an officer's wife in the same state. Considerable alarm, was in consequence excited, and a vessel hired for the purpose of carrying an express to headquarters with the melancholy intelligence and requesting further medical aid, one of two medical officers there already suffering under it and the hospital being crowded with numerous sick. She arrived here on the 26th, and I was immediately despatched in her, along with an acting hospital assistant, Mr McAvoy,[3] arrived there on the following evening the 27th and remained until March following. The disease, in the interim, had received some check and been moderated in its course among the troops by judicious steps very properly adopted for the purpose. New barracks that were erecting in the immediate vicinity and on a similar site with the old ones, but more roomy and airy were though not quite dry, fortunately so far finished as to afford accommodation for the troops who were accordingly removed into them, and the old ones appropriated for the reception of convalescents from the hospital, those ill of other complaints than the prevailing fever, and a separate one for the sick women and children for whom there was no fit place in hospital. The number of admissions daily and, of course, that of deaths was in consequence much diminished, though at the same time spreading more extensively and generally through the town, but had not yet appeared among the sailors on board the English ships in the bay, who however were not destined to continue long exempt from it, but soon shared the same fate with the others and suffered in an equal degree. A hospital was then opened for them ashore, at the expense of the colony, but which from the unhealthiness of the situation, being an empty house that had been deserted on that very account and communication between the sick in it and the well on board not having been prevented so effectually as could have been wished, it did not prove so useful as it otherwise might have done.

In the country some few cases occurred, but none so far as I heard (and I believe I heard nearly of all the white community being so very small) unless after communication with others ill of it, principally in the town, and to which it might be fairly ascribed. For instance, a manager a few miles from town whom I saw dying with black vomiting and purging, on inquiring how he had been exposed to it, was told that on the Sunday preceding his attack, he had attended the funeral of a friend of his who died of it in town, happening at another time to be at Dr Panting's when a gentleman called there to receive medical directions for the treatment of his brother lying ill of the fever, in a distant part of the country and whom he was just going down to attend. On expressing my surprise how it could have reached him there, he mentioned his having been in town a few days before being taken ill and having imprudently called to see and been in the room with a Mr Row then dying of it. I heard soon afterwards that the brother was also ill but whether of the same disease I cannot pretend to say.

The governor who resides a few miles from the town and garrison when he found that he actually had the disease at once said that he caught it from visiting the barracks and garrison when the fever was at its height there. The governor was the first of his family taken ill. Thus, it was confined to no particular place, no class or description of persons, but affecting equally the soldiers (and their officers who by the by had been healthy young men) on the summit of the hill, the inhabitants at the foot of it, and the sailors on board the ships in the bay, not simultaneously but successively and as chance seemed to direct it in its course, by bringing fresh subjects from different directions under its baneful influence and where it was once introduced, it ran through in its usually destructive manner. The higher classes enjoying every ease, comfort and luxury were not more exempt than the lower under every hardship and deprivation. The governor himself had a severe attack, which he very narrowly escaped and lost one daughter by it. The president of the council, Dr Cummins, lost his wife, a resident for more than twenty years in the West Indies, and it ran in a remarkable manner through nearly the entire of that family, mostly natives of the island. The collector of customs and his wife died of it. In the garrison, by 24 December, twenty-six persons, according to the hospital expenditure returns of that date, had already died of it, and of whom John Harrison only was an African negro, between that and 24 January, sixteen and in the month ending 24 February, six more died of it.

Among the civilians, as far as it extended, it was fatal in a still higher degree. Throughout, it was characterized by a strongly marked malignity, the danger always being considerably greater than could be portended from any of the symptoms unless the actually fatal ones occurring in the latter stage.

In a disease so generally affecting the entire system, much variety in the appearance of symptoms was to be expected according to the diversity of constitutions, and the various states of different parts of the system, according to which in individual cases some parts were more likely to be affected in a more remarkable manner or degree than others.

It is unnecessary for one to enumerate a long list of febrile symptoms fully detailed in every book on the subject. I shall, therefore, confine myself to a few of the most remarkable ones and the various appearances they assumed. The attack in some was sudden so as it were immediately to knock down the patient and confine him to bed. In others, it was more slow and gradual, and the disease seemed to take time for its formation. The first was well instanced in the case of Mr Bullen, the collector, who called on me on a Thursday in good health and spirits and remained conversing a longer time than was convenient for me to attend to him. He was suddenly taken ill the same evening and after the most usual symptoms, black vomiting having appeared a short time before death. He was interred on the following Monday at the very time he was to have expected a large party to dinner. The governor was an instance of the latter who fell unwell and complained of wandering pains for which he used warm baths for some days before he was obliged to confine himself to bed. The febrile accession that usually appeared at first and prevailed during the early period varied a good deal in intensity and in a few odd cases from what I shall state hereafter I have reason to think was altogether wanting. The pain in the fore part of the head in some was very severe, and I observed at the same time in many to be not at all proportioned to the degree of increased vascular action or accelerated circulation of the blood. Others complained most of pain in the small of the back, while in more it was principally felt in the limbs. In Mrs Bullen's case, who was taken ill a few days after her husband and was buried on the following Monday, they were so severe that I was told she likened them to labour pains. The redness of the face observable in several was not of a bright vivid but rather dusky hue and reminded me of the appearance which the skin puts on in some dependant parts of the body when the blood begins to lodge and settle in the last moments of life. The pulse though increased in frequency tolerably full and expanded I found on application of the finger to yield to the slightest pressure and to be soft and compressible. In no instance did the blood (which I had an opportunity of seeing in numerous cases) appear at all cupped or buffy – but, on the contrary, in rather a lax and dissolved state. The pulse of the governor towards the commencement of his illness was more full and firm than I felt in any other, and he seemed to derive immediate relief and benefit from a moderate bleeding. But I was informed that at the same time with Mr Bullen the fever was remarkably high, pulse very full and yet bleeding after a full and fair trial proved unsuccessful as well as in other similar cases. One of the earliest I witnessed among the civilians was that, I think, of a Mr Row, whom I found a handsome, interesting young man lying in a dozing state but easily roused, and answered questions put to him rationally. No delirium, black vomiting, yellowness of the skin or other the usual precursors of death present. But on applying my hand to his wrist, I found his skin cold and damp, his pulse not to be felt, and that he was evidently gradually falling into an eternal sleep, which happened in a few hours afterwards. I was told it was the third day of his sickness, that his fever had been very high, and that the Lancet had been used freely to moderate it.

While the above were instances where the fever ran high, the following is one where it was altogether absent. On visiting the hospital one day, I was distressed to find admitted amongst the fever patients one whom I conceived free from any symptoms of it; his pulse regular, skin natural and only complained of pain in his back with general debility. I had him immediately removed into a separate room. But on the following day, I found him weaker, affected with convulsive twitching of the muscles of his face and arms, his eyes and skin becoming yellow, slight delirium came on, and the matter of black vomit was found in his stomach after death. From the course and result of this case and the great general and long continued debility attendant on another of an old man at the same time in hospital who only complained in a similar manner of pain in his back, without any other febrile symptom and from which he very slowly recovered, I am led to suspect to have been of a similar nature. While the attack and early symptoms thus varied, the approach to death and the appearances immediately preceding were not less various and uncertain.

In the fatal cases, black vomiting though by no means universal, was far the most frequent of these appearances, and in some of those who had not at all suffered from it, on examination of their bodies after death, the black vomit was found contained in the stomach, while in others in whom this symptom had appeared, though relieved and the vomiting entirely restrained by medicine, yet the patient continued to sink under the disease and which notwithstanding soon proved fatal.

I only saw one instance of recovery after black vomit had actually appeared, which was in the case of a serjeant in the Royal York Rangers, who had it in but a slight degree, having vomited the black matter but once or twice and which was of the floccular kind. The matter of black vomit was not always the same in appearance. In some, it was floccular – small, distinct flocculi plainly perceivable floating in the fluid, which seemed to give colour to it and adhered to the sides of the vessel that contained it or to the inner coat of the stomach as was observed on dissection. In others, it was a dark turbid mixture as if from coffee grounds or even soot or gunpowder mixed up with the contents of the stomach. In one, an African who had been attendant on the sick in hospital and died of a disease, what was found in the stomach had a very peculiar appearance, being of a thicker consistence, and a more uniform mixture than usual, not inaptly compared I thought by a person present to diluted or thin mercurial ointment. A purging of the same kind of matter generally attended the black vomiting, but also frequently appeared independent of it, and was then by no means so fatal a symptom, many having recovered after it and in some such cases when the stools changed their appearance, I observed them put on a red bloody one, and to continue so for some time before they assumed their natural state or colour. Haemorrhages from different parts of the body not infrequently occurred in the latter stages. I have in different cases seen the blood running from the corners of the mouths and on having them opened, and inspecting internally could not perceive it flowing from any particular point, but rather appeared as a general oozing. This has happened in some whose mouths were affected by mercury and also in others who were not in the least touched by it. The nose has bled in the same stages. I have before mentioned the black stools changing into red and bloody looking ones, the same kind of stools have also appeared in other cases and on dissection, I have repeatedly seen the internal surface of the small and large intestines covered with the same kind of red bloody matter. On the thighs of some subjects stripped for examination, I have seen the dried blood that had dropped from the point of the penis. Captain O'Keefe's wife in whom labour so speedily succeeded to the fever that I may say it supervened on it, I was informed died of haemorrhage from the uterus, and I understood hers not to be a singular case. Some persons recovered that were affected with these bleedings from the nose or mouth, or the red bloody stools, therefore though very unfavourable symptoms, they are not to be considered as absolutely mortal ones. Though yellowness of the skins was certainly evident in several, yet I think in the majority, even of fatal cases, not the slightest tinge was perceivable, and in not very many was it a prominent or very remarkable symptom. Therefore, and as the same appearance is so generally observable in other very different kinds of fevers and diseases, where there is an increased secretion of bile, so frequent in this climate, I conceive a more improper term could not have been well hit on for a distinctive appellation of this disease, and which must evidently lead into endless error and confusion. Dysuria in some was troublesome, the governor suffered a good deal from it. Delirium was not a frequent symptom. It came on in some towards the close of life, in one (Captain O'Keefe's servant), a strong robust young man, it rose to a higher pitch and lasted longer than I witnessed in any other, during the violence of which he contrived to cut his throat, but not effectually, as he survived it a few days and then seemed to die of the fever itself. In a few cases, convulsions closed the scene. The death of Mr Row before mentioned was not ushered in by any of these severe symptoms, without the intervention of them, after a couple of days' fever, life quietly ceased, he having gradually dozed off into an eternal slumber.

The duration of the disease varied, many were carried off by it in two, three or four days while in many others, it was spun out to a longer period. One young man whom I had an opportunity of seeing frequently, having been placed in an empty house near where I lived under the care of a black nurse, it was protracted till towards the close of the third week, having assumed a typhoid character, from which he gradually recovered though it had been attended with very unfavourable symptoms – bleeding from the mouth and nose, irritability of the stomach and black stools.

Appearances on dissection, though some might be observed more frequently than others, were by no means so constant uniform and certain in their appearance, or so peculiar to this disease as might be supposed by some, and from what I shall presently mention appeared rather in my opinion as consequence or effects of the disease itself, than as immediately connected with or indicating the cause. In the head, in a few cases, there appeared slightly increased vascularity, in most on turning out the cerebrum and cerebellum and dividing the medulla oblongata as low down as possible, there remained in the base of the skull about from half an ounce to an ounce of serous fluid. How far this may be natural or not I cannot say, not having examined in this manner a sufficient number of heads after other complaints to be certain. In one man, a dropsical subject from Trinidad, who died of this fever, every part of whose body was found remarkably pale, and almost every cavity inundated with serous fluid, a much larger quantity remained in the skull. In the thorax, the lungs in some were found red and rather dense as if gorged with blood, in which cases I had observed dyspnoae in a more remarkable degree than usual to have for some time preceded death, and which therefore seemed to have been more immediately induced by the effusion of blood into the substance of the lungs. In the abdomen, the morbid appearances were more frequent and uniform though also not without exceptions and variations. The stomach and intestines were very frequently found loaded with the black kind of matter already stated to have been vomited and purged, and even in some cases where this had not happened before death. In others, the inner surface of the intestines was covered with the red bloody-looking matter before mentioned to have been passed by stool. The blood vessels of the stomach and intestines, in many parts, were very much dilated so as to give a red and vascular appearance to such parts. This was very general but not universal even when the stomach contained matter of black vomit. All persons that die in General Hospital here, with very few exceptions indeed, are examined after death; and I have made it a point for some years to examine the stomachs particularly for which purpose I have then taken out of the bodies and laid open from one orifice to the other, along the lesser arch so as to expose to view the entire inner surface, very generally I have found one part of the stomach on the posterior side, towards the lesser arch, and the cardiac orifice vascular in a remarkable degree. In one man of the 3rd W.I. Regiment who died suddenly, while standing sentry in this hospital, in consequence of the diseased state of the coats of the aorta which formed a pouch on one side ulcerated in different points, one of which having suddenly given way caused his immediate death. This stomach which contained a hearty meal half-digested on examination the following day was found vascular in an extraordinary degree, and in some parts dark coloured, so that it struck me at the moment, had he died of fever, it would have probably been considered as inflamed and gangrened. I was therefore not so much surprised at the vascular appearances of the stomachs, which I meet with at Tobago. In a few, the entire inner coat appeared as if stained with the dark-coloured fluid lying on it, in some others it was only so in patches, or points which gave it a variegated or mottled appearance. In a few, small spots of blood were observed effused under the external coat of the intestines, having the appearance of Ecchymosis, in several where the coats of the small intestines being distended with wind were thin and transparent, the contents appearing through, gave them a dark appearance, but on cutting into them the cause was at once discernable. In no instance did I find the coats disorganized or their texture injured so as with any propriety they could be considered to have gangrened.

 In the very first subject I examined at Tobago, there was no increased vascularity of stomach, though it contained the matter of black vomit, nor indeed any other satisfactory appearance to account for death, in talking over this with Mr Panting afterwards he related an instance of a child, whom he had examined before my arrival, whose stomach was found to contain the black matter, with a similar want of any appearance of increased vascularity. I have myself also witnessed a few other similar instances. It is, therefore, manifestly not essential either to the production of the fever or the appearance of black vomit, from which and considering the nature of the symptoms in the early stage, that if present would indicate it, those actually appearing in the latter stage which are more correspondent, and the effects of the means used, I conceive when it does take place, not to be of a primary but of a secondary nature, and the effect of the disease itself, in the same manner as we observe in parts under view at the same period passive haemorrhages to occur from we may suppose a similar dilatation of the smaller blood vessels. In a few where Dysuria had been troublesome (independent of any application of blisters) and which was also a late symptom, I was led to look into the bladder and found a similar dilatation of the blood vessels observable there.

In seeking for a sufficient cause to account for the production and prevalence of this disease, could I be content with the favourite doctrine of marsh miasma being the sole cause of all such, and were the circumstances attending it compatible with such a supposition. I should have an easy task to perform. Were all the endemic and epidemic fevers of warm climates so nearly allied, as to have but one common origin and cause, they should possess a similarity of character, and require an agreement in the mode of treatment, but which medicine would be much simplified and made easy to those practising it. I am well aware, I know by experience that wherever this cause exists, it is constant uniform and certain in its operation and effect, that of producing fever of a peculiar kind even to a destructive degree, and which is in consequence the constant endemic of such situations. I mean the term miasma in a more limited sense than it is now generally received, that from evident marshy and uncleared grounds usually neglected by man, where in consequence from heat and moisture there is a constant round of rapid vegetation, growth, decay and putrefaction sensible from the offensive smell occasioned thereby, particularly in the mornings and evenings. I cannot mean any exhalation caused by mere vegetation, which as far as chemistry informs us, has a salubrious useful tendency, in causing noxious gases to be absolved and disappear, and more pure and vital ones essential to life to be emitted. But on the contrary, that arises from decay and putrefaction. While man appears to be thus deservedly punished for neglect and indolence in not tilling and applying the ground to its proper use, it is hardly reasonable to suppose that in return for his labour and industry properly applied he should receive pestilence and death as the fruit of it. Indeed, from the general acceptation of the word miasma and the ideas which prevail on it, no part of the earth cultivated or not would be free from the imputation of causing sickness by the supposed production of such.

Certainly, very convenient for the physician who would always thus have a ready cause at hand to account for any sickness that might occur. I am led into these remarks from the stronghold, that what I conceive to be very erroneous ideas seem to have taken off the minds of many persons. A medical gentleman walking near a cane field, on his observing the canes growing luxuriantly, though no weeds or moisture was to be seen on the ground, turned up his nose thinking that he perceived miasmata. Another looking at a field to windward of his quarters which was dry and cultivated and where even vegetation was scanty, asked me if it was not apprehended that deleterious miasma would arise from it. Such theorists by a little ingenuity of reasoning (and it certainly requires some) contrive to extract miasma to suit their purpose from the arid Rock of Gibraltar and even onboard English ships of war to form artificial swamps (very artificial ones indeed) by means of the solid timber cut down for fuel, so as to constitute (in their minds) hot-beds for the production of miasma, when necessary for the occasion of accounting for sickness.

In perfect conformity with what I should have expected from such considerations has been the result of my observation as far as it has gone, wherever marshy ground was to be found in the vicinity and to windward of a station or town, whether on a height as at Morne Fortune, St Lucia, at very trifling elevation above the sea as in the gorge between the Cabrits of Prince Ruperts, Dominica, the low town of Basseterre, Guadeloupe, all the low country about Pointe-à-Pitre of the same island, and I understand the very low sands of Demerara and Berbice. The constant and uniform consequence is the prevalence of an endemic of the intermittent kind, requiring the determined use of bark for its treatment, and which though sometimes under aggravating, or particular circumstances perhaps of season, or concentration and intensity of cause may assume the continued form, and rival in severity the worst kind of fever. Yet when in such cases it does not prove early fatal, in general gradually, it runs into and terminates in the intermittent form, requiring bark for its removal, apt to recur on every slight occasion, and to be complicated with every complaint that may attack the patient at an after period of life frequently rendering the treatment of such excessively delicate and difficult, so certain and correspondent are the effects to the cause, that on visiting a hospital and seeing the kind of fevers in it, may be at once determined whether marshy grounds are to be found in the neighbourhood so formed or situated as to have any effect, and vice versa on examining the country around can be certainly seen, whether intermittents are frequent or even at all to be met with in the hospital.

In this island Barbados, throughout cleared and cultivated, where as far as I have seen, nothing like marshy ground is to be found, but in some sandy patches (I allude principally to Oistins) close to the seashore, where the water seems to have free ingress and egress, sensibly rising and falling with the tide, therefore not stagnant nor attended with putrescency. The fevers whether of the ordinary kind constantly occurring, or the malignant one in its occasional visitations, never put on this appearance. But one of an acute nature speedily terminating either in recovery or death, ceasing of themselves without the use of bark and even less apt to recur after an attack than before.

How then can diseases evidently so widely different in their nature, and requiring such different treatment, with any plausibility or appearance of truth or reason, be considered to be the same in kind, and to have the same cause and origin, even in direct opposition to the very testimony of our senses. While therefore it is most freely admitted that wherever such cause actually exists and in such places, it is obvious and evident to the senses, it is pernicious by the production in consequence of the miasmata, emanating there from, of an endemic constantly prevailing, though in different degrees and wherever it predominates greatly, so highly so, as to render some such places even uninhabitable.

The remarkable fever in the island of Edam mentioned by Mr Johnson[4] appears to have been of this kind, as he mentions in page 176 of his first edition "several of them changed into obstinate Intermittents at sea with great derangement of the liver, spleen and bowels" which is supposed to have been the case with nearly all that were not early carried off by it from the sentences immediately preceding the one quoted – viz "several officers, seamen and soldiers were sent on board from this island in hopes that change of air might mitigate the disease, many of even the worst cases of these would promise fair for a few hours in the forenoon; night always dispelled our hopes for then the patients relapsed as bad as ever; they almost all died. But their fate was considerably procrastinated, many of them lingering out a great length of time, sinking at last from the consequence of the fever rather than from the fever itself". The last sentence but one points our pretty clearly the nature of the fever by the distinct remissions or intermissions of the morning and the evident exerbations[5] or paroxysms or relapses as they are termed of the night and the first quoted one stated the consequences that proved fatal to the more procrastinated cases mentioned in the last. Of course, there are sufficient facts and evidence to prove that this fever was not contagious. Is it, therefore, philosophical to suppose or argue, that there can be fever from no other source and that this must be the sole one of all kinds and descriptions of fevers, even of wide spreading epidemics breaking out at uncertain, perhaps distant periods, in its progress not sparing even the driest situations and those usually most healthy, preserving and maintaining the same uniformity of symptoms and character different from that of the former, and the same destructive malignity in all places however differently situated, even on board ships at sea if any [infected individuals or sources] are once received into them. On looking over the history of the epidemic of those islands, particularly of Barbados, given by Dr Bancroft, I find the first one noticed to have been in this island in the year 1647, more than twenty years after its settlement, having suddenly broke out in the month of August, and in a short time proved so destructive "that the living were hardly able to bury the dead" stated to have been "very infectious" to have extended to St Christophers, the French islands, and even "our plantations in America" as has also happened in more modern times, and then again to have ceased for another very long period. This perfectly corresponds with the usual accounts of contagious epidemics but is altogether inconsistent with all we know of marsh miasma. Thus for more than twenty years, when any miasma that the island was capable of producing may be fairly supposed to have been most abundant, from the uncultivated, uncleared and neglected state of it and the inhabitants but newly arrived from a cold climate, unassimilated to a warm one, therefore particularly disposed and liable to be acted upon by such, yet it was only after this long period had passed over that it was supposed to operate in so severe and violent a manner, and then again to have ceased acting, and to have lain dormant for many more years. Wherever swamps at the present day are to be found capable of emitting miasmata injurious in a high degree as at Pointe-à-Pitre, Guadeloupe, Prince Ruperts, Dominica, they are pretty uniform and constant in their operations and effects every year. For from the well-known regularity of the return of the wet and dry seasons in every year, there are few or none, in which there are not periods of continued and excessive drought or moisture during their respective seasons or of any intermediate states, which joined with the uniformly high temperature so generally prevailing in this climate may be best suited to give the highest degree of activity or virulence to the miasmas proceeding there from.

    I know of no swamps acting in this extraordinary manner, remaining inactive for many years, then after distant uncertain intervals suddenly bursting forth, throwing out their noxious miasmata as if in an explosive manner, so as to prove highly destructive for a short time and soon to rest again for another long period, thus resembling volcanoes in their eruptions. Many other similar reflections from the history of these epidemics occur to my mind too tedious for the limits of this report. I shall, therefore, content myself with concluding that from very numerous facts and circumstances it appears to be fairly established, that endemic fevers constantly prevailing in the vicinity of marshes, evidently proceeding from marsh miasma and the epidemic ones occasionally raging in these as well as in others, even the most dry and healthy situations to be two very distinct diseases, and to proceed from very different causes. I believe that it is an undoubted fact that for some years previous to 1816 no fever as an epidemic prevailed in any of the islands and in consequence the new regiments that arrived within that period. The York Chasseurs then but lately raised, and 4th Battalion 60th which arrived in 1812 after being entirely newly formed in England in 1811 did not suffer in any remarkable degree nor did the seamen on board the ships of war of the squadron under the command of Sir Charles Durham that came to and served in the command during the same period. But since then, the scene has completely changed a malignant fever having broken out at Guadeloupe about the latter end of May or beginning of June in 1816, which soon spread over that island and from thence to the neighbouring one Antigua, and the other French one Martinique, afterwards on the removal of troops on surrendering that island to the French to some of the ships of war that conveyed them, and to some other English islands that they were conveyed to, as this one and Grenada, which caused great havoc among the seamen, troops and inhabitants and according to every account at least fully as much to the French as English.

The following year, it reached Dominica, which I have before reported on, and Trinidad affecting however only the inhabitants the troops very properly by the advice of the late Staff Surgeon Safe[6] having been kept out of the way of it in the country at St Joseph. But on being quartered in town the following year 1818, after a few months it reached them, and they also suffered in a similar manner while the inhabitants who had gone through it the preceding year, I understood retained their ordinary state of health. This year 1818 was the period also of its attacking Tobago, though I am more immediately concerned of its prevalence at St Christopher's in its usually destructive manner, even at that generally healthy station, Brimstone Hill. I am also informed of its committing dreadful ravages on the Spanish Main. Having thus in the course of these three years traversed successively most of these islands and in each running its course in a short space of time, in all preserving the same malignity of character, showing the same train of symptoms and producing the same direful destructive effects, I hope it may now have closed and terminates its career here, and that by proper precautionary measures for the future its reoccurrence may be prevented, which I conceive to be very possible.

It is melancholy to reflect on the number of lives that have been lost, that might have been saved could it have been arrested and put a stop to early in its progress. At Tobago to windward of the garrison at a short distance lies the Bacolet Swamp, and in consequence fever of the intermittent kind is the prevailing endemic there, but the swamp not being great in extent and in a sandy soil (which however I was told was rather artificial from having been one filled up with sand) and near the sea beach, does not appear to have been productive of very noxious miasma or pernicious in any very high degree. That the fever I am now treating of, and which is the subject of this report, did not proceed from this cause and was [in no] way connected with it, but on the contrary, of the same kind as the epidemic malignant that had been spreading from island to island, and had already affected the neighbouring ones, I infer from the following considerations. Had it merely proceeded from the miasmata of the marsh rendered particularly noxious and pernicious from any peculiarity [the same would] have happened to the other marshes of the island at the same time and in an equal degree, so as to have produced similar and simultaneous effects in different parts, contrary to what was found to be the case as before stated.

It is to be observed that the northerly winds had set in as usual at that time of the year before the fever commenced, and continued to blow steadily during the entire prevalence of it from the northward of east while the swamp lies to the southward of east at least E.S.E. of the garrison [so that] none of the miasmas from it could therefore have then reached the town or garrison. But while the character, symptoms, progress and effects were perfectly corresponding to those of the malignant fever when prevailing in the other islands they differed altogether from those usually appearing in or attendant on the endemic of this one. Though in some of the soldiers old Trinidad subjects liable to frequent recurrence of intermittent fever from the slightest cause, paroxysins[7] of it were observed to succeed the other and come on during convalescence from it, in many others as the civilians not thus prone to it this was by no means observable. On the contrary, I have mentioned the case of one young man where the fever was protracted too far in the third week which put on the typhoid character preserving the continued never changing to the intermittent form and which perfectly coincided with what happened in all other such cases that might be fairly considered as pure ones of this particular kind of fever. And I have observed even in some cases where the intermittent did succeed, a distinct interval between the termination of the one and the commencement of the other, so that the latter seemed to come on during the debility of convalescence from the former and not like a continuation of the same disease by the one gradually running into the other without interruption. From the annexed abstract of the returns of sick at Tobago during twelve successive years may be seen the effects of the ordinary endemic fever constantly prevailing there from the operation of ordinary causes.

Here follows the statement:

Table 12.1: Sick at Tobago

Date	Corps	Strength	Admit	Died	Remarks
1806	Royal Artillery	21			First inserted in the monthly ordnance
	1st Battery Royals	207	276	13	
	1st West India Reg	109	58	5	
		337	334	18 1/18*	*of the strength
1807	Royal Artillery	26	46	2	
	1st Battery Royals	250	252	20	"
	1 W.I. Regiment	103	170	5	
		379	468	27 1/14	

Date	Corps	Strength	Admit	Died	Remarks
1808	Royal Artillery	25	27	3	
	1st Battery Royals	272	405	12	"
	1st W.I. Regiment	87	60	1	
		384	492	16 1/24	
1809	Royal Artillery	21	21	2	
	1st Battery Royals	273	350	11	"
	8 West India	90	40	2	
		384	411	15 1/25 ½	
1810	Royal Artillery	21	16	1	
	1st Battery Royals	289	450	15	"
	8 West India	89	20	0	
		399	486	16 1/25	
1811	Royal Artillery	20	25	1	
	1st Battery Royals	273	467	15	"
	3rd West India	58	16	2	
		351	508	18 1/19 ½	
1812	Royal Artillery	18	29	1	
	1st Battery Royals	200	82	5	
	2nd Battery 60th	296	410	18	"
	90 Regiment	105	42	0	
	3rd West India	55	3	1	
		674	566	25 1/27	
1813	Royal Artillery	17	16	0	
	2nd Battery 60th	92	95	0	
	90th Regiment	105	142	6	"
	3rd West India	77	57	2	
		291	310	8 1/36 ½	

Reports from Tobago

Date	Corps	Strength	Admit	Died	Remarks
1814	Royal Artillery	20	21	0	
	2nd Battery 60th	91	111	5	
	Royal York Rangers	106	307	7	"
	3rd W. India	75	32	0	
		292	471	12 1/24 1/2	
1815	Royal Artillery	19	9	0	
	Royal W.I. Rangers	240	222	10	
	4th Battery 60th	183	141	2	"
	3 West India	74	50	3	
		516	422	15 1/34 1/3	
1816	Royal Artillery	14	23	1	
	4 Battery 60th	179	63	1	
	York Chasseurs	420	637	21	"
	Royal York Rangers	191	163	14	
	6 West India	173	61	1	
		977	947	38 1/25 2/5	
1817	Royal Artillery	19	19	3	The numerous deaths this year, I was informed, arose from the many sick sent from Trinidad to this island for change of air affected with dropsies. Dysentery, intermittent fevers and other chronic complaints of which they died in hospital.
	Royal York Rangers	256	461	59	
	6 W. India	162	105	3	
		437	585	65	

In 1805, when the malignant epidemic is known to have prevailed in other islands, I find that the 1st Battery Royal Scots or a detachment of it 236 strong, which had but just arrived from some other island, lost between 21 October and 20 November, twenty-four men; and

21 November and 20 December, twenty-two; and 21 December and January, seven, in the course of three months, fifty-three, nearly one-fourth of the entire, similar to what happened lately. On its thus breaking out there last December, the symptoms, appearances and manner of spreading through individuals were so very different from what Mr Panting had been in the habit of seeing for several years before, that in his very first communication on the subject previous to my arrival he announced it as a distinct disease from ordinary ones and to be highly contagious. The opinion and evidence of an officer of such long and extensive experience in the West Indies in general and that island in particular and so highly respectable ought surely to have no small weight. I annex the answers to my queries on these points of Assistant Surgeon Palmer Royal York Rangers*, a gentleman that had been at least four or five years in the country and has had experience even in his own person of some of the principal diseases, in 1815 at Basseterre in Guadeloupe having suffered severely from acute fever terminating in obstinate intermittent in consequence of which for change of air he moved to Beau-Soleil and afterwards to this island Barbados.

Copy

*__Query__ – Do you suppose the fever that has proved so fatal here to be the same as that ordinarily prevailing every year, only differing in degree from it or different in kind?

Reply – As far as my own observation has led me to form an opinion, I have no hesitation in saying that it is essentially different in kind.

Query – From your observation in hospital do you suppose it to be contagious?

Reply – I have not the smallest doubt of its having been communicated by contagion amongst the patients in hospital as well as some of the orderlies

Signed
C.J. Palmer
Assistant Surgeon
Royal York Rangers

He was very early attacked by the malignant fever at Tobago in a very severe manner and which did not terminate like the former one. Mr McAvoy from casual remarks I have heard him make I am pretty confident entertained the same opinions, but I did not wish to draw any from him a young man just entering the practice of the profession but rather leave them to be matured by further experience. Among the inhabitants generally the same opinion prevailed and which I believe contributed in no small degree to shorten the duration of the disease, having from the precautions adopted saved many from it. Of the civil practitioners that I had an opportunity of conversing with, I did not hear a single one offer a dissenting opinion, and as for myself, I can only say that the numerous facts I witnessed there only tended to corroborate and confirm the opinion formerly given by me, having in the first instance originated in and been founded entirely on facts that fell under my observation before I had hardly given the subject thought, but the correctness of which I am fully satisfied of by much varied subsequent experience. Where the occurrence of fever was not unusual and the first cases not being necessarily the most severe, fatal or even strongly marked ones, and as it came on in an unexpected manner, not suspected until it had appeared in all its violence. It is not so easy to point out the first cases even of admission into hospital from it. I find by the expenditure return of 24 December that on the 1st of that month, one man, Corporal Doyle, died of fever, after having been twelve days in hospital and two others were dismissed same day viz John Jacob marked common continued fever, seven and Thomas Canes Quotidian intermittent fourteen days in hospital. On the 4th were admitted two fever cases that terminated favourably; on the 6th James Primrose marked the first day of admission for ulcer and the second for thin fever of which he died on the 10th of the month. The number of admissions after this became more numerous; the disease may be considered as decidedly in the hospital and [as it] began to spread to the other patients. Serjeant John Hunt lingering in hospital under other ailment was suddenly attacked with an accession of fever bearing the character of this one, which carried him off on the 9th.

Private B. Raddock, who had been in hospital since the 21st of the former month on account of ulcer, was attacked with fever on the 11th of this one and died on the 19th, with the regular black vomit. Mr Palmer the medical officer in charge and attendance on the hospital was about this time also taken ill with fever, from which after a most severe attack he very slowly recovered. I requested Mr McAvoy to make out a return for me of all persons that he could learn that were employed about the sick, stating whether attacked with the fever or not and any remarks as to their length of residence in the climate or previous attacks of fever that he might clearly ascertain, a copy of which I transmit annexed.

Table 12.2: List of Persons Employed about the Sick in the Garrison or Hospital, Tobago, between November 1818 and March 1819

Names	Occupation	Remarks	Period	Remarks
Serjeant I. Gioran	Steward	Not attacked	Native	A coloured man; had fever in Barbados in 1808
P. Jas Thompson	Orderly	Attacked and recovered	10 years	Had fever in Guadeloupe in 1811
William Prowse	Ditto	Attacked and died	3 years	Had been 6 months at Grenada and 2 yrs at Tobago
A. Curry	Ditto	Attacked and died	8 years	Had fever in Barbados time not exactly known
William Lockhart	Ditto	Attacked and recovered	3 years	Was only two days orderly when taken ill with fever
Corporal Barnes	Clerk	Attacked and recovered	7 years	Had been in the islands of Grenada, Guadeloupe and Martinique, and 3 years in Tobago. Had 3 attacks of intermittent fever last year
William Greenhalsh	Cook	Attacked and recovered	7 years	Had intermittent fever in Trinidad
G. Bourdearsy	Orderly	Not attacked	7 years	A native of the East Indies
B. Sinicher	Ditto	Not attacked	7 years	Had fever at Barbados shortly after arrival in W. Indies
I. Bennet	Ditto	Not attacked		Orderly but for two days

Reports from Tobago

Names	Occupation	Remarks	Period	Remarks
Jno: Foy	Ditto	Attacked and recovered		
Jno Hydeck	Ditto	Not attacked	7 years	Had fever in Trinidad
P. Callaghan	Cook	Not attacked	5 years	Had fever in Trinidad
Jo Parsons	Servant	Attacked and died	3 years	Attended the Lieutenant
Flora	Washer-Woman	Attacked and recovered	Africans	Washed the hospital linen
Victoria	Ditto	Attacked and recovered		
Mr Power	Servant	Attacked and recovered		Was servant to Lieutenant Fothergill
M. Burke	Servant	Attacked and died	7 years	Was servant to Captain O'Keefe
L. Daly	Servant	Attacked; still in hospital	8 years	Servant to Captain O'Keefe
S. Chander	Servant	Attacked and recovered	5 years	Was servant at Government House when the fever prevailed there
Mrs Beneditt	Washer-woman	Attacked and died	African	Washed for the convalescents previous to their going into Bks
O'Connor	Orderly	Not attacked	African	A negro

Names	Occupation	Remarks	Period	Remarks
Ins. Harrison		Attacked and died	African	
Ins. Bateman		Attacked and died	African	
Isaac Newton	Pioneers	Attacked and recovered	African	Attended the sick and slept in hospital
I. Hancy		Attacked and recovered	African	
I. Steward		Attacked and recovered	African	
Clifton			African	
Andrews			African	
O'Brian			African	
Blankly			African	Employed about the out work of the hospital in cutting wood for the cooks carrying water rations, provisions and so on from town
Bruce	Pioneers	Not attacked	African	
Moffatt			African	
Kemil			African	
Kennedy			African	
Yankee			African	
Boyer	Servant	Attacked and recovered	African	Attended Mr Palmer when ill with fever
Morton	Pioneer	Attacked and recovered	African	Servant at Government House during the illness there

From this may be seen the number attending on the sick that were in consequence soon afterwards themselves attacked with the disease, but particularly deserving of attention as strongly corroborative in proof of the highly contagious nature of it are the deaths and attacks among the few African negroes that on account of the press of sickness were taken into the hospital to assist the orderlies in waiting on the sick and who as I was particularly informed by steward remained and slept in it at night. John Harrison died of it before my arrival I was told with the usual black vomit, Bateman I was myself present at the dissection of and have mentioned the black matter found in his stomach, three others mentioned in the return as in like manner exposed were attacked and admitted as patients with it, as was also the black washer-woman Flora. Mr Palmer's servant boy an African apprentice suffered from a severe attack during his master's illness and a black pioneer about Government House during the prevalence of sickness there while a remarkable immunity from it was particularly manifest throughout the numerous others, who from their employment as labourers were much exposed to the weather as well as any moisture or miasma that might be supposed floating in the atmosphere. They were quartered in barracks adjacent to the hospital, separated from it but a few yards by being advanced a little in front to Windward and being in a line of direction parallel to a continuation of that of the hospital it has therefore no advantage over it in point of situation. It is to be admitted that on the opposite side of the question there were a few individuals freely exposed to the contagion of the disease without being the least affected by it, Mr McAvoy who diligently attended the sick in hospital and who assisted at the dissections, and Lady Robinson who was most assiduous in her attentions to her husband and the child who died of it while ill without suffering are instances. But I believe similar ones are to be met with in other diseases allowed by all to be contagious and which only prove where a cause prevails so generally as to produce an epidemic that such subjects were not susceptible of being acted on by that cause whatever it may have been, but nothing whatever as to the particular nature of the cause itself. It will be asked from whence the contagion more immediately reached this island.

There are strong reasons for supposing from the Spanish Main various accounts from thence mentioned the severe ravages it was making there and communications with it are more frequent than with any of the islands. While I was there scarcely a week passed without some arrival from it. Mr Panting having heard of some seamen that were landed and left behind sick by a vessel that came from thence and who was suspected of having introduced the disease. I went with him to see and examine them and having made them out with some difficulty being in one of a group of poor small dwellings found two in a poor reduced state after the severity of fever, and from the account they gave of the sufferings of the crew from sickness, think they may have had this fever on board. But which also might be accounted for from other causes, as they mentioned that having cattle on board, they had frequently to go on shore to cut grass for them in damp marshy places and so on, and at all events the date of their arrival turned out to be a little subsequent to that of the commencement of the fever. Therefore, though I fully acquit them of having introduced it, I mention the circumstance to show the possibility of its having been thus introduced and which was likely to have remained a secret as a vessel thus landing and leaving behind sick seamen was by the laws of the island liable to a penalty and which was intended to have been inflicted on the vessel these men belonged to whenever it should again call there. Having heard Captain Knox mention in conversation some interesting circumstances on this head I requested him to state them in writing to one which he has been kind enough to do, and though not referring to this island but being much to the point in question, I forward annexed the copy of his letter on the subject.

Copy

St Ann's Barbados

Dear Sir

In compliance with your request, I beg leave to acquaint you that I was quartered with a detachment of my corps, the Royal W.I. Rangers, stationed at Brimstone Hill, St Kitts during 1818 at which time the fever raged violently in the garrison and throughout the island. Its first appearance in the garrison to the best of my recollection was in the latter part of the month of May, Gunner Neilson of the Royal Artillery died on 26 May. Prior to this death there had been frequent communications in the way of traffic between the small-town Sandy Point, St Kitts and the five islands so-called, laying between St Bartholomew's and St Martin's. At this place the patriotic fleet rendezvoused with such captures as they made in those seas. A fever had broken out at the island of Margarita, the depot of the patriotic army, and from whence several of the officers and soldiers came to the five islands, and from thence to Sandy Point, St Kitts to avoid the fever and distress which existed at that island (Margarita). I recollect an instance of one of the soldiers of the Venezuelan army having died at Sandy Point and several came over in a sickly state. This man Neilson of the artillery had been in the habit of visiting Sandy Point (about a mile and a half from the garrison) associating and receiving visits from some of his friends which were in that army, and I have no doubt but in his case the fever proved contagious.

Bombardier Watson visited Neilson during his sickness. Watson took the fever as also two of his children who died. Mrs Watson took ill immediately after, and two more children, all of whom died in the course of one week. In an adjoining hut to the late Watsons lived Gunner Bell who attended the deceased Mrs Watson and children. Bell took sick and died and in [a] few days two of his children died. In hospital it raged violently. I cannot say the number of deaths. Captain Stratton's (Royal Artillery) lady took ill on 5 October died on the 9th. Mrs Montgomery, wife of Ensign Montgomery, 1st W. I. Regiment who visited Mrs Stratton after her death took ill and died on the 17th. Captain Stratton died on the 23rd. Dr Morgan,[8] 1st W. I. Regiment who lived [in the] next room to Mrs Montgomery took ill after visiting Mrs Montgomery. He went to Basseterre for [a] change of air and died on the 24th. Various other instances I could adduce to prove that this fever is infectious but there have many instances occurred with different constitutions and habits of body who are not susceptible of this contagion that does not prove it is not so.

Arthur Esq.
MD
I have the honour to be
Signed *John Knox*
Captain 1st W.I. Regiment

According to reports among the inhabitants that had not experienced a similar visitation since 1801, when their loss and suffering from the same kind of fever was fully as great as lately, I was told by Dr Cummins that it was then generally considered to have been brought from Berbice in an American vessel which had lost several of her crew by it. They, therefore, seem not to have participated with the troops in their sickness of 1805 so short a time having elapsed (an interval of but a few years since they very generally passed through it themselves, similar to what happened last year at Trinidad).

In a former report on the malignant fever at Dominica in 1817, I adduced many instances showing a marked malignity of that disease causing excessive mortality wherever it has appeared though under great diversity of treatment, characteristic of an essential difference between it and the ordinary fever of dry cultivated situations, the common ardent fever or *causus*.

In instances [where] the two kinds of fever having prevailed at successive periods in the same corps, the 2nd or Queen's and to have attacked the same individuals in like manner, and again at the very same period and at the same place to have appeared in different bodies of men. Each kind of fever steadily preserving its uniformity of character under all circumstances and the difference between the two being marked and manifest though under similarity of time, place and treatment, having been treated by the same medical officer, the late Dr Wray in the same hospital. The one, in some cases, with high fever and apparently were symptoms but tractable yielding to treatment, attended but with little mortality and proving non-contagious. The other with perhaps less fever and apparently milder symptoms at first, extremely intractable under every mode of treatment that I have known attended with great mortality and proving highly contagious. Knowing the great faith that is generally put in the efficacy of bleeding in the treatment of all kinds of fevers in warm climates, which is certainly a very successful and the principal remedy in the one. I wished to show that notwithstanding its free use, in the other nearly the usual unvarying mortality attended it. I stated several facts in proof of this, and by chance having obtained was able to give a copy of a table that was made out of the practice in one hospital where during the prevalence of the epidemic some cases were treated with and others without bleeding with pretty equal success. In stating these facts, I intended merely to point out a marked and decided difference in the character of the two diseases and which I have since seen further strongly exemplified.

About the middle of last year, a batch of recruits principally or entirely from Porchester Castle, England, came out to join the regiment. They were destined for service in the command, when they got their liberty on shore and received some money, they gave loose to their inclinations committed every excess and irregularity and the rainy season being set in, frequently exposed themselves to the changes and inclemency of the weather. In consequence, fevers became rife amongst them, and I had soon two wards in General Hospital under my charge filled with fever cases from them, but which were totally devoid of malignity so that though several of them were in appearance sufficiently severe, they all yielded to treatment and terminated favourably, not one death occurring amongst them. As I am sensible, it may be said, and perhaps with some truth, that many would have recovered from the efforts of nature alone with little or no aid from medicine and that therefore so serious a remedy as bleeding was unnecessary. I feel it due in favour of it to mention the following remarkable circumstance, and which at the same time, I pointed out to Staff Surgeon Dr Hughes,[9] who was then here. Two men in rather advanced stages of fever were admitted from on board ship; they had not been bled at all during their illness though they had been previously, as a preventive (as to the utility and necessity of which I am by no means satisfied from this as well as other facts and circumstances). They recovered but very soon after, they suffered relapses which proved very severe, and from which they very narrowly, and with much difficulty, escaped. They were the only two fever cases out of two wards full then in hospital not bled.

The above fever in character and result corresponded pretty nearly with what I had witnessed for a succession of years at St Pierre, Martinique, as well as during different short periods that I served in this island before. But how widely different from what I met with the latter end of the same year and beginning of this one in the epidemic malignant at Tobago; where notwithstanding the utmost efforts of medicine, so very large a proportion of cases from it proved fatal, even among the healthiest subjects of which description were some of the soldiers and nearly all of the civilians. Perfectly similar to the effects and result from it in every situation wherever and whenever it has appeared.

The mischief caused by it in the other islands more recently must be fresh in the recollection of all, and may be yet remembered by many the devastations committed by it on four occasions, for instance in 1804 at Antigua, when General Dunlop, the officer commanding there, and of the 70th Regiment, quartered on the heights; thirteen officers, including the surgeon and upwards of two hundred men were quickly carried off by it, and in the following year in this island, the 15th Regiment six hundred strong suffered in an equal degree, having in the course of July, August and September, lost also upwards of two hundred. The fate of General Myers and his family about that time cannot be forgotten – the 96th on the heights of Antigua were equal sufferers, and the 90th, divided between Fort Charlotte and Dorsetshire Hill, St Vincent, suffered also severely though in a less degree, having lost more than one hundred men.

I have just before me the report of Mr Mortimer Naval Surgeon published in the 13th no. *Medico Chirurgical* journal and reviews page 13, where he details some of the effects in the Navy as follows: "In the Naval Hospital, Antigua during the months of October, November and December 1810. Of 622 Fevers, 127 died in December alone. Of 360 fever patients, 133 died." This will receive further elucidation by reference to a few particular ships the *Paerlin* before and after the commencement of the quarter was visited so severely by sickness that according to the report of the surgeon, the diminution of sickness seemed only influenced by the diminution of numbers.

Table 12.3: Deaths of Non-commissioned Officers and Privates in the Army Serving in the Windward and Leeward Colonies for 12 Years, from 1 January 1796 to 31 December 1807

Years	1-Jan		January		February		March	
	White	Black	White	Black	White	Black	White	Black
1796	15.457	491	67	0	75	0	100	0
1797	14.458	251	600	0	289	3	286	1
1798	12.722	928	148	0	139	6	110	6
1799	8.752	3.657	119	11	86	14	90	6
1800	8.971	4.387	63	20	75	15	60	21
1801	9.435	4.997	120	23	114	13	49	13
1802	4.841	4.706	110	18	106	17	83	10
1803	8.501	3.556	54	20	39	15	33	15

Reports from Tobago

Years	1-Jan		January		February		March	
	White	Black	White	Black	White	Black	White	Black
1804	7.849	3.861	124	10	86	9	90	8
1805	7.467	3.991	91	19	78	20	49	9
1806	8.279	4.861	159	16	84	50	64	22
1807	7.717	5.91	81	48	49	27	54	29
TOTAL			1736	185	1220	189	1068	140

Years	April		May		June		July	
	White	Black	White	Black	White	Black	White	Black
1796	200	1	365	1	370	3	485	2
1797	334	2	131	2	215	1	234	7
1798	165	1	78	13	129	5	180	22
1799	73	15	91	16	84	20	75	14
1800	55	20	89	27	187	35	184	22
1801	87	14	221	24	280	22	347	35
1802	67	100	61	14	54	17	95	28
1803	72	13	57	12	46	14	72	12
1804	93	13	107	32	125	14	235	17
1805	64	24	92	37	88	15	172	15
1806	43	24	57	14	56	17	65	23
1807	47	41	48	18	70	36	76	41
TOTAL	1300	268	1397	210	1704	199	2220	238

Years	August		September		October		November	
	White	Black	White	Black	White	Black	White	Black
1796	922	8	949	6	1273	0	894	1
1797	344	1	331	2	370	7	534	6
1798	156	30	143	28	190	17	191	15
1799	57	33	96	30	71	19	96	20
1800	162	29	123	34	115	29	111	13
1801	312	26	312	22	334	32	196	26
1802	87	27	127	8	109	21	68	15
1803	100	10	108	15	156	15	138	23

Years	August		September		October		November	
	White	Black	White	Black	White	Black	White	Black
1804	301	26	222	17	151	10	174	23
1805	347	13	237	16	298	62	165	38
1806	101	32	107	23	68	20	99	39
1807	105	47	126	33	124	42	83	30
TOTAL	2994	282	2881	234	3259	274	2749	249

Years	December	
	White	Black
1796	905	3
1797	378	2
1798	160	16
1799	68	36
1800	106	21
1801	122	26
1802	49	15
1803	118	16
1804	105	33
1805	219	14
1806	86	34
1807	81	21
TOTAL	2397	237

(The following note was attached to the above Table)
"The same thing will appear from the following Table of Deaths in this command alone for 12 years during which this disease prevailed so frequently and extensively being kept up or reviewed in various places by the constant [arrival] of fresh subjects and the frequent reinforcements and changes of troops. Compared with the well-known state of the West Indies as to health for a long period of several years, before the commencement of it in 1793, as well as during a subsequent one between the close of 1810 or 1811 and the reappearance of this disease in 1816 at Guadeloupe."

The *Thetis* in November sent 182 to hospital, of whom 84 died. The *Nyaden* about the same time lost thirty-three of ninety-eight sent to the same place and immediately afterwards fourteen on board and ten out of thirty-four sent to hospital on arriving at Barbados again. Yet out of twenty men constituting nearly the whole of the crew of the *Grouper* sent to hospital, eight died, of thirty-four from the barracks eleven died, of seventeen from the *Forrester*, six died, of nineteen from the *Demerara* ten died, of fourteen from the *Laura*, seven died and of six from the *Balahou* three died. This statement is certainly intended to prove the unhealthiness of the situation of that hospital. Was the effect more constant and uniform, I would readily admit the cause assigned and should only wonder that such a situation could have been first chosen for a hospital or that it should have been so long occupied at the present day by the military for the accommodation of the sick, of all the white troops at Antigua, without such sad effects being produced and that also it was not productive of such to Admiral Durham's squadron, I am led to imagine that the excessive mortality stated must have proceeded from other sources. Not inapplicable is the account that Mr Halcrow, late gunner of the *Childers*, who died in this hospital of consumption, gave [of] one of the different fevers he had laboured under in this climate, which I requested him to do, when he mentioned that he had been on board the *Childers* all the time the fever raged in her so violently, even when cleaning out at Antigua without being at all affected. He stated that in 1805 at Trinidad in His Majesty's Ship of War, *Dart*, he suffered severely from fever, when the captain, surgeon and fifty-three others in all died out of ninety, the total number on board and that in 1807 he had a brain fever, as he termed it, attended with high delirium on board His Majesty's Ship *Northumberland*, and that at the same time others had the same fever, but none died of it and that these were all the fevers he had during fourteen years' service in the West Indies. The former, a good instance of the malignant with great mortality, and the latter of the common fever from ordinary causes with strong symptoms and but trifling mortality.*

He, at the same time, mentioned the case of the *Nyaden*, already alluded to in extracts from Mr Mortimer's report, which he mentioned to have been attacked with the fever off Suriname (where according to his statement it seems to have commenced and not at Antigua) and between there and Antigua and others, out of 210 to have lost

116 persons including the captain and the lieutenant of marines and also that another vessel one of the Danish frigates that was afterwards made into a troop ship but the name of which he forgot was attacked soon afterwards at the same place in a similar manner and with as great loss there, on the passage thence and at Antigua, which I suppose they resorted to when such alarming sickness broke out, for the convenience of the hospital and which would thus account for the great number then in hospital there.

I would, therefore, divide under three distinct heads the principal fevers to be such with in warm climates particularly among the whites commonly confounded together under one common appellation yellow fever. First, that arising from marsh miasma, prevailing at least some time every year in the neighbourhood of marshes and only to be found in such situations. [It manifests] of the intermittent kind, though varying in type and form, requiring in some part of its course before its termination, in cases, in general, the use of bark for its removal. After being removed, [it is] remarkably apt to recur so that persons having once laboured under it became more liable to subsequent attacks than they were to the first one; [this fever] is non-contagious.

Second, the causes of ardent fever, the common endemic from ordinary causes in dry situation, of the continued kind (according to Dr Cullens's[10] division of fevers) with a tendency to terminate spontaneously, not requiring the use of bark for its removal, and after thus terminating, not leaving any aptitude to. But on the contrary, rather some security against its recurrence, so that a person once affected becomes less liable to subsequent attacks than they were to the first one, non-contagious and devoid of malignity, though attended with high fever and apparently severe symptoms usually yielding to treatment and particularly to the use of the Lancet so as to be attended with mortality in no high degree. This may properly be subdivided into two varieties that arising from slight causes in those lately arrived or as they are termed newcomers, and that in older subjects requiring a stronger cause to operate on them and in whom from the usual habits, particularly among the soldiers in this country, it is apt to be complicated with diseased viscera.

Third, the epidemic malignant fever appearing only occasionally, at uncertain, sometimes distant periods, spreading successively through all different kinds of places and situations, as chance directs it, by bringing subjects from or those destined to such situations, under the influence of its contagion, attended with extreme malignity so as even under milder appearances uniformly to cause great mortality, proving highly contagious and from which I have not known a single well authenticated instance of second attacks.

Those not attending to such distinctions, but who jumble together all under one common head of yellow fever can, of course, produce innumerable. In my report on the epidemic malignant at Dominica in 1817, I mentioned a few positive instances of persons that had passed through the disease before and who were then again exposed to the cause of it, without being affected. I mentioned the governor in whose family the disease had appeared, his nephew, secretary to him having been sick with it, without his being affected having had it before. The older practitioners of medicine who, in the course of their daily avocations, must have been fully exposed to whatever may be considered as cause escaped, while the younger ones not having had it before suffered.

I have now to instance Mr Panting and myself again, he having had it in the year 1795 or 96 at Martinique when it raged there so severely and I had it in 1810 at Gibraltar Bay in the transports from Cartagena in consequence though engaged among the sick from early in the morning until late at night, for some days unable to sit down to our dinner until after 9:00 p.m., and then not without interruption, consequently not without experiencing no small degree of personal fatigue and mental anxiety yet throughout escaped. Mr Halcrow in the *Childers* the circumstances of whose case I have a little before related is another strong instance. I am also able to add [the] remarkable circumstance of Captain Hyde, 1st W.I. Regiment and his wife escaping it at St Kitts last year, though most freely exposed to it there (as he told me) in repeatedly visiting the hospital while it prevailed, acting frequently as officer of the day, nearly all the others being sick, in visiting and assisting his brother officers when ill with it, which he said he did freely, not being apprehensive of any ill consequences from so doing and she also in visiting their wives who were ill and some of whom died of it. I mentioned him in my report on Dominica as having taken the disease by going from Prince Rupert's to Rousseau on a court martial while the fever prevailed there in 1817 and having gone there regularly through it. I understand his wife was also attacked by it soon after her husband and also went through it there, as they both informed me.

Could I offer any mode of treatment as certainly successful or that would reduce the mortality from this kind to a level with that from some other fevers as the endemic causes for instance, I should consider myself extremely fortunate and would derive no small degree of satisfaction and pleasure there from.

Persons that have at different times experienced great success in the treatment of the ordinary fevers to be met with in many situations in this climate particularly, have deceived themselves in believing them to be of this malignant kind, and have thus led others astray by confident assertions on this supposition. Some of the first cases that occurred at Tobago last year on being examined after death exhibited the vascular appearance of the stomach and the bowels which was supposed to indicate inflammation of these parts, it was therefore believed that the true nature of the disease was clearly ascertained, that the appropriate and certain remedy was equally manifest, and from which being carried fairly and fully into effect they entertained the fullest confidence of complete success from the positive statements of authors leading them to form such expectations but unfortunately to be disappointed. It was found to fail in some of the cases that seemed to bid fairest for it and the mortality notwithstanding still continued extremely great. On my arrival, I learned that they had found it necessary to restrict their bleedings within narrow bounds, in quantity not to exceed between twenty or thirty ounces, and to be very cautious how they repeated it in any case.

As far as my own experience warrants me to speak of it as a remedy in the fevers of this climate, I would say that in the common ardent fever of dry situations from ordinary causes it may be used with freedom and confidence, that it is the principal remedy and that much success may be expected from its proper use. In fevers of the intermittent kind at the commencement when in the continued form, in many cases I have seen it of use by moderating the fever and inducing remissions or intermissions during which bark might be administered thus tending towards the cure of, while at the same time I have seen in distinct paroxysms of this kind of fever followed by complete intermissions that high degree of fever and arterial action present which in the former would indicate the necessity of free venesection. But in this would be the height of rashness to interfere with and would have, I am convinced, the contrary tendency to that just stated, and which I apprehend I have actually seen happen. So much the more necessary is it to attend to the particular character and nature of the fever than to any particular set of symptoms and which should be held in view in the application of this remedy at any period in this kind of fever. In the malignant kind, I believe it may be used but with prudence, caution and moderation, as a palliative and to aid and promote the operation of other medicines as to be hereafter stated.

The use of mercury, the next principle and disputed remedy while recommended in the strongest manner by some as one of the most efficacious, [is] condemned by others as useless or even pernicious. A remedy not long since in the highest vogue for a variety of complaints, now fast sinking into disrepute, neglect and contempt. Thus, apt are medical men in particular to run into great extremes – I must say that while I have heard those who had been in the habit of using it freely speak highly in commendation of it, those loud in its dispraise were persons that from prejudice had never been partial to it or given it a fair trial, but who appeared to have been constantly on the lookout for opportunities to carp at and find fault with it. I never knew any person that had been once favourable and in consequence in the habit of using it freely, ever give it up from observing it, either inefficacious, or injurious, when used only with proper discretion.

In fevers of the intermittent kind and when in the intermittent form I have seen it show, I may say an anti-febrile effect, the disease having yielded to the bark as the mouth became affected which had before resisted it, and when in the continued form, as the mouth became sore, the fever intermitted, and in some few seemed to have ceased, but recurring again and becoming obstinate as the mouth got well.

In the common, continued ardent kind of fever I have been

likewise in the habit or using it as a purgative to open the bowels at first, throughout to keep them free and also so as to effect the system generally, I believe with good effect; as a purgative, the use of it is pretty generally admitted, and I certainly know none more convenient or efficacious that plain Calomel, or if necessary, followed and aided by saline purgative, the use of it also so as to affect the system in that variety of it complicated with diseased viscera is pretty generally allowed.

In the malignant kind in which we have to complain of so great a want of efficacious remedies, I would not readily give up so active a one likely to be of any use judging by analogy from its effects in the other kinds of fever, where the testimony in favour of it is so strong and one which can be conveniently used without interfering with the others. It was used freely in the fever at Tobago. I must admit that some whose mouths were fairly and fully affected, notwithstanding, died. However, the proportion of such was very small. Of course, the usual caution is necessary in the use of so active a medicine. It is unnecessary to excite ptyalism to a high or severe degree. The effects of the medicine on the system are frequently turned on the bowels producing there extremely painful symptoms and sensations resembling dysenteric ones and which if mistaken for part of the disease itself and the medicine pushed further, might terminate most unfavourably, but which on discontinuing the medicine and administering warm opiates, etc. are most certainly relieved and removed.

I have also seen the mercurial *erythema* with the fever and irritation attending it during the use of mercury for that malignant fever at Tobago. But which on discontinuing the medicine and from proper treatment disappeared as the disease itself had done. From any possible ill effects that might arrive from it this way, it is not right to argue against the proper application of it. It is not fair to argue against the use of a medicine from the abuse of it. The most violent poisons properly managed may be the most useful remedies.

Soon after my arrival, Mr Panting informed me that he had found warm bathing answer better than cold bathing or dashing with patients ill of this fever and which I could very readily suppose from what I observed of their states – cold bathing or dashing requiring a certain stamina or strength of constitution to produce a reaction in the system necessary for the beneficial consequences to be expected from it, but which appear deficient in general in these patients. The state of their bowels was throughout attended to being kept free and open. So that the usual course of treatment with these patients when admitted was first to have the head shaved ready for a blister as this was the part in many most complained of. They were bled until they felt relief in the head, etc, which was in general from a very moderate quantity seldom exceeding twenty-four oz or at furthest, thirty oz. This also relaxed their skin which was further promoted by their being immediately immersed in a warm (I may rather say vapour) bath for their means of heating water being but small and their bathing vessel merely a large wooden tub of an elliptical form, the warm water in it not deeper than a few inches which, however, being made as hot as the patient could well bear, he being laid supine in it and rug thrown over the top to confine in a great measure the steam, it answered extremely well, and produced general relaxation of the skin and a free perspiration on being taken out and covered up in bed.

After the bath a large blister was laid over the entire head and a dose of ten grains of Calomel administered to open the bowels, if necessary, followed by salts to produce that effect, and afterwards given in smaller quantities to keep the bowels free and affect the system. In many, the fever was immediately moderated, relief evident, and recovery generally progressive from this. In others, the fever continued with but little alterations, some of whom finally recovered, others died. In such, the mercury was pushed by being applied externally as well as administered internally so as to affect the system as speedily as possible. To relieve, after symptoms as vomiting, I have found Camphor and Opium, five grains of the former to one of the latter, effervescing draughts, blisters over the pit of the stomach, and a repetition of the warm bath sometimes successful. With Burke, Captain O'Keefe's servant before stated to have delirium to such high a degree and long continued, I had cold dashing applied very fully and repeatedly, but the issue of the case was unsuccessful.

The result of the above practice, considering the nature of the subjects I had to deal with was a very fair proportionate success, as

I find from the expenditure returns for January and February that of sixty-three patients in the garrison, forty-four of whom are distinctly marked as *Febris Continued (sic) Icterodes*,[11] that were taken ill between 1 January, about which time I commenced the superintendence of the treatment of the sick in hospital to 24 February, the date of the last of these returns, sixteen died.

Signed
John Arthur, MD
Physician to the Forces

Half-Yearly Report of Sick of the Troops at Tobago to 15 December 1818, by Staff Surgeon S. Panting

Tobago – 25 December 1818

There has been no change in this garrison since the last half-yearly report. It has been constituted as it then was by 15 men of the Royal Artillery, 200 of Royal York Rangers and 150 military labourers. The character and description of the York Rangers, has not improved such of the men as formed the detachments from Trinidad and who have survived the twelve months, since their arrival here, still retain the same cachectic appearance, have the same disposition to general and local dropsy, particularly of the chest and are capable of but little duty. The whole is almost without exception, dissolute and drunken; there is a great reluctance to punish both in the regimented officers and in the general commanding, but such is the enormity of their offences, that notwithstanding this, there are constant courts martial and frequent punishments, and nothing but the difficulty of assembling officers in this country, has preserved them from the severest sentences. This regiment is in daily expectation of being embarked for Canada and there to be disbanded. The military labourers are quiet and orderly; no discontent has been shown at their reduction as soldiers, the labour of the garrison, whether in building or in ordinary fatigue is entirely carried on by them and great cheerfulness.

The face of the country around the fort is the same as heretofore; no steps have been taken towards draining the swamp at Bacolet which remains as far as I can observe stationary. Within the last fortnight, much of the brush to windward has been cut down, and burnt by Fatigue Parties of the military labourers, and this it is intended continue.

The new buildings at the fort continue but slowly, the large Brick Barrack for the crew is just completed and now occupied by the Rangers. It is built upon arches six feet in height, is dry, and well-ventilated, and bids fair to be a healthy quarter. The aspect of the long front is south-east. The new hospital is but little advanced. The principal walls are furnished, but the roof is still wanting and it will require many months to complete it. No foundation is yet laid for the officers' barracks, the houses for the staff officers or any of the other buildings which are projected within the fort.

There have been, at all times, medical inspections in this garrison, more or less frequent, according to the health of the men. The object of these inspections has been to prevent soldiers from concealing their complaints or having sores out of hospital. The convalescents in barracks are paraded daily and either dismissed to their duty or returned there as the surgeon judges necessary.

By perseverance and care, the ulcers have been reduced to nothing. The chronic diseases of the crew from Trinidad have occasionally been troublesome, several of this description have died, worn out, and perfectly exhausted by long suffering.

The weather during the greater part of the period has been sultry and oppressive. From June to November there was no diversity; the thermometer in the shade stood generally at eighty-nine and was often during the night at eighty-three. The winds were light and southerly. The rains were general and frequent, and sometimes during the night violent there was more thunder and lightning than is usual in this island. No planter had witnessed so favourable a season, or one that promised such abundance towards the middle of November, the weather became cooler, and there was more rain, but the winds were still southerly.

In the first days of December, there was a sudden and perhaps remarkable depression in the temperature of the atmosphere, the thermometer sank to seventy-four and seldom at any time rose above eighty. The wind became northerly, rain fell at intervals nearly the whole of the day and night. The air was damp and chilling and conveyed a more uncomfortable sensation, than can well be imagined in this country. This still continued upon the 20th. There is nothing extraordinary in this change, except in the degree of it. Something of the same kind generally occurs at this season, when the north winds set in and is commonly much dreaded by the negro population; from the number of severe inflammatory complaints which it gives rise to. This year the north winds were much later than usual.

With respect to diseases, the general disposition to fever, during the last six months, has been such as to absorb all our attention, and nearly to exclude the consciousness of any other disease having existed. The low fever, which was stated in the last half-yearly report, to prevail among the artillery at Courland ran through the whole of that detachment, and their families, in the course of a few days. Each individual was in the greatest danger, through only two men and one child died.

These fevers, as I before observed, began with symptoms of little apparent danger, but suddenly ran into those from which everything serious might be expected. The fatal termination of the first case aroused our attention, but notwithstanding the advantage of a post-mortem examination, it was impossible to cut short the disease.

Each case ran a determined, and a pretty similar course, apparently with equal danger, the only morbid appearances were an effusion serum upon the brain and within the ventricles. Topical bleedings were alone admissible, and these with repeated blisters were made use of to the greatest extent.

I have examined with great attention the influence of this disease, and am persuaded that it was not contagious, because none of those who were not exposed to the same local causes were affected by it. I attribute the whole to the malign influence of the post which was probably at that time in increased activity. Courland has since this period been abandoned, as far as respects European troops, and is now guarded by a few black soldiers. The common sources of diseases, are so multiplied round this post, and are so much out of the reach of military control, that there is no safety but in flight.

The fevers which originated at headquarters near the same time, all partook of the same low character, though certainly not in an equal degree; and although there was no death among them, still there was sufficient to mark the same disposition under perhaps a less powerful excitement, and which is another evidence against its being connected with contagion. This terminated about the middle of July.

From that period there were many cases of remittent and intermittent fever. Frequently varying their type, and in almost every instance combined with hepatic affections. Many of them were severe, but only one terminated fatally, where a large abscess had formed in the centre of the liver, and nearly destroyed the whole of that viscus. General bleeding from evacuation, blisters, and mercurial function were always successful. This was the state of the garrison when reported in September, and nothing occurred during the next two months to disturb our tranquillity. There were fewer admissions than usual, and the fewer was still the prevailing disease, and in almost every instance accompanied with hepatic affection, it produced but one casualty, was readily subdued by the same treatments, and excited no alarm.

The uncommon heat of the weather was of itself sufficient to explain the general tendency to hepatitis, when coupled with the exposures, which the duties and the impudence of a soldier always tried to produce.

Early in December a remarkable change took place, and the remaining part of the period of this report from 6 to 20 December, will form an important epoch, as far as respects the diseases of this island. I shall confine myself in it, to such general circumstance connected with the history of the disease which prevailed, as took place either within or without the garrison, and reserve the particular description of the disease itself, until the next quarterly return when I trust it will have terminated, or when at all events a less imperfect account of it may be given than at the present moment.

At this period a fever, at once alarming and destructive, made its appearance among the troops, the symptoms were rapid and decisive, often terminating fatally with the black vomit upon the third day. This with the post-mortem examinations left no doubt as to the nature of the disease. It was decidedly the fever. *C. Icterodes*, in a very aggravated form, by whatever channel this fever was conveyed into the garrison, the first cases appear to have originated in hospital, and for nearly a week after its commencement, to have been pretty exclusively confined to it.

The progress was as follows: about the 5th or 6th two men of the Rangers who had been admitted into hospital for other diseases were attacked with fever and both died upon the 9th. Upon the 11th, an orderly man complained, as well as several of the patients, most of whom came under the head of surgical cases, and had been admitted either punished or with ulcers. Some of the slight cases of fever also, already in hospital, began to put on a morose appearance, or rather assume the character of the prevailing disease.

About the 13th and 14th, it began to show itself in different parts of the garrison, and to affect persons of every description. At this time Mr Palmer, the assistant surgeon in charge of the hospital was attacked as was Lt. Campion of the Rangers and Serjeant Hemming, the regimental schoolmaster, who kept school in a part of the same quarter with him. These were all severe cases. Serjeant Hemming died upon the 3rd and Lt. Campion on the 6th day. Between the 14th and 18th, Captain O'Keefe and his wife, an officer of artillery, and two inhabitants of the Rangers (the whole who resided with the fort) were affected with fever, and two of them eventually died. The women and children attached to the artillery and York Rangers, were most of them taken ill at the same time, so that with the exception of the large barrack and convalescent ward, every part of the garrison was infected with the disease.

On the fifteen[th], two men of the rangers and two of the military labourers were admitted. The serjeant of artillery, who was also admitted upon this day, had been attended in quarters, as a dysenteric patient for many days previous. He died with well-marked symptoms of the reigning disease upon the 19th, a day memorably fatal to the garrison, and on which no less than nine persons fell victims to the same malady – one of these was a military labourer.

On the 16th and 17th, four cases of fever were admitted, one an orderly man in hospital. On the 18th, two of the Rangers were admitted, one of them an orderly, who had but a slight attack. On the 19th, five of the Rangers and four of the Royal Artillery were admitted and upon the 20th, one man of the Rangers. At this period which embraces only the space of fourteen days, from the commencement of the disease we had lost one officer, and eighteen men out of about forty who had been admitted, one woman and two children. The appearances both in and out of hospital, were at the same time of the most alarming nature. Almost every case admitted was a severe one, and the minds of the men began to be extremely affected. In this state, it was judged necessary to appraise both the commander of the forces and the inspector of hospitals, of our situation, and an express for that purpose was sent to headquarters.

The few African soldiers stationed at Courland were all healthy, as was the officer of the Rangers who commanded these. Unfortunately, the mortality at the fort made it necessary to withdraw him. He was soon after seized with fever and died with the black vomit three days after he was attacked.

I have as yet only spoken of this fever as it prevailed among the troops, but its appearance within the fort was secondary. It is true that the nature of the disease was first ascertained and defined there, but I can without difficulty trace several cases to have previously occurred in town, two of them so early as 24 November. One of these died on the 27th with every symptom of the highest gastric inflammation, and that peculiarly distressed respiration which occurred with many of those who died early in the disease, and where the erisypelatous[12] inflammation of the stomach was most vivid, and if we excepted the dark colour of the duodenum, the only morbid appearance, the other died upon the 30th with black vomit.

After 6 December, when the garrison became affected, continual cases were occurring in town, but some, I believe, extended beyond it, and even these were confined to a few families. In one house, a young man of twenty and two children were attacked, at an interval of three days between each. The eldest child after a severe struggle recovered, the other two died. The stomach of the child was full of the black vomit but without the slightest appearance of inflammation either within or without, nor did any part of its contents adhere to or seem to depend upon the villous coat. The child had been ill three days and was seventeen months old. The family were creoles.

A great proportion of those attacked in town died. They were generally young Europeans, but not exclusively so; one lady who died had been twenty-five years in the country, without quitting it, and several of those attacked were creoles or long residents. A few people of colour were affected also and a still smaller number of blacks – they generally did well. A weakly mulatto man, whom I saw upon the fifth day of his disease, had the black vomit, but with little heat of skin or fever. He recovered.

There has been no epidemic in Tobago of equal magnitude with the present, since the year 1801. At that time, more than one-half of the garrison died, and out of sixty-three persons who were attacked with it in town, two only recovered. The black vomit was then a principal feature in the disease, but I am informed, from medical authority that there was no erisypelatous inflammation of the stomach. No person connected with the hospital, was at that time affected with the disease.

In 1805, some cases of this description of fever certainly occurred here and the surgeon of the York Light. Infantry volunteers who had lately arrived from Europe died with it, but it did not extend beyond the garrison. With respect to the mode by which this fever was introduced and continued in the country, I am aware that there will be more than one opinion. I have never entered into the question of contagion and have never been induced to believe that there was much of it in the general population of this country; beyond what individual neglect and inattention sometimes creates. It was impossible however to refer this disease to any increased activity of local causes, when the contrary was the fact. I was disposed to consider it therefore as one of those which a combination of natural evils had conspired to produce. The first rudiments having been generated during a long and unusually hot season, were now called into action by a sudden and great depression in the temperature of the atmosphere, which has been considered essential to the production of this fever. All these facts fully existed, but they were insufficient to explain the phenomena, and I was led to believe from observing them that in whatever manner the disease had originated, it was kept up by contagion. There were numberless circumstances which I thought it impossible to reconcile in any other way. For example, first it was almost entirely confined to the fort and to the town. Second, the general infection of almost all those who were connected with the hospital, even to the Black Pioneers, and the women employed to wash for the sick, one of whom died. Thirdly the whole of the officers being attacked particularly the one recalled from Courland, and this being followed by the illness of all the servants who attended them; and by the death of some.

Among the inhabitants many circumstances occurred to give weight to the same opinion, such as wives being attacked when attending upon their husbands, and relations and friends upon each other. The governor's was almost the only house in the country, in which the disease was known, and that was only a short distance both from town from the fort. Sir Frederick Robinson after having visited the garrison, was the first person attacked there, and very narrowly escaped. Two ladies in the house, and several of the domestics followed shortly after. One of the ladies died. The intercourse between this house and the garrison was constant and could scarcely be avoided. The shipping suffered in no part of the island but in the principal bay near the town. Two vessels that were affected before any precautions had been taken, infected every man that came on board, while the rest who were placed under better regulations nearly escaped altogether. If the principle of contagion is admitted in this matter, it is not difficult to support it in every stage.

There were at this period several arrivals from the Spanish Main, where a disease apparently the same, had destroyed a great part of the population of several villages. In Saint McGill's not ten out of five hundred remained. I conversed with some of the seamen who had belonged to these vessels, and found that several of their men had died on board with black vomit, that many were landed who died soon after, and that others among whom were themselves, still remained sick on shore. Through the medium of these men, I have reason to believe that the disease was first introduced into the two vessels I spoke of, and those who are acquainted with the easy communication between all description of people in the West Indies, will have little difficulty in imagining the rest.

The two and fort have at all times free intercourse, but in the present, it was more than accidental; the wife of the ordinance armourer was I believe the first resident attacked; she resided in town. I saw her on 24 November, and she died upon the 27th. The serjeant of artillery was upon the most intimate terms with this family. His wife attended the woman who died, during her illness, and afterwards carried her family to the fort. Someone or other from the garrison was constantly in the house of this person, and although the first well-marked cases there, certainly occurred in hospital, yet it is equally certain, that the wife of the serjeant was herself attacked with some kind of fever, soon after her return, and had not recovered from it when her husband was attacked. The first moment that circumstances and observation led me to believe, that this disease was contagious, I reported it to the general commanding, and every means was instantly adopted to counteract its extension.

The new barrack was fortunately ready, and capable of receiving the whole of the York Rangers; they were removed into it, and the old barrack converted into a convalescent ward to allow every man discharged from hospital a probationary period before they were returned into quarters and thus prevent all danger from relapses. All communication was denied between the hospital and the garrison, nor was anyone admitted into it, but such as were affected with the prevailing disease.

I had a regular inspection of every man not in hospital, twice a day, and fumigations of some kind or other were constantly going on; both within and without the buildings. The guard was withdrawn from town, and all intercourse with the inhabitants prohibited. White orderlies in hospital were permitted as little as possible for though we had sufficient evidence that the African constitution was susceptible of the disease, when strongly exposed to its influence, yet there appeared no question but that it was much less so than the European.

Signed
S. Panting
Surgeon to the Forces

Half-Yearly Report of Sick of the Troops at Tobago to 20 June 1819 by Staff Surgeon S. Panting

Nothing has occurred in the external relations of the fort, that could in any way influence the health of the troops, since the last half-yearly report. The Swamp at Bacolet remains untouched, but does not appear to increase. The lowlands that surround the fort are in the same state of partial cultivation as before, intersected on all sides with dikes of stagnant water, and masses of decayed vegetable matter. The brush in its immediate vicinity is occasionally cut down with the exception of a part of the windward quarter, which is the property of private persons. The buildings within the fort are the same as when last reported.

The new barrack which was first occupied by the York Rangers in December last now accommodates the two companies of the 4th Regiment who relieved them. It has no gallery which is a great disadvantage in this country but is dry, well-ventilated and in every other respect comfortable.

The new hospital is very nearly finished, and could be occupied if the out-buildings were erected, but there is no prospect of them at present. The sick of the European Corps are accommodated in the large ward of the old hospital. The new ward since the arrival of the 4th has been appropriated to the sick of the artificers and military labourers, and much advantage has certainly been derived from our having been able to separate them.

Our numerical strength upon 21 December 1818, was 14 of the Royal Artillery, 200 of the York Rangers, and 150 of the military labourers.

It will be remembered that the island was at this period under the influence of a violent and apparently contagious epidemic – the *Febris Continua Icterodes*. It had then existed about a fortnight, during which time forty cases had been admitted into hospital, eighteen of whom had died. At this period also, almost every officer in the garrison had become affected with it; and two of them if not actually dead, were beyond all expectation of recovery. In the adjacent town several cases of the disease had terminated fatally, and in many of the merchant vessels at anchor in the Principal Bay, it ran through the whole of the crew with dreadful malignity.

The 15 to 30 December was the most aggravated period. It continued, however, with great violence, through the whole of the next month, during which fifty-six new cases were admitted, from that time it gradually subsided and about 24 February had ceased altogether, a period of something less than three months from its commencement and during which the garrison had lost five officers and forty crew, four women and four children.

A number equal to one-fifth of the white troops within the Fort, and as one to two and a half of those attacked with the disease – during this time the crew stationed at Courland were perfectly healthy – the officer who commanded there, was unfortunately ordered to Headquarters. He very soon contracted the disease, and after three days' illness, died with the most aggravated symptoms.

It was only within the Fort, the town of Scarborough and among the ships at anchor in that Bay that this fever was known. The country with the exception of two or three cases, which were certainly contracted in town, escaped altogether. In the town and within the fort, it ceased nearly at the same time, but among the shipping, it was exceedingly difficult to eradicate. I am persuaded that nothing but the establishment of an hospital on shore and the strictest regulations could have effected it. Their mortality was much greater in proportion than either with the garrison or the inhabitants; the garrison again, considering the number who were attacked, suffered much less than either – this is perhaps not difficult to account for, and it appears to me that in the West Indies at least, all serious epidemics will have the same results.

By the military arrangements the promptest attention is paid to the first appearance of disease, and the readiest obedience given to whatever is suggested. The progress of symptoms is more carefully watched, than it could be in any other situation, while the post-mortem examinations put us in more complete possession of its precise nature. Independent of this the attendants are more experienced, and attentive, than any that can be obtained in private life, and all the requisite theories and comforts being upon the spot, facilities are afforded, that no other situation can command. This never was more apparent than in the present instance, and I had much opportunity of observing it.

Of the nature and progress of this fever, I have said all that I believe there is occasion to say, in my reports for December and March last which were nearly devoted to the subject. With respect to liability of attack, I could observe no distinction. The York Rangers, who were the principal subjects of it, were not new to the climate or immune to the diseases. They had suffered severely on almost every station in the command; still they were, generally speaking, vigorous and effective, and certainly very few of them, in that reduced health, which might seem to invite disease; though in their moral habits they are vicious to an extreme.

Individually, the robust and the delicate appeared to have an equal chance. Whether it is possible to be twice infected with the disease, I am not prepared to say. I believe that it is possible, but am at the same time inclined to think, from what I have observed in myself and others, that the susceptibility is much lessened by the first attack. Whatever difficulty there may be with respect to the origin of this fever, there can be no question but that it was afterwards propagated by contagion, both within and without the garrison, supported by innumerable facts, and I have no doubt but that its progress was checked, and its influence much circumscribed, by the alarm which existed and by the precautions that were everywhere taken in consequence.

In the fort, nothing was omitted that was considered likely to eradicate infection; the hammocks and blankets of the white troops, the bedding and flannel dresses which they had worn in hospital during the sickness were all condemned and burnt at the instance of the inspector, by a special board of survey. At the same time, every means was made use of, to cleanse and purify the buildings.

From the second week in March, the Rangers became healthy, and remained so until they were relieved, with the exception indeed of a few intermittents, but this appeared to be a general disposition throughout the island, not only with the European inhabitants but also with the coloured natives, attended in many cases with severe negative affections.

Upon 14 April, the York Rangers embarked for Canada to be disbanded, and were relieved in this garrison by two companies of the 4th Foot, consisting of 3 officers and 113 crew. This regiment formed one of several, which had very recently arrived in the West Indies, and as they were all new to the climate, the greatest anxiety was respecting them. Every indulgence consistent with their military duty was extended to them, and a number of regulations were established at headquarters for their general and particular guidance; all intended to protect them, as far as possible, not only from the danger of service in this country, but from their own inexperience and independence.

These views were fully entered into by the general officer, commanding in this island, and no precaution has been omitted, that could, I believe, in any way contribute to this object – their military duties have been rendered as light as possible, they furnish no parties of fatigue, a number of covered sheds have been erected to protect them from the sun, wherever they mount guard.

Their parades are short, and at an early hour they have few courts martial, and still fewer punishments. Their walks and outdoor amusements are restricted to proper hours, and there are daily health inspections which are minutely performed.

The soldiers of the 4th are, generally speaking, stout and of a healthy appearance, still they have more invalids amongst them, as well as crew of a certain age, than might have been expected, in a selection for the Peace Establishments. Upon their first arrival, in reference to the fever which had so lately prevailed among the York Rangers, a general and thorough purification both of hospital and barracks took place, before they were allowed to enter them: new dresses, bedding, and utensils were issued, and the large ward of the hospital was entirely appropriated to their sick, that nothing which promised their advantage might be withheld.

The results, I am sorry to state, have not been proportionate to the pains that were taken – the new troops have been and remain much unhealthier, than we anticipated, but as I have already noticed both their complaints, and our treatment of them, in my quarterly report, I shall contend myself in this with a general view.

During April, but few were admitted, and these were generally slight cases of continued fever, but always accompanied with biliary derangement, and a yellow tinge of the skin. This continued until nearly the end of May, when the long, dry season broke up, and was followed by excessive rains.

From that period to the present, their diseases became more important, and although but two casualties have occurred yet, since the beginning of May, a full third of the detachment has been constantly in hospital. The form of disease has been generally fever, either continued or remittent, but the great and alarming part of its character has been the constant and violent local determination to the head, the stomach or the intestines, attended in a number of cases, with the mildest and most frantic delirium although the febrile action was seldom high, and the hepatic character of the first cases entirely lost.

In treating these several complaints, there was a manifest distinction – while the hepatic character prevailed by moderate bleeding, and a steady mercurial phlegm, adapted to the urgency of the case, they all recovered.

When the head, the stomach and the intestines became affected, the principal indication was general and local bleeding. In many instances, this was carried to an extraordinary degree, and always with proportionate advantage. The temporal artery was frequently opened several times in the same subject, to relieve local symptoms and the only two cases in which we have been unfortunate, were those where from the fears, or peculiar constitution of the patient, but little blood could be abstracted.

The post-mortem appearances strongly showed its necessity, in the principal case. The other patient had been an invalid from his arrival. The cause of this sickness among the new troops, notwithstanding so many precautions had been taken to prevent it, is a question of much importance. Some part of it is certainly to be ascribed to the independence and irregularities of the crew themselves; for though they have few of the other vicious propensities of the York Rangers, they are at least equally intemperate, this alone in a climate so new to them, and so little favourable to health, cannot be without its effect, but the great cause to which so many inflammatory complaints are probably to be referred, is the unequal temperature of the day, and night, in the high and exposed situation of the fort.

This evil so long as continues needs to be posed, it is impossible to obviate – little can be added. I believe to the existing regulations by way of prevention, and certainly no duty is exacted that can be dispensed with. The detachment at Courland has been singularly healthy, nor has any officer in the garrison been sick since the *Febris Icterodes* disappeared.

During the month of January, the weather continued to be cold, wet and uncomfortable. In February and March, it became fine and pleasant, but the thermometer which had been remarkably depressed from the early part of December did not hastily recover itself. It generally ranged from seventy-six to eighty through the day, which it seldom exceeded. The winds were high but always hanging to the northward. The nights were cold and bleak. From March to June, it was dry, hot and oppressive. The thermometer ranged as high as 89 through the day but fell during the night to seventy-four. With May, as is usual the dry season terminated and from 1 to 20 June there was a constant succession of rain. Still the days were most oppressively hot and the nights cold and chilly.

Of these changes, those who are exposed to them within the fort are particularly sensible. The children and such crew of the garrison, as could not substantiate their having had the small pox, have been from time to time vaccinated, particularly the military labourers. This has been also pretty general through the island, but has not always been judiciously conducted, and I am persuaded that much future evil will arise out of it.

Signed
S. Panting
Surgeon to the Fort

Extract of Half-Yearly Report from Tobago to 20 December 1819 by Staff Surgeon, S. Panting

The smallness of the garrison and the recent epidemic which terminated only in February last, might have promised a healthier close to the present year, but since the first month after the arrival of the new troops, which was in April last, there has been a constant succession of disease. The number of sick at any time has seldom been considerable, but there has been no interval of health, one severe case has so constantly succeeded another, and the management of them has been so arduous and perplexing that the duty of attending has been more than usually painful.

The description of the disease has been uniformly fever, generally remitted with violent determination to the head, stomach and intestines. These cases have seldom united all the symptoms of the *Febris Icterodes*, but have for the most part, so nearly resembled it, that I can only consider them varieties of the same disease. The mortality as must be expected under such circumstances, has been considerable, and the detachment of the 4th alone has within the period of this report lost eleven men, few of them by acute disease, this is a number nearly equal to one tenth of the detachment.

The officers of the garrison have been exceedingly healthy. With the exception of Lieutenant Beer of the 4th (who has been long Pulmonic), no one has been sick. It is difficult if not impossible to account not only for such constant disease amongst the men of the 4th Regiment, but also for the extraordinary nature of the disease itself. These men have every indulgence which can be extended to a soldier, there is no duty exacted from them that can possibly be dispensed with, and every prudent restriction is enforced, as far as it can be, without having recourse to corporal punishment, which is scarcely known in the regiment.

The men as far as regards themselves, are extremely imprudent, and many of them intemperate, but again it is a truth and a melancholy one, that our mortality has generally fallen upon those who are best disposed and least addicted to excess. The sentinels have each of them a long shed to walk under by day, and a box to retire to at night; but the situation of the fort is certainly unfavourable to night guards. The hill as you ascend it becomes bleak and chilling, and the wind from the sea collected through a large drain is often poured upon the sentinel with great violence, and which notwithstanding the precautions which have been adopted, must be injurious to health, but will it be supposed that this exposure alone can generate diseases so peculiar, or uniformly create this violent erythema in the stomach, which is so destructive of life.

The inspections which were instituted upon the arrival of this detachment for the detection of acute diseases in its first stages, have been constantly, and regularly continued, with more or less frequency, according to the prevalence of disease. The military labourers, through the hot months, had [a] number of men sick, with ardent fevers, many of them of great severity, and attended with local affections very nearly resembling those of the white troops. Much of this must be referred to the nature of their occupations, so different from the military duty in which they were formerly employed.

Amongst the white inhabitants, there has been nothing beyond the usual casualties of the climate. The black population has suffered exceedingly throughout the whole of the year. In the early months the whooping cough was very destructive amongst the children. In July and August, there was a strong disposition to ardent fever, with severe affections of the head, and abdominal viscera. These again were succeeded by diarrhoeas and by acute and chronic dysenteries, and such was their prevalence and severity, that upon many estates very nearly the whole of their numbers were infected.

Towards the end of September, we were alarmed by the appearance of yellow fever, on board a merchant vessel at anchor in the Principal Bay near the town. She had arrived about a month before, from Europe, and was loading to return thither. The second mate and every foremost man, who slept in the forepart of the ship, were affected with the disease, and nine out of nineteen of them died, and all with the black vomit. The captain, his son and the first mate, who slept in the cabin, escaped it altogether.

Every enquiry was made as to its probable origin but without effect. It did not extend farther.

Stephen Panting
Surgeon to the Forces

Supplementary Report to 20 June 1820 Follows Mr Arthur's for December 1820 by Ralph Green Inspector of Army Hospitals

Tobago – 25 December 1818

The half-yearly remarks on the diseases of the British army in the West Indies to 20 June 1820 were incomplete, Tobago, Demerara and Berbice having been omitted; no reports having been received from those colonies until nearly the close of the year to enable one to give a summary of the medical occurrences at those stations at the usual period of making the return. I shall, therefore, include in the present report on the diseases at those stations such as appeared during the whole of the year; and in the others the last six months to 20 December.

At Tobago, the two companies of the 4th forming its garrison had lost a considerable number of men from their arrival there in April 1819 to the end of that year. In the stomachs of three of the fatal cases, matter resembling black vomit was found. The first of these was private Sirson who died on 5 June 1819 – three days ill. The disease however did not spread farther for twenty-two days when another case something similar was admitted (24 June) – Private I. Heams. He died on the twelfth day of his illness on 4 July. Happily, no other similar case occurred until 4 November when Private Leonard Kemp was admitted on 5 November and died on the 14th. He, however, had but little irritability of stomach throughout and it may be much doubted whether his disease was *Typhus Icterodes*. The two first to the best of any judgement were decidedly so, although the duration of Heams's illness was unusually protracted.

In recurring to these solitary cases I have been induced from the consideration that it is much to be doubted whether yellow fever had really disappeared among the inhabitants as it had carried off a considerable number of them during the latter part of 1818 and the first months of 1819. The last case in the garrison was 19 February when it ceased and until the embarkation of the detachment of the Royal York Rangers, which had formed it on 11 April when the two companies of the 4th were landed there in perfect health to relieve them previous to which all the hammocks and blankets used by the York Rangers, had been burnt by my recommendation and the barracks and hospital thoroughly purified by whitewashing; and new hammocks, blankets, hospital bedding and dresses issued to the fresh garrison.

To get accurate information of the state of the public health in any town in the West Indies is almost impossible. Many poor Europeans and strangers die unknown and unattended when yellow fever prevails excepting by the poorer class of coloured people, and thus the disease may lurk in obscure places for some time after the epidemic has generally ceased among the higher classes of the white population – and it can easily be imagined that it was possible and probable at Tobago, when neither infected bedding or clothing was destroyed upon any occasion by the inhabitants, and which would retain the contagious virus for probably a much greater length of time than the interval between 19 February and 2 June, that fresh accounts might appear among newly arrived Europeans if exposed to its influence, and from their arrival on 10 April 1819 to 15 February 1820, the admissions into hospital of fever, were numerous, some of which were of a most suspicious character. Fourteen of these were fatal. It was not however until the 15th of that month, that any of the cases appeared in the decided form of contagious yellow fever, when one of Sir Frederick Robinson's servants, a soldier of the 4th was admitted and which soon spread rapidly among the other servants at Government House and finally carried off his son (and A.D.C.) and a beautiful girl, his daughter.

I shall add the information received in Staff Surgeon Panting's own words. "You have been aware from every report which I have made how nearly allied all our severe complaints were to the epidemic which caused such distinction among the York Rangers in the early part of the last year. Still, they were insulated cases, and there was no suspicion of contagion. Upon 15 February a soldier of the 4th was admitted from Government House. He died upon the 19th with the black vomit. In a few days afterwards, two soldiers of the 4th, a private servant from England and the wife of a soldier were all admitted from the same quarter. The soldiers both died upon the first instant (March) and both with black vomit. Their bodies were so offensive when opened, that I had difficulty in being present at the examination. The orderly who attended us was taken ill next morning, and is dead. Lieutenant Duthey of the 4th, who lately arrived here from Grenada, died upon the 8th after five days' illness. He very imprudently went into the dead-house where the bodies lay after I left the place. Assistant Surgeon Palmer was attacked upon the 6th, and is now so ill that his recovery can scarcely be looked for. Ensign Clarke is also threatened with an attack, and I was this evening sent for to see Mr Robinson, son and Aide-de-Camp to the general, at Government House, who seems to be affected pretty much in the same way with the rest."

From this date to the embarkation of the remains of these two companies for Barbados only eight individuals out of the whole number escaped the disease, and the mortality was most dreadful. I shall annex a copy of the return of the number of officers, servants, orderlies and patients admitted into hospital for other diseases who were attacked there. To reason upon such positive facts is unnecessary, and the individual must be most sceptical who will deny contagion on this occasion. All the fatal cases which occurred being almost without variation attended by the same symptoms and same appearances that is headache, great irritability of stomach ending in black vomit, dark coloured or tar-like (frequently fetid) stools, and excepting when bleeding had been resorted to, and the irritability was sometimes wanting, but the stomach on examination after death was found to contain the black vomit in considerable quantities and the gall bladder duodenum and small intestines loaded with the tar-like matter.

From 15 February to 6 April, no attempt was made to arrest the progress of the disease, either by separation or by removing them, during which period fifty cases had occurred and four officers, twenty-seven non-commissioned officers and privates and two women of the 4th, and one military artificer had died. At this period the white men and women in the barracks were encamped with the exception of the artificers, but it was now evidently too late as the whole mass was infected and as might be expected, cases of fever continued to be sent in from thence to 22 May when they returned into barracks. Thirteen of the number sent in died. At this time, the disease appeared to be arrested for not a case occurred in barracks until 7 June – sixteen clear days – when it again commenced its ravages, and continued with unabated violence, as far as the diminished number would allow to 2 July – in fact these two fine companies were reduced by death, at this time to about one-third the original number which had landed at Tobago in the preceding year. On 2 July, Sir Frederick Robinson again attempted to arrest its further progress and removed the remains to Courland – a post on the other side of the island – but here they also suffered, as eight cases were admitted from thence to the 7th when it ceased altogether. But it might be remarked that only one officer, two non-commissioned officers and five Privates had escaped an attack.

Table 12.4: Return of a Detachment of the 4th Regiment Stationed in the Island of Tobago – with the Deaths during the Time of Remaining there, from 6 April 1819 to 9 September 1820 When They Embarked for Barbados

Original Strength and Losses	Officers	Non-comm. Officers and Privates	Women	Children	Total	Remarks
Effective strength	6	123	11	6	146	Of the number attacked 8 were officers' servants of whom 7 died. 5 were orderlies in the hospital of whom 4 died, and 7 were patients admitted for other diseases of whom 4 died and 3 recovered
Lost by sickness	5	84	8	3	100	
Total remaining	1	39	3	3	46	
Number not attacked with yellow fever	1	7	3	3	14	

Captain Fletcher remained with this small detachment at Courland from this period until 8 September whereas all the men had continued perfectly healthy from 8 July when the last case of yellow fever died, they were embarked from thence to Barbados, and sent to a distant quarter in the island to prevent their having any communication with the garrison at St Ann's. Here, they continued perfectly healthy to 22

November, when they embarked for Grenada to join the headquarters of the corps, where they now serve.

Signed
Ralph Green
Inspector of Army Hospital

Return of Officers' Servants, Hospital Orderlies and Patients Admitted into Hospital with Other Diseases Who Were Subsequently Attacked with Yellow Fever at Tobago from 1 March 1820

Officers' Servants:

No. 1 – Joseph Tillett had been servant to Lieutenant Duthey who died upon 8 March, and attended him constantly during his illness. He was attacked with fever upon 23 March, and had the disease in a very aggravated form, but eventually recovered.

No. 2 – Edward Lofts had been servant to Ensign Clarke who died upon 23 March. He attended his master during his illness. He was attacked himself with the disease upon the 25th and died upon 27 March.

No. 3 – Edward Clarke had been servant to Lieutenant Beer who died upon 26 March. He attended his master during his illness, was unwell two or three days before he reported himself admitted into hospital upon 4 April and died upon the 8th.

No. 4 – John Garrett was servant to Captain Fletcher, had frequent communication both with Ensign Clarke and Lieutenant Beer during their illness, and constant intercourse with the servants who attended him. He was admitted into hospital upon the 28th and died upon 29 March.

No. 5 – John, a negro boy of ten, a native of Tobago, was servant to Captain Fletcher. He was greatly attached to Garrett and could not be prevented from visiting him in hospital. He was taken ill upon the 2nd and died on the 5th.

No. 6 – James Rockett was servant to Captain Fletcher, was admitted into hospital upon the 4th May and died upon the 8th.

No. 7 – Thomas Serjeant, servant to Captain Fletcher was admitted into hospital upon the 11th and died upon 16 May.

No. 8 – Edward Scantlebury, servant to Captain Fletcher was admitted upon 19 June and died upon the 25th. His symptoms for the first two days were those of colic. This was not an uncommon mode of attack.

It is singular that Captain Fletcher who was so constantly exposed to the disease should so entirely have escaped it. Three officers of the 4th and a hospital assistant died within a few yards of his quarter literally under the same room with him, and he lost five servants by each of whom he was attended to the last moment of their admission into hospital. All these servants in succession occupied the same room – it was part of an old barrack, appropriated to the use of the married soldiers of the 11th Regiment. It has since been abandoned.

Hospital Orderlies

No. 1 – Joseph Wilson had been employed as an hospital orderly since the arrival of the 4th at Tobago. He was attacked with fever upon 1 March, shortly after having assisted at the dissection of Milner and Reid who died upon that day with *Febris Icterodes*[13] – but he had felt a little unwell for a day or two previous. His case terminated fatally upon 8 March.

No. 2 – Stephen Parks, an hospital orderly was ill twice between 19 March and 25 April. His complaint was not severe, on either occasion, but evidently allied to the prevailing fever. He remains still an orderly, and is the only hospital attendant belonging to the detachment of the 4th that has outlived the disease.

No. 3 – Thomas Cornwall had been first a convalescent, and then an orderly in hospital. He was attacked upon 11 June with the prevailing fever and died upon the 15th.

No. 4 – A. Westlake had been very long employed as an hospital orderly and has passed through all the diseases that occurred there without being affected by it. He was attacked however about 25 June, with prevailing fever and was apparently in a state of convalescence when a second attack took place of which he died upon 9 July.

No. 5 – Serjeant Hinksman was employed as hospital steward and resided in the hospital. He was attacked about 24 March with *Febris Icterodes* and died upon the 30th.

No. 6 – Mrs Hinksman, the wife of the hospital steward, lived in the hospital with her husband, and was attacked there about the same time with *Febris Icterodes*. She died upon 27 March.

No. 1, 2 and 3 – **Africans** – Camden, Guriara and Brough, three military labourers were attacked with *Febris Icterodes*. Employed as orderlies about the hospital, they went through the disease with more or less severity of symptoms but all ultimately recovered.

No. 4 – Thomas Saoler, an African, a mason employed to whitewash a ward in the hospital after some men of the 4th had died there. Whilst employed upon this duty he was attacked with the same fever. It proved a severe case and he recovered with difficulty.

Patients in Hospital

No. 1 – John Adams had been in hospital from 14 March in consequence of ulcerated legs. He was attacked upon the 18th with symptoms of fever and died upon the 23rd.

No. 2 – Corporal Watkins was attacked in hospital about the middle of March with fever. He had been admitted some days before, with a severe pain below the shoulders, extending through the chest – apparently a hepatic affection. It proved to be a severe case but terminated favourably.

No. 3 – N. Lambkin was admitted into hospital upon 6 April and died upon the 21st. The fever with which this man was admitted ran a mild course of seven days, and he was not discharged at the end of that time, because there was no intermediate quarter between the hospital and the barrack. Upon the 17th, he decidedly had the *Febris Icterodes*, and died upon the 21st.

No. 4 – Robert Bee was admitted into hospital upon the 6th and died upon the 22nd April. This was a case of *Febris Icterodes* from the commencement, but he was perfectly convalescent with an exceeding sore mouth upon the 17th. He died however with coma and the black vomit upon the 22nd.

No. 5 – James Serrun was convalescent in hospital and attacked with *Febris Icterodes* upon the 5th May. This case was a severe one, but terminated favourably.

No. 6 – William Jones was also a convalescent in hospital and attacked upon the 7th May. His case also proved severe but had a favourable termination. This man had a former attack of the same disease upon 20 March.

No. 7 – Mrs McSheffery lost her husband with *Febris Icterodes* upon 27 March and a boy, her son, upon the 17th June. After the death of her husband, she lived with a man of the same regiment of the name of Clarke, who died also with the same disease upon 2 July. Upon the 1st July, she was herself admitted, had the disease in a very aggravated form and died upon the 4th.

Respecting its supposed origin, she gave to the Hospital Steward the evening before her death, the following account. That being particularly desirous of seeing Clarke, she contrived on the night of 30 June to get secretly into the ward in which he was laying with another man of the name of Jones and continued there for some time. It was the fourth day of his illness. She said that she found his breath extremely hot, and offensive, and from that moment felt herself sick.

To these perhaps a few other cases might be added. Still, as they were not immediately under my own direction, I cannot state them with sufficient accuracy to do it from myself, but during the whole time this fever prevailed. It is remarkable how few cases of a different nature presented themselves. It must not be inferred, however, because some doubtful one were admitted into hospital that they were exposed to all the malignity of the worst cases already there; the greatest caution was exercised to rescue them from unnecessary risk.

They were placed in a ward distinct and remote from the rest, and quite unconnected with every other patient.

Signed
S. Panting
Surgeon to the Forces

The Following is a Sketch of Such Cases of Febris Icterodes as Occurred among the Officers of the 9th and 21st Regiments and Their Servants While at Tobago in 1820 by S. Panting, Surgeon to the Forces

Mrs Jewoise, wife of Captain Jewoise of the 9th Regiment, about twenty-five years of age, and of a delicate habit, arrived in Tobago upon 9 September. She had previously passed a year in St Vincent and supposed herself within a few days of her accouchement. She passed the first week at Courland and then removed to a small house on the side of a deep ravine at the bottom of the Fort Hill. She was perfectly well until the 18th when she was suddenly seized with intense headache, violent pulsation of the arteries of the neck and head, weakness of the knees and acute pain of the back and limbs. Her face was scarlet, her pulse full, strong and throbbing. She was bled upon the first and second day to the extent of forty-two and a half [ounces]. The febrile symptoms subsided, but in such a manner as to give the impression that nature was not relieved, but over-powered. The retching was incessant, as was her thirst. She was delivered late in the night of the 21st of a dead child, and died on the morning of the 22nd, having had the black vomit for more than eighteen hours.

James Stone – Upon the 24th September, Captain Jewoise's servant, a soldier of the 9th Regiment was taken ill with all the usual symptoms of *Icterodes*. He refused to be bled and took nothing but evacuants and warm baths. He remained near Captain Jewoise's quarters until 2 October, when he was perfectly free from fever, and so far, recovered as to be able to walk to Courland. He was, however, again attacked there upon the 3rd and died on the 6th.

Captain Jewoise – 9th Regiment, a strong healthy man about thirty years of age. He was attacked and soon upon 27 September with headache, burning of the eyes, weakness in the back and limbs. He gave himself up at once, and he was bled to one pound. His headache was relieved, and his febrile symptoms to all appearance trifling. There was no throbbing of the arteries, but the irritation at the stomach was constant and distressing. He was blistered and well evacuated. The head of skin and pulse sunk gradually, and he died upon 1 October, after having had the black vomit for 36 hours previous, and so collected and aware of his situation, that after having made what arrangements he could respecting his child, he requested that a coffin might be ordered for him.

Assistant Surgeon Colvin[14] – of the 21st Regiment about twenty-eight years of age, and of a spare habit was seriously attacked upon 16 October. He had been about five weeks in Tobago, and had several times within the last fortnight, been confined for a day or less with slight attacks of fever and biliary derangement, so that he had begun to endeavour to affect his mouth with mercury. From this attack upon the morning of the 16th he never rose – he had one very severe rigour, followed by nausea and intense headache – he had constant thirst. Some the little increased heat of skin, and a quick small and irritated pulse. His retching was the most prominent and distressing symptom. He was not bled but his head and stomach were more than once blistered. He was well evacuated and used mercury both internally and by friction. His mouth was not sore. He died upon the 22nd with black vomit.

Major Cameron – About twenty-six years of age, young vigorous and active, commanded the detachment of the 21st. Upon 20 October, he had felt unwell through the whole of the day, but although I had met him abroad twice during the forenoon, he made no complaint. He was walking about his room in great agitation, and complained of violent pain in his back, head and limbs. He had had no rigour but retched incessantly and brought up a thick ropy matter which afterwards became brown and bitter. Having had a warm bath and his bowels opened, he appeared to be considerably relieved, but as his pulse full, face flushed, and there was a very considerable throbbing of the arteries of the head and neck, I bled him from the arm to one pound, which he bore but indifferently, and the bleeding was not repeated. His head and stomach were largely blistered, and every effort was made to affect his mouth with mercury. Upon the 21st, he was evidently labouring under stupor – his eyes were constantly shut and he did not speak until roused. His heat of skin and fullness of pulse had subsided, but the pain in the head and throbbing of the arteries remained. He used applications to the head and had warm baths repeatedly; the cold effusion distressed him. His bowels were opened still more freely and as he complained of much pain in the abdomen that was blistered also, injections were given and the mercurials were continued. The pain in his head gradually subsided but his thirst and retching continued. The stupor increased and his pulse became gradually lost. Upon the 22nd, he had that heaviness and apparent partial paralysis of the hands and lower limbs, which is so frequent in this disease and so uniformly a fatal symptom. His face, neck and arms were early livid, but not yellow; and upon the 24th, he was delirious. The last pain he appeared to feel was in the intestines, and that very severely. If these had been examined, I have no doubt that they would have been found gangrenous. He died upon the 25th.

Lieutenant Lindsay – Of the 21st Regiment, about twenty-six years of age, and of a very robust habit, was attacked during the night of the 20th with symptoms of a common cold, his eyes were suffused with tears and his face much flushed. He had some pain [in] the head, but more in the back and limbs and rather a tendency to fever than actual fever itself. His symptoms however soon increased in violence, the pain in the back and head became excessive – the retching constant and overwhelming. He was not drowsy, but it was as severe a case as I had seen, and it was evident from the commencement that there was little chance of his doing well. He was bled twice to the extent of one pound each, was blistered early, upon the head and stomach, and was freely evacuated. He retained his senses until a few hours before his death, but for the last two days he had the black vomit and passed a similar matter in appearance by stool. He died early upon the 25th.

Lieutenant Waller – 21st Regiment. About twenty years of age and of a spare habit. From the period when the other officers were affected, Mr Waller was complaining. He had derangement of the stomach and some inclination to fever. For this he several times took medicine, but never I think perfectly recovered. He was at Courland with his men and I saw him but seldom. I was called over to him by signal upon 3 November. He had every symptom of *Icterodes* in the second state. His headache was nearly gone but his eyes were coloured and injected. He was dressed and not in bed. He died upon the morning of the 4th with black vomit. He had been very assiduously attended by Mr Warner, a private practitioner who resides at Courland. He had no suspicion of his own danger. Mr Waller was not bled.

Lieutenant Fairweather – of the 21st Regiment. Upon the 23rd September, he complained of nausea and very considerable uneasiness about the region of the stomach. He had some tendency to fever, and as the disease advanced, threw up quantities of that ropy mucous matter which generally attends *Icterodes*. He continued in this state for two or three weeks, always expressing general pain and uneasiness although it never amounted to very serious, at least to very dangerous illness. His mind was greatly depressed. He often changed his situation as to place, but never perfectly recovered until he left the island.

James Mulver – 21st Regiment. October 30. Habit strong and robust, servant to Major Cameron, and while in attendance upon him, was on the evening of the 23rd September attacked with the usual symptoms of *Icterodes*. He was much dejected, had constant irritation of the stomach, violent pain in the head and back, great heat of skin and throbbing of the arteries. He was bled immediately to a pound from the arm, and afterwards to the same extent from the temporal artery; had his head and stomach blistered, and warm baths frequently repeated. When his mouth became affected, his febrile symptoms left him. He was long convalescent but ultimately recovered.

Charles Murray – 21st Regiment. October 28. Spare habit. Was servant to Mr Fairweather. Had felt unwell for some days with pain in the head and sickness at the stomach, but endeavoured to dissipate it by drinking. Upon the 27th, he reported himself. His pulse was weak and quick. His heat of skin was natural. Upon the 28th, he appeared to be much relieved. His blisters upon the head and stomach had risen well. His bowels had been freely opened, and he took nourishment with some appetite. Towards evening however, he became restless and during the night wildly delirious. His senses never returned. He gradually sunk till the morning of the 30th when he died. He was not bled nor had the black vomit.

John Marshall – 21st Regiment. Had been servant to Mr Colvin and was in quarantine with the other servants when attacked. This was upon the evening of the 8th of November. His head and back were principally affected. His stomach was not irritable. His head was shaved and blistered. He was bled to a pound and a half and his mouth was affected with mercury. He had a short convalescence and was discharged.

Thomas Monaghan – 21st Regiment. October 30. Strong habit. Was servant to Major Cameron and in quarantine with the rest. He was attacked with great severity upon the evening of the 9th and reported himself next morning. His face was extremely flushed. The throbbing of the temples excessive, the pain in the head extreme and the retching incessant. He was bled both generally and from the temples, and had repeated warm baths. His head and stomach were blistered, and mercury used internally and by friction. His symptoms never relaxed or for a moment gave any hope of his recovery. He died upon the 14th.

John Eversley – 21st Regiment. October 25. Strong habit. Was servant to Mr Waller. This man had been at Courland with his master and left it upon the 5th to perform quarantine with the rest of the officer's servants at the Fort. He was taken ill upon the evening of the 9th and died upon the 12th. His symptoms did not vary from the rest. His head and back were principally affected. His stomach exceedingly irritable, and his mind reduced from the highest daring to the lowest state of despondence. His stools were brown and watery, but never black. His skin had no tinge of yellow, indeed this seldom occurred, but his face and arms had a livid hue, which was much more common and always a fatal symptom. He was bled to two pounds from the arm and the temporal artery. In other respects, he was treated as the rest.

George Cameron – 21st Regiment. At forty spare habits. Was also servant to Major Cameron, and performed quarantine with the rest. He had been sent for when Einsley was taken sick without my knowledge, and as he had slept all night in the room with the Major it became necessary that he should remain there. He was attacked upon the 12th with the usual symptoms and in a severe way, but as he was delicate and apparently not in natural good health, he was bled only to twelve ounces from the temporal artery. His mouth became early affected, and after a long convalescence he recovered.

James Bayley – At twenty-two strong and robust habit was groom to Mr Waller. He had seen but little of his master while sick but was brought in with Einsley to perform quarantine at the Fort. He was strong, robust and surly and very impatient of his confinement. He remained quite well until the evening of 19 November, when he was most severely attacked. His skin when admitted was hot and dry. His tongue white but not parched. Thirst excessive; Great pain and fullness about the head as well as most acute pain at the back and across the region of the bladder. He vomited occasionally. He was bled to three pounds from the arm and the temporal artery, but nothing but the heat of the skin was relieved by it. He was blistered and freely evacuated, but the vomiting increased, and a profound stupor from which he was not easily roused took possession of him. He died upon the 23rd but had no black vomit. His skin was nearly a lead colour, but not yellow.

This case completes the list of officers, and the servants of the 9th and 21st Regiments who were attacked with *Icterodes*. Two servants only escaped the disease. There were Captain Jewoise's second servant, but who did not attend upon his master when he was sick, although he lived constantly with his comrade.

In the history of these cases if we had a satisfactory explanation as to how the disease commenced with Mrs Jewoise, a very strong argument might be drawn from them, in favour of contagion. As it is it will perhaps be regarded as a confirmation of the opinion that the disease is most frequently in the first instance, generated by particular local influence and afterwards supported by contagion. The circumstances which have at different times occurred in this garrison probably can be reconciled in no other way.

Signed
S. Panting
Surgeon to the Forces

Extract of Annual Report on the Diseases Which Prevailed in the Garrison of Fort King George, Tobago from 1 April 1839 to 31 March 1840 by Charles Stewart,[15] MD, Assistant Staff Surgeon

This unfortunate increase of mortality has been chiefly occasioned by Phthisis and a severe visitation of yellow fever. The latter assumed a very malignant character and prevailed epidemically among the white people, both civil and military.

Fevers, bowel and chest complaints have always been the principal causes of the sickness and mortality at this station. Fever especially within the last five months predominated it assumed the epidemic character occasionally presenting itself in the continued form but more frequently the remittent and so generally did it prevail among the troops (white troops eighty-three) that no white man escaped its influence except 17. Demerara, Barbados and St Vincent suffered from fever about the same time and whatever its type might have been, the mortality according to accounts has been very serious. The last epidemic fever that assailed this colony prior to the one under consideration occurred in years thirty-six and thirty-seven, but the one which bore the greatest resemblance to the malignant character of this fever was described by Dr Panting; it broke out at this station in 1820 and quickly carried off four-fifths of the whole European troops in garrison. The mortality has been great enough on this occasion, but perhaps less than anywhere else, the proportion of deaths to cases have not exceeded 1 to 9.

Detailed Notice of Any Epidemic Which May Have Visited the Station in the Course of the Year, Stating the Circumstances Under Which It Appeared, Its Subsequent Progress, and If It Was Attended by Any Atmospherical Phenomena

During the first half of the period occasional cases of fever used now and then to take place among the troops as well as amongst the white civil population, but rarely proved fatal until (the month of October) that the disease assumed a very malignant character and began to spread epidemically. Then the mortality gradually increased, especially amongst the civilians, and at one time was so alarming that everyone attacked died, and that generally on the fourth day of the disease, yellow suffusions frequently showed itself so early as the second day; passive or active haemorrhage or black vomit, sometimes both on the third; and death on the fourth.

The troops were assailed in the latter end of October. It commenced first with the officers, women and children; next the men were attacked right and left and in less than two months, the half of the whole European troops had passed through the usually but formidable febrile ordeal. The remainder were immediately encamped at some distance to the interior of the island, but their new locality altho' considered the healthiest part of the colony, failed to afford the slightest protection against the epidemic influence. They were violently attacked wherever they went, and it will be seen by the annexed return of that epidemic that only 24 Europeans escaped fever out of a strength [of] 117 (officers, men, women and children) that 93 persons of that number were attacked; that 12 of them had relapses, making in all 105 cases of white troops. It will also be seen by the same return that 13 of the black troops were treated for the same fever which had all its symptoms clearly developed with the exception of yellow suffusion haemorrhage and black vomit. Hence, it appears that the number of cases treated in all has been 117. That 104 cases were conducted to a favourable termination; whilst only 13 proved fatal. It is proper also to remark that no strange atmospheric phenomena appeared during this period, except perhaps an unusual degree of atmospheric humidity and dampness very probably aggravated by the frequency of northerly winds and heavy falls of rain. This severe fever occasionally presented the continued form throughout until followed by collapse, but the remittent type prevailed most.

This epidemic seemed to owe its origin to a combination of evident causes particularly malaria, which appears to have been abundantly disengaged from the windward marshes especially when vegetation was at a stand and animal and vegetable matter rapidly passing into a state of decomposition. The Bacolet swamps seem to be the most prolific in the production of febrific miasmata, and which if not soon remedied by draining and so on, must inevitably prove highly prejudicial to the health of the troops in garrison.

Nine years have elapsed since the grounds in question were cleared by drains and open ditches, which having now choked up with mud, vegetation and stagnant water, aided by the heavy muddy nature of the soil, malaria of a highly morbid character may be exhaled without the presence of much surface water. The flatness of the ground and which is worse being in parts below the level of the sea, naturally precludes the possibility of applying a satisfactory remedy. At all events the open ditches ought to be cleared and the banks of the almost stagnant rivulet which leads through the ground divested of their soil, to prevent a return of luxuriant vegetation. Should this not be attempted a *wooden* or *iron barrack* would require to be built to enable the troops to be removed to healthier localities, when the fort becomes suffocated with malaria wafted thereto.

Detailed History of Such Cases as Any Have Been Particularly Worthy of Mention, with Symptoms, Diagnosis, Modes of Treatment and Post-Mortem Examinations

The only cases most worthy of notice among the medical occurrences which took place at this station during the last year belong to the class of fevers, of which the remittent type predominated. This fever prevailed epidemically among the troops, the civilians and even the black and coloured population. The phenomena presented in the different cases, although admitting of slight variation to be ascribed to the influence of age, sex, constitution and habits capable of diminishing or increasing the intensity of morbid action, were invariably so uniform, that separate details do not appear necessary. Presuming therefore that a general description may suffice, let it be commenced by remarking that the duration of the paroxysm averaged seventy-two hours from the period of accession, that evening exacerbations continued to annoy for some days after the remission but in no case except such as proved fatal, were subsequent paroxysms allowed to return.

The general symptomatology of the disease seldom deviated from the following. The patient for a couple of days previous to the development of other symptoms used to experience a loss of appetite attended with a sense of chilliness, oppression and a disagreeable sense of constant coldness at the epigastrium. The night slumbers were disturbed by a series of disagreeable dreams, the mouth felt clammy and uncomfortable, the bowels were confined, the evacuations scanty and of a broken down tarry black appearance. The pulse was slightly accelerated, and rather feeble. The skin cool and as it were contracted; the eyelids itched; occasional giddiness could often be fancied, a general feeling of languor and lassitude soon gave way to general pains and extreme prostration of strength; at length the patient compelled to his bed, naturally calls for some warm drink, now the skin relaxes and the whole surface is quickly bedewed with a cold clammy perspiration, and the skin itself might be well pinched without occasioning much inconvenience. The tongue is of a yellowish white cast relaxed and unusually cold, the gums are noticed spongy and, in many cases, ulcerated. Some degree of pain now commences in the forehead and temples as also at the epigastrium, the stomach irritable and breathing oppressed, by this time alternate flushes of heat and chills are frequent, until at last the former predominates, and the skin becomes uniformly hot and arid, the pulse is excited, and to this succeed the remainder of the phenomena peculiar to the second or hot stage.

The uniform aggravation of the general pains especially the epigastric and that part of the headache confined to the bottom of the orbits, the eyes are also painful, suffused and injected; nausea and dizziness are felt the moment the head is raised; the thirst is urgent; the tongue dry; the mucous membrane lining the mouth inflamed especially where it covers the gums; by and by the contents of the stomach are ejected;

the bowels continue torpid until the liver is acted on and up to that period a dead doughy feel is conveyed to the hand when laid on the abdomen. The urine becomes scanty, high coloured and afterwards suppressed, the features will be fully expanded and occasionally the countenance is flushed, the thirst on the increase, and the smallest quantity of fluid swallowed was immediately rejected, loaded with thick bile resembling marshed greens. And instead of coldness and oppression as formerly felt at the *scrobiculus cordis*[16] the heat and pain in that region are almost insupportable; the skin now conveys to the physician's hand a stinging hot sensation and the pulse averages 120 but seldom regular in its other characters. It frequently happens now that the epigastric pain spreads over the whole abdominal cavity; but the most frequently affected region is the hypogastric over the urinary bladder, the right and left hypochondriac regions occasionally suffer and posteriorly the renal. The extremities are always severely pained and often seized with agonizing cramps; the tongue is tremulous and occasional twitches among the facial muscles may be frequently noticed. The next change that follows is an aggravation of either the cerebral or gastric symptoms, which never fail to bear the onus of the disease; they are the most urgent as well as the most difficult to subdue. The tendency is to continue gradually increasing in intensity until relieved by a favourable remission in the remittent type, or a salutary cessation of febrile action as in the continued, and if this anxiously looked for crisis be not established at the end of seventy-two or eighty-four hours, the sufferer has cause to apprehend the utmost danger. For the one or the other of the two trains of symptoms will quickly assume the most aggravated character. If the cerebral, the headache and ocular pain will be the most excruciating soon followed by yellow suffusion of surface. Muddiness and want of the natural lustre of the eye itself; throbbing of the temporal and carotid arteries and other evidences of determination of blood to the head; the neck becomes flushed and tumefied[17]; the occipital region exceedingly hot, swollen and even ecchymosed[18]; the pupil of the eye dilated; the patient talks incoherently or falls into a state of furious delirium; sometimes coma supervenes, but more frequently life is extinguished by the occurrence of one or two convulsive fits. It may also be remarked that at the very time [at] which the brain suffers most, the patient to the inexperienced would appear evidently improving. The irritability of stomach from torpidity of its nerves, arising from the diseased and compressed state of the brain having ceased the patient is enabled to eat and drink and retain both. Now false hopes of recovery are once more entertained, but to be quickly disappointed by a sudden and unexpected death.

In other cases when matters are so reversed that the gastric symptoms predominate, the *sensorium*[19] rarely suffers any great molestation and the patient continues sensible to the last. It cannot be said but the head symptoms may give occasional annoyance, but nothing beyond what local applications can readily relieve, whilst gastric and abdominal symptoms are gradually on the increase and sometimes perfectly intractable the pain and irritability at [the] stomach, with almost constant retching are most distressing, the thirst is insatiable, the fluid vomited (consisting of bile mucous thread-like matter) and the fluid begins to assume a darker colour and every subsequent ejection a shade darker than the one immediately preceding, until at last it has acquired the appearance of coffee grounds, and constitutes what is termed black vomit. The biliary salivating put on the phlegmonous blush and continued to ulcerate. The alvine evacuations assumed a dark broken down appearance and frequently composed of nothing else than the fluid known by the appellation of black vomit, the surface is exceedingly yellow; the *tunica sclerotica*[20] the same. Now every sense of pain is seldom much longer felt, the stomach becomes retentive and the patient expresses himself perfectly well, with the exception of a feeling of sinking at the *praecordia*, which is always complained of; the pulse is scarcely perceptible; the extremities become cold, the countenance collapses; the breathing oppressed and the patient sinks almost insensibly and without a struggle. There is a third termination of this fever in which active or passive haemorrhage of blood puts an end to the scene.

A fourth termination is a crop of *furunculae*.[21] A fifth is the production of carbuncles. A sixth is visceral lesion laying the foundation of subsequent disease without occasioning immediate death. The third termination proved fatal in two instances, but in both black vomit had its full share in the internal ravages; in the other termination it did not appear, and no deaths occurred thereby, the sixth excepted to which two or three deaths might safely be attributed. These terminations then, it is needless to say, were both frightful in appearance and dangerous in consequences, and which when superadded to the exanthenatous and ulcerated state of the gums (before a grain of Calomel had been given) and the highly aggravated aspect of all the ordinary symptoms were sufficiently characterized to distinguish the disease from the ordinary fever of the colony.

It is due now to remark that a remission was generally established at the lapse of seventy-two or eighty-four hours that this happy deliverance was uniformly preceded by very profuse sweating; and that shortly after it became general, all the symptoms even the most ardent began to abate and continued declining until the remission was fairly established. Exacerbations continued to recur but, in many cases, the second paroxysm was warded off. In others the remission presented a less perfect character and subsequent paroxysms followed and either occasioned death or a protracted convalescence. In a third set of cases the paroxysm continued without scarcely any abatement of symptoms, until life expired; and in a few other cases the paroxysm terminated in health without leaving the slightest inconvenience to complain of except weakness in which the mind participated equally with the body.

The greatest anomaly perhaps connected with the disease was the recovery of a woman belonging to the 74th Regiment – a Mrs McDugal – after having suffered a severe attack of fever and decided black vomit for nearly forty-eight hours. And the discovery of evident black vomit as it were in the urinary bladder of a man of the same corps. The preparation is carefully put up and exhibits in a very satisfactory manner the dark bluish jelly coating of the mucous membrane, peculiar to the existence of the fluid termed black vomit.

With respect to the pathology of this fever it must be acknowledged that although pathological enquiries may be considered of the greatest importance in the investigation of disease, whereby its nature and origin are more likely to be detected and more applicable remedies suggested that such researches cannot always avail us of success, nor even to fulfil our anxious expectations. So it happened in the victims of yellow fever where the morbid appearances after death so far from throwing a light on the nature and causes of the disease, in some cases failed, even to correspond with the character of the symptoms, and much less to account for sudden dissolution as will hereafter appear. In the generality of the cases which proved fatal at this station, death supervened on the 4th or 6th day of the disease; and so little variety presented in the post-mortem appearances in each class, that a description of the general appearances met in each is deemed preferable to separate and individual details.

Port-Mortem Appearances of Men Who Died on the 4th Day of the Disease

External appearance: – body muscular, deep yellow suffusion of the whole skin and *tunicae scleroticae*; marks of blistering and occasionally cupping; the blistered surfaces either erysipelatous or in a state of gangrene, a discoloration and puffiness of scalp over the occipital region and the same dark bruised like appearance not infrequently extended itself over the whole posterior or inferior surface of the body and extremities. The body being moved to any extent black vomit issued from nostrils, mouth and anus. The animal heat, although the utmost tendency to decomposition prevailed, was retained a very unusual time after death.

Head – On cutting through the scalp much dark grumous blood in general issued from the divided vessels. The *calvarium*[22] being removed the membranes of the brain appeared unusually vascular, and the *meningeal*[23] vessels highly distended. Further dissection displayed a highly congested state of the *plexus choroidei*[24] of all the sinuses.

Thorax – Nothing remarkable of a recent nature presented except a more or less congested state of the lungs.

Abdomen – The stomach, bowels and urinary bladder externally presented considerable vascularity and the organs having been emptied of the contained fluid denominated black vomit. The mucous membrane was covered over by a dark bluish jelly of some consistence and depth, this being removed the villous coat itself presented a highly vascular appearance, and in parts displayed numerous arborescent darkish red patches of an erysipelatous[25] character.

The blood exhibited a thick dark broken down appearance; the gall bladder generally contained dark viscid bile. The liver assumed an unusual light-brown appearance and in parts a yellowish aspect. The spleen generally oozed with blood and softened in texture. The kidneys, notwithstanding the suppression of urine (but often retention) in consequence of inflammation and thickening of mucous membrane of bladder and urethra, never showed the slightest morbid appearance.

When the head symptoms predominated the morbid appearances were more fully developed, and less destruction of mucous membrane resulted, and the vice versa.

Signed
Charles Stewart MD
Assistant Staff Surgeon and P.M.O.
In charge of garrison detachment hospital
Fort King George, Tobago

4 April 1840

Extract of Annual Report of Prevailing Diseases in the Garrison of Fort King George, Tobago, from 1 April 1841 to 31 March 1842, by S.H. Hardy,[26] Staff Assistant Surgeon

A Detailed Account of Any Epidemic Which May Have Visited the Station during the Year, Stating the Circumstances under Which It Appeared and Its Subsequent Progress

Remittent fever of a low and malignant form was epidemic amongst the white troops here during the months of April, May and June, the symptoms each of which will be detailed under the head fever.

It was, I conceive, consequent on the dryness of the season for immediately on the setting in of the rains in July and August, the admissions became less frequent and the disease was of a milder and more manageable character. The following table is annexed:

Table 12.5: A Return of the Number of Cases and Deaths from the Epidemic Remittent Fever at Tobago from 1 April to 31 July 1841

	White Troops						Black Troops		
	Strength	Treated for fever	Relapses	Died	Recovered	Escaped fever	Strength	Treated for fever	Recovered
Commisd. Officers	13	6		1	5	7			
Non-Com Ditto and Privates	89	93	23	14	79	19	112	3	3
Women	12	10			10	2	17		
Children	14	8	1	1	7	7	19		
Total	128	117	24	16	101	35	148	3	3
Whites Proportion of Sick to Well $117/128$ Ditto Deaths to Treated $16/117$									

The following tables will elucidate the queries on this head.

Table 12.6: Military Unit Strength and Mortality Report by Age

Classes of Ages	Strength of each Class	Admitted	Died	
15 to 20 years	$1^{1}/_{6}$	2		
20 to 25 „	$14^{7}/_{12}$	29	3	Did the sickness or mortality most affect young soldiers or those advanced in life, and has it fallen in a higher proportion on those recently arrived than on those long resident etc?
25 to 30 „	16	46	5	
30 to 35 „	34	64	7	
35 to 40 „	$9^{2}/_{3}$	15		
40 to 45 „	$3^{5}/_{12}$	11	2	
45 to 50 „				
Above 50				
Total	$78^{10}/_{12}$	167	17	

Table 12.7: Military Unit Strength and Mortality Report by Period of Residence

Period of Residence	Average Strength of each Class	Admitted	Died
Under one year	$10^{10}/_{12}$	8	
1 to 2	$57^{6}/_{12}$	138	16
2 to 3	$8^{10}/_{12}$	20	1
3 to 4	$^{6}/_{12}$		
4 to 5			
5 to 6			
6 to 7			
Above 7	$1^{1}/_{12}$	1	
Total	$78^{10}/_{12}$	167	17

Vaccination

Six adult privates in the 1st Regiment were vaccinated but all without success; it was practised in the cases of four children in three of whom it was successful. A case of *variola*[27] has not occurred at this station during the past year.

Febris Remittens – 106 cases of this form have been treated, 14 of which proved fatal. An asthemic[28] and malignant form of this species prevailed epidemically amongst the white detachments here during the months of April, May, June and July 1841; the symptoms were as follows: on admission the patient complained of general lassitude, pain in the back and limbs, headache and thirst, the skin was generally hotter than natural but not to a great degree; the pulse varied from 90 to 112; the tongue was coated and yellow, and sometimes red at the edges and thick; the bowels were sometimes constipated, sometimes lax and occasionally regular; in about twenty-four or thirty-six hours a remission came on followed by two or three accessions of fever, till about the fourth day, when fever ceased to recur and the patient with care became better. The stomach was usually very irritable; this was the course in the more favourable cases, but in others a new train of symptoms set in about the third or fourth day, characterized either by obstinate irritability of stomach; the fluid evacuated being of an inky colour and genuine black vomit, or by excessive prostration of strength with extreme restlessness or by haemorrhage of an atomic nature from the kidneys or by the appearance of *petechiae*[29] or *vibices*[30] on the skin which were observed in one case.

The fatal cases exhibited some one of these last-mentioned symptoms which terminated in coma and death. The occurrence of haemorrhage was not invariably a fatal symptom as one recovered who had it from his kidneys and another who had it from his *nares*[31]; it was more frequently observed in the relapses. Death generally took place about the fifth day.

On examination after death, the mucous membrane of the stomach was invariably found in a state of inflammation, varying in intensity and kind in different cases, it was generally in patches, some of the florid others copper colour and others of a dark grumous[32] tinges. The mucous membrane of the intestines was also found inflamed and sometimes ulcerated and frequently very livid and containing a blackish unctuous[33] fluid.

The liver was enlarged friable and of a yellower colour than natural. The gall bladder sometimes contained a dark green fluid and sometimes a fluid like tar, and in one case it was nearly empty. The spleen was generally congested and softer than natural. The heart, lungs and brain exhibited but slight traces of disease. In a case which died with haemorrhage from the kidneys, the mucous membrane of the pelvis of these viscera was intensely ecchymosed[34] and contained some fluid grumous blood.

Signed
S.H. Hardy
Staff Assistant Surgeon
1 April 1842

Extract of Annual Report of the Medical Occurrences in the 92nd Highlanders at Tobago from 1 April 1842 to 31 March 1843 by C.J. Palmer, Surgeon, 92nd Highlanders

This fatal variety of febrile disease has not prevailed so extensively as at former periods of the service of the regiment in the command and altho' the aggregate appearing on the numerical return as having been treated in the course of the year amounted to thirty-nine it may be proper to remark that twenty-six of the number remained at the end of the preceding in a convalescent state and were eventually discharged free from complaint and thirteen recent cases were admitted during the present. One of these occurred in the first mentioned and the other twelve during the last four months of the year, December being the period of its greatest prevalence and in the course of which eight cases took place and four in January, February and March. They were derived from various sources – seven from the Brick Barrack, one (an officer's servant) from a part of the town called The Bay, two were hospital orderlies and three patients in hospital who had been originally admitted with bowel complaints. Of the three last mentioned, two had a fatal termination accompanied with black vomit. The three men attacked in hospital were all taken ill in the lower ward. It was also in this ward that one of the fatal cases under the head of *febris cont: communis*[35] was attacking. Cases of fever of an aggravated type appear to have taken place at former periods in the same ward and in another on the same flat on the opposite side of the passage in which no less than thirteen cases of yellow fever of a highly aggravated character lately occurred amongst the patients of the 46th Regiment. The two hospital orderlies were attacked to this ward but they had committed previous excess in liquor [and] had lain in the open air a whole night. The men admitted from the barrack were some from the upper and some from the lower flat of the building and had been employed in their ordinary military duties. The febrile excitement was generally preceded by the usual premonitory indications and the heat of surface in most instances of a very ardent character. In two of the number, the disease was attended with slight cough and pain and oppression in the chest, in a third with marked derangement in the hepatic system and in a fourth with the last mentioned together with severe enteric irritation, delirium with a strong marked typhoid diathesis foul and parched tongue and incrustation or sores about the teeth. Indeed, the typhoid diathesis was a constant accompaniment in all generally attended with a great degree of lethargy and apathy during the continuance of the acute symptoms and followed on remission by much depression of strength and a peculiarly slow languid and sluggish pulse. Yellowness of the surface was also a constant attendant tho' not in general. Except in two cases and in these it subsided slowly.

C.J. Palmer
Surgeon 92nd Highlanders

13. Reports from Trinidad

Preview: Only two reports were recorded from the period 1818 to the 1840s for Trinidad. Of special note is the appearance of detailed medical prescriptions in the earlier report. These are written in Latin and every effort has been made to have these translated. It is quite possible that the appearance of these prescriptions reflects the professional training background of the doctor who makes them up. Again, as in the other reports that we have transcribed, the case notes that have been included are invaluable in getting a sense of the prevailing philosophies of medical practice that characterized the period under study.

Staff Surgeon Sharp's[1] Half-Yearly Medical Report from Trinidad from 21 June to 20 December 1818

June
From the 23rd to the 29th, there were daily heavy falls of rain alternated with calms and much thunder. From this until 4 July, the weather was more moderate and drier, when the rain again commenced and continued at intervals to the 20th. The wind was, in general, steady from the south-east
Average range of the thermometer, Morning 73°.
Noon 81°; Evening 78°. Highest observation: 88°, Lowest 71°.

As is usual in the Royal York Rangers who were quartered during the period in the huts at Orange Grove, cases of fever occurred amongst them, but the disease was of a mild remittent type, yielded to venesection, followed up with the use of evacuating remedies, the occasional application of the cold effusion or hot baths, and a strict antiphlogistic regime. Out of the 25 admissions of fever, only one case proved fatal, and this man's condition was very much injured by intemperance in rum drinking.

At this period, thirty cases of acute dysentery also occurred amongst them, and although nineteen of the number were men who arrived in the island from Europe on the 1 and 12 June, the symptoms even in them were equally as mild as in the assimilated soldier, and the disease yielded to the common remedies – viz – bleeding when the state of the vascular system appeared to indicate the use of it, but in general, saline purgatives in small and repeated quantities were only necessary with small doses at bedtime, of Calomel and Opium, infusion of ipecacuanha[2] or Dover's powder,[3] and this with tonics, moderate use of port wine and a light farinaceous diet generally and speedily accomplished a perfect case.

A coloured man, upwards of three months in hospital, with a large sloughing ulcer, which extended over all the toes of the right foot, died during this month. He had had repeated attacks of inflammation of the lungs. In dissection, they were found tuberculated, and the cavities of the chest, pericardium, and abdomen contained a large quantity of water. The following are the symptoms, treatment [and] appearances on dissection of the fatal case of fever that occurred during this month.

Sergeant Gillan of the Royal York Rangers, *aetatis anno* 39, of a phlethoric habit,[4] and much addicted to intemperance, assimilated to the climate by a servitude of about ten years – was admitted to Hospital at Orange Grove on 24 June 1818, seized yesterday with headache pain at the *scrobiculus cordis*,[5] *hypogastrium*[6] and general soreness. Symptoms on admission: pain at the *scrobiculus cordis*, considerable irritability of the nervous system, vessels of the aorta turgid, pulse 120 and fluttering, skin hot and covered with profuse diaphoresis[7]; stomach irritable, excessive thirst, tongue foul and tremulous, two dark coloured stools during the last twelve hours – *Vespere* –

Capiat Hydrargyri submuriatis g^r x v statim[8]

The 25th passed a tolerable night. Pulse expanded, bowels not sufficiently opened, otherwise as yesterday. *Capiat Jalapo Radicis*

*Contriti ʒfs statim*⁹ — 26th — Had a good night; pain at the *scrobiculus cordis* relieved, pulse quick; skin hot, considerable despondency, stomach extremely irritable, thirst, tongue foul, bowels open — *Capiat Hydrargyri submuriatis Ði statim et Haustus effervescens pro re nata — applicetur Empl/[astrium]: Lyttae Ventriculo — Vespere.*¹⁰ Three or four alvine dejections since morning, stomach retentive.

*Rep[etitu]r Hydrargi (sic) submuriatis ut supra*¹¹

27th: Had several stools and rested tolerably during the night, pulse frequent and rather small, heat natural, skin soft, thirst much less, tongue foul.

Capiat Infusi Calumbae fl ℨii
*quarter in die*¹²

Vespere — Complains of heaviness across the anterior part of the head, eyes inflamed, pulse as morning, skin warm and dry, bowels open.

R_x *Hydrargyri submuriatis Ði*
Pulveris Jacobi Ðfs
Mucil Acacroe Gummi q: s: ad
Fiat massa in Pilulae sex distribruenda statim sumendus
*Appl: Empl: Lyttae nucham*¹³ —

28th — Rested well and feels better this morning, head better, pulse tolerably regular, skin moderately warm, bowels open.

*Cont[inuetu]r Infus. Calumboe ut antea*¹⁴

3⁰ 30" *Post Meridiem*. Seized suddenly with languor, pulse quick and feeble, skin warm and covered with profuse diaphoresis, countenance anxious, breathing laborious, no stool since the early part of the morning.

R_x *Otheris [sic, recte etheris] Rectificati fl Ðfs*
Tincturae opii ɱxx
Aquo Puro — ℨ1 M[isce] fiat Haustus
pro re nata sumendus, habeat
Enema Purgans statim et
applicetur Empl[astrium]: Lyttae amplum
*Pectore*¹⁵

Wine and Brandy Toddy are to be given frequently, and bottles filled with hot water are to be applied and frequently repeated to the axillae and feet. *Vespere.* Considerable inaction of the sanguineous system, pulse scarcely perceptible at the wrist, surface cold and covered with clammy sweat, pupil contracted, much anxiety depicted in the countenance, intellect's clear, but is unable to articulate, appears to suffer no pain, had a trifling faecal evacuation since the enema – *Cont[inuetu]r. Eadem Medicamenta et habeat Enemate Stimulantia.*[16]

The treatment was assiduously continued until midnight, when he expired. <u>Dissection.</u>

External surface livid.

Head – Turgescence of the vessel of the brain – effusion of serum into the left ventricle – a large proportion of bloody serum in the base of the cranium.

Thorax – considerable congestion in the lungs – a large quantity of serous fluid in the pericardium – Heart flabby – Abdomen – Liver considerably enlarged and gorged with blood – gall bladder – distended with vitiated bile – spleen much enlarged and sphacelated – internal coat of the stomach destroyed by gangrene.

From the commencement of July to 20 August heavy showers of rain, accompanied as in the former month with much thunder, continued to prevail.

Average range of the thermometer: Morning – 73°. Noon – 85°.

Evening – 81 °. Highest- observation 88 °. Lowest – 70 °.

During this month, only ten cases of fever remitted and continued occurred in the Royal York Rangers at Orange Grove, and the disease was equally as mild, its symptoms as in the former period and only one case after a lingering illness of twenty-three days proved fatal. Sixteen cases of dysentery also occurred and, with one exception, soon yielded to the same remedies and applications as were adopted in the former month.

A detachment of the Royal Artillery consisting of seventeen men, only a few months from Europe, and six, who had been for four years and upwards in the West Indies, accompanied by six women and fifteen children, arrived at Orange Grove barracks on 12 April, where they remained until 26 May on which day they were removed to a room in the Sea Fort of Port of Spain. – Fever on 21 July suddenly made its appearance and first commenced in a small and miserable hovel which was allotted for a few married families, and in the space of a few days, four women and four children fell victim to it. – On its first appearance, the detachment was immediately removed to Orange Grove barracks. However, it was too late. The disease, in a day or two, became general amongst it and assumed a most malignant and marsh type, and out of the detachment – eleven men, four women and five children have died.

That the locality, bad construction and ill-ventilated state of the barrack operated as the only exciting cause of the disease in the detachment cannot be questioned. My only surprise was that they remained so long in it healthy as they did. The room fourteen of them occupied is only twenty feet in length by sixteen, and twelve in height, and one small window with gratings opening to the north and two to the South. Consequently, it never admitted the free circulation of the trade or east-wind. The site of the barrack, likewise as I have already reported, is not only exposed to the influence of the extensive east swamp but is also exposed to the putrefactive exhalations from the ditches which surround it and the shallow and foul bed of the gulf on which it is immediately situated, the offensive exhalations from which at low water is severely felt by those whose occupations lead them at that time to pass it.

The wooden shed in which the married families live is erected at the end of this room, the gable and windward end of which answers as a support for its roof. It is out of repair. In rainy weather, they were completely drenched in it – and more equally exposed to all the vicissitudes of the climate, and not one who occupied it escaped an attack of the fever. The fever they were attacked with was, in general, ushered in with a headache, violent pains of the back and limbs, and considerable prostration of strength. In some, the face was flushed, heat rather above the natural standard, and the pulse accelerated, but more commonly, the body was covered with clammy perspiration. The pulse was feeble. The powers of life, even in some newcomers previously of a most robust and healthy appearance, rapidly sunk. The tongue from the commencement was black and furred in the middle; at the edges, it had a fiery red appearance. The pupil became dilated, delirium succeeded, the skin became in general of a dirty, livid colour, and the body emitted a most offensive smell. Hiccoughs and black vomiting in every case at this period occurred and soon put an end to the patients' miserable sufferings.

Evacuating the bowels formed the natural and primary practice adopted. However, the low stages so rapidly succeeded that stimulants, both externally and internally, were obliged to be had recourse to, freely and largely. In some cases, where the head appeared particularly affected, I was induced to sanction venesection to be tried, but in no case in this detachment, during the prevalence of the epidemic, did it succeed. The convalescence was lingering and, for weeks and months, never became perfect – of the seventeen newcomers, only two escaped an attack of the epidemic; of the seven who had been for years in the West Indies, three were attacked, and one died. The following detailed cases will elucidate the symptoms and general mode of practice adopted, with the appearances on dissection –

John Anderson of the Royal Artillery, of a plethoric habit: five months from Europe, *aetatis anno* 28, was admitted to Hospital at Orange Grove on 25 July 1818 – Symptoms seized last night about gunfire with rigour, which left him and recurred. This morning, attended with severe headache and considerable action of the sanguineous system; pulse 100 and full, eyes inflamed, face flushed, skin hot and arid, preternatural thirst, tongue foul and dry, bowels open

> *Capiat Extracti Colocynthidis comp: ℈i*
> *statim et postea solut: Magnesiae*
> *Sulphatis ad effectum detrahatur*
> *Sanguis e Brachio ad ℔ iifs*[17]

Vespere. Several stools since admission; headache continues but in a lesser degree; symptoms as morning.

> *Capiat Hydrargyri submuriatis ℈i*
> *Et Pulv: Jacobi ℈fs statim*[18]

26th Had some sleep during the night and appears somewhat better this morning; pulse less frequent, skin moderately warm and soft, less thirst. Tongue foul and moist, bowels open.

> *Habeat Hydrargyri submuriatis Ðfs*
> *Pulveris Jacobi qr viii statim*[19]

Vespere. Felt tolerable well during the fore part of the day, but became extremely low towards evening; pulse small, irregular and frequent, skin cool, countenance dejected, bowels open.

> *R$_x$ Misturae Camphorae fl℥ ifs*
> *aetheris Rectificati*
> *Liquoris Ammoniae compa a[n]a fl ʒ fs [:] M[isce]*
> *fiat haustus 2nda quaeq[ue]: hora*
> *capienda*
> *Applicetur Empl: Lyttae inter*
> *scapulas et tibibus internis et*
> *Cataplasmata Capsic: frutescens*
> *Plant: ped: Wine and Brandy freely.* —[20]

Post Meridiem. Has been extremely restless through the day, with no material alteration of symptoms

> *Cont: eadem Medicamenta et adde*
> *Tincturae opii ⋅ xL.*—[21]

27th: Passed a restless night, considerable anxiety of countenance, yellowness of the conjunctiva, pulse quick and feeble, skin cool and covered with clammy diaphoresis, stomach irritable, tongue covered with a dark fur and dry, bowels open.

> *R$_x$ Camphorae Ammoniae Subcarbonatis*
> *Baccae Capsici frutescens a[n]a gr v*
> *Extracti opii qr I syrupi q: s: ad*
> *f[ia]t. Bolus [ter]tia quaq[ae]: hor: sumend:*
> *Applicetur Empl: Lyttae Capiti*
> *et Scrobiculo cordis* – Wine and Brandy continued[22]

He continued in nearly the same state until the afternoon of the following day and expired. – *Sectio Cadaveris*[24]: External surface livid.

Head – increased vascularity of the brain and its membranes, adhesion along the falciform process of the dura mater – *Thoracic* viscera natural – *Abdomen* – Liver enlarged, indurated, and gorged with blood – gall bladder empty, inner coat of the stomach highly inflamed.

Thomas Simpson of the Royal Artillery, *aetatis anno* 38, of a full habit, about five months from Europe, was admitted to Hospital at Orange Grove on 25 July 1818. Symptoms on admission; headache, pains across the loins and in extremities, pulse accelerated, skin hot and dry, much thirst, tongue foul, bowels regular. *Capiat Pilulae Cambogiae comp: scrupulum*[24] – on the next day, headache, increased turgescence of the vessels of the conjunctiva, pulse quick and hard, skin hot and bowels open. He was bled to two pounds, and blisters applied to the anterior part of the head and nape, also cold affusion.[25] *Hyd: submurias et Pulv: Jacobi*[26] were given. Towards evening, his pulse became quick and feeble, countenance anxious, stomach irritable. A blister was applied to the epigastrium, and stimulants such as Camphor, ammonia, wine and ardent spirits were given without effect. He died on the afternoon of the 27th, after three days in hospital.

Sectio Cadaveris – A general livor over the surface – *Head* – Turgescence of the meningeal vessels, slight adhesion along the falciform process – *Thoracic* viscera natural – *Abdomen* – Liver considerably enlarged but of healthy structure. The gall bladder empty, and the inner coat of the stomach is highly inflamed and, in some places, gangrenous. The spleen is in a state of sphacelation.[27] This man's wife and child were in the hospital at the time with the same type of fever, and both died on the following day.

John McMurray of the Royal Artillery, *aetatis anno* thirty, of a robust habit, five months from Europe, was admitted to Hospital at Orange Grove on 26 July 1818 with the following symptoms: Considerable headache, pulse quick and rather small, skin warm and dry. Face flushed, vessels of the adnata turgid, preternatural thirst, tongue foul, bowels costive, *Hydr: Submurias et Pulv. Jalapi*[28] were given in combination and afterwards *sulphas magnesiae*.[29] 27th, passed a restless night, pulse quick and feeble, skin cool, countenance anxious, stomach irritable, tongue morbidly red and parched; headache with same confusion of intellect, bowels open. Blisters were applied to the head and epigastric region. Camphor, ammonia and capsicum were given in combination. Effervescing draughts were exhibited, also wine and brandy largely. He died about 2:00 p.m., two days in hospital.

Dissection: External surface livid. *Head*. Serous affection on the surface of the brain, adhesion along the falciform process. *Thorax* – Contents natural. *Abdomen* – Liver enlarged, gall bladder full of bile of a dark bituminous appearance; inner coat of the stomach highly inflamed and, in parts, running into gangrene.

John Ellis of the Royal Artillery, *aetatis anno* twenty-six – of a delicate habit, five months from Europe, was admitted to Hospital at Orange Grove on 5 August 1818. Symptoms on admission – Bowels obstinately costive, free from fever, *Pilulae Cambogiae comp: scrupulum et postea solute magnesiae sulphas*.[30] 6th. constant vomiting occurred, pulse quick, skin warm and dry, tongue covered with dark fur, bowels open. A blister was applied to the stomach, and effervescing draughts were given. The stomach became easy, and a complete remission of fever took place on the 9th. His bowels became confined, and a scruple of *Pilulae Cambogiae comps*[31]: was given with effect. The next day, he became extremely low, pulse small and frequent, skin cool and countenance collapsed, vomiting a dark fluid resembling coffee grounds. Another vesicatory[32] was applied to the epigastrium and *Mistura Camphorae* combined with *liq: Ammonia comp*[33]: were given with wine and brandy freely. Blisters were also applied to the legs and sinapisms[34] to his feet but without effect. He died at about 3:00 p.m. on the 11th, seven days in hospital.

Sectio Cadaveris: Nothing extraordinary in the external appearance. *Head*. Turgescence of the vessels of the brain and its membranes, adhesion along the falciform process. *Thorax*. The right lobe of the lungs is tuberculated. *Abdomen*. The stomach contained a large quantity of fluid similar to that vomited, its internal coat gangrenous. This man's wife and child died at the Sea Fort of the present epidemic and [he] was the first who was attacked by it.

Meteorological} from the 21 August
Observations} to 20 September

At the commencement of this period, a sudden change in the state of the atmosphere took place. Rain fell in torrents with much thunder, calm, and a perfect stagnation of the atmosphere succeeded. The heat became most oppressive, and the thermometer in the coolest part of the Orange Grove barracks stood for hours, daily as high as 93°.

Sickness about 27 August commenced amongst the men of the Royal York Rangers, and in the course of the monthly period, we admitted sixty-seven cases of fever. Five remained on the 20th. Out of this number, seventeen died. Twenty-four of those admitted were out of the hundred and ninety-two men who joined the regiment in June from Europe. The remaining forty-three were men assimilated to the climate. Nine of the former and eight of the latter died, and also two of the artillery, one a newcomer, the other an assimilated soldier, years in the country.

The fever was very different to what occurred in the Royal Artillery last month. It put in a most formidable and inflammatory appearance from the commencement, partaking little or none of the appearances which characterize the marsh type of Trinidad. The head was violently affected, the eyes were inflamed, the pulse was full and, in general, hard. The bowels were obstinately constipated. A general soreness was felt over the body, and the calves of the legs were particularly affected with spasms.

In those who were habitual drunkards, the progress towards a fatal termination was most rapid. In those surgical cases who were attacked with the epidemic in hospital, the symptoms assumed a more formidable and aggravated type than in those who were admitted from barracks – Bleeding to the extent of two or three pounds with mercurial and saline purgatives, the application of liquor, *Ammonia Acetatis*[35] to the head, previously shaved, the cold affusion in so far as our limited means of obtaining it allowed; Diaphoretics: – viz, saline julep[36] with other *Nitricum*[37] or *Liquor Ammonia Acetatis* with *James's Powder, Submuriate of Mercury*[38] and the use of blisters, particularly to the nape of the neck, were the primary remedies employed when remissions became complete. Cinchona was used with advantage. In the low stage of the disease, brandy with stimulants such as *capsicum*, *Camphor* and *ammonia* were largely and freely given.

From the local situation of the huts and barracks at Orange Grove, it has clearly been given as the decided opinion of some experienced men, and particularly by Dr Fergusson, that the European soldier, at such a season of the year, could not long withstand its pestiferous exhalations surrounded to the east by a chain of mountains which completely obstruct the free circulation of the trade wind, exposed to the marsh influence of the eastern swamp to the putrefactive bed of the river in which it is situated, also to the effluvia of annual and vegetable matter with which it is in every direction surrounded. These decomposed, particularly by the action of such a vertical sun as we then had, and more especially after such heavy falls of rain as preceded it, it might perhaps be hazardous to say that annual and vegetable miasmata were not alone the immediate and exciting cause of the fever which occurred, but to those who witnessed the scenes of irregularity and drunkenness in which the men of this corps indulged themselves at this period, this conjecture may be problematic.

During this period of excessive heat and perfect stagnation of the atmosphere, the men, heated by intemperance in drinking, no doubt suffered much from the crowded state of their habitations, as [no] fewer than seventy, on average, being heaped together, if I may use the expression, in a hut of only fifty-four feet in length by twenty-six in breadth, without galleries or jalousies. When rain occurred, the few blinds they [had] been kept shut during the night. The consequence was, and it is known beyond contradiction, that more than a third, particularly those who were in a state of inebriety in general, slept outside of them, exposed to the chilling damps of the night and all the vicissitudes of temperature.

At my request, exertion was made to remedy this evil, but I suspect with very trivial success or attention. To remedy their crowded state was also tried, but no house for their reception could be found in Port of Spain.

Our considerably ill-ventilated and worse constructed hospital, without baths, remote from the source of obtaining water, without out-houses, even a kitchen except the one in common allotted for the Barracks, was at this period crowded – often eighty patients, all labouring under acute disease, occupying one ward a hundred and thirty feet in length by twenty-six in breadth.

It necessarily followed that our exertions were much cramped and, in fact, rendered abortive. It was witnessed by every medical officer in attendance that during the oppressively hot state of the hospital at this period, men who were apparently and actually in a favourable state of recovery were attacked with irritability of the stomach, low-muttering delirium and cold, clammy sweats, extreme debility succeeded and in the generality of those so affected, death was the consequence.

After some difficulty, on 4 September a house was at last obtained and rented in Port of Spain, capable of containing about thirty patients into which I ordered surgical cases and convalescents.

The advocates for contagion at this time would have had a fine field open to their observation of assisting them in establishing and supporting their doctrine on this subject.

Out of the nine orderlies employed this month in the hospital, not one escaped an attack, and three of them died. Some of those who recovered have had a second attack. Assistant Surgeon Cochrane[39] of the Royal York Rangers, O'Connor of the artillery and Mr Stewart,[40] hospital assistant, all in attendance at the hospital, were likewise severely attacked, as well as almost every surgical patient who was in it previous to their removal to the hired house.

Example of a Fatal Case – The cases of acute hepatitis and the three dysentery admitted during this month were extremely slight, and the greater proportion of the latter cases in hospital were discharged perfectly cured.

Details of a Fatal Case – 18 September: **Henry Clay of the Royal York Rangers**, *aetatis anno* 30 of a full habit and assimilated to the climate by a residence of more than six years, has been an Attendant in hospital for the last fortnight. He was seized yesterday with severe headache and pain in the inferior extremities, pulse quick and full. Eyes inflamed, face flushed, tongue foul, thirsty, bowels costive: (1)

> *Capiat Pil: Cambogiae c[ompositae]* ℈i *statim*
> *Et post horas duas Magnesiae*
> *Sulphatis* ℥ifs *detrahatur Sanguis*
> *E Brachio ad* ℔ *ii*[41]

Vespere. Vomited considerably after the bleeding, but the stomach is at present retentive, headache less severe, pain in limbs continues, pulse quick and rather small, skin hot and dry, bowels opened. [2]

> *Capiat Hydr: Submuriatis ϶i statim*
> *affusionem frigidum Capite raso*
> *applicetur impl: Lyttae et habeat*
> *Statim post balneum Haust: seq[ent]tis*
> *R$_x$ Liquoris Ammoniae Acetatis*
> *Aquae Menthae Piperitae a[n]a fl ℥ i [:] misce*[42]

19th: Passed a restless night, complains of severe headache, pains in the extremities, pulse full and quick, skin hot and dry, thirst excessive, tongue parched, slight muttering delirium, bowels rather slow.

> *Habeat Pil Cambogiae Comp ϶i statim*
> *detrahatur Sanguis e Brachio ℔ j*
> *et ex Arteria temporale ℔ fs*[43]

Vespere. Headache and pain relieved, pulse quick and small, less heat of skin, tongue moist, several alvine evacuations since morning.

> *R$_x$ Misturae Camphorae*
> *Liquoris Ammoniae Acetatis aa fl ℥ ii,*
> *aetheris Rectificati,*
> *Nitrici aa fl ʒfs M[isce] f[iat] Haustus*
> *Hora somni sumendus*[44]

20th – Had a tolerable night and passed several bilious stools, pulse small and quick, skin cool, countenance expressive of anxiety, considerable prostration of strength, had a little Madeira wine in the night, which he vomited, tongue moist, bowels painful.

> *Capiat Misturae camphorae fl ℥i*
> *omni hora cum Tinct. Opii. ♏xx in*
> *primo dosis applicetur Empl: Lyttae*
> *Ventriculo et habeat Vini fl ℥ii omni hora*[45]

Vespere. Appears much better, pulse more expanded, has no pain, stomach retentive, dislikes the wine for which reason it was vomited, and brandy toddy in small quantities substituted.

> *Rep[etitu]r, Misturae Camphorae et supra*⁴⁶

21st – Slept well in the night, vomited this morning, pulse small, skin cool and of a yellow hue, much anxiety, bowels open, tongue clean.

> *R$_x$ Misturae Camphorae fl ʒi*
> *Liquoris Ammoniae Comp: fl ʒj M[isce] f[iat] Haustus*
> *Omni hora sumendus applicetur*
> *Empl. Lyttae nuchae colli.*⁴⁷

Brandy and wine are to be given in as large quantities as the stomach will retain. He continued to sink until one o'clock p.m. and expired.

Sectio Cadaveris: External surface yellow, head meningeal vessels turgid, strong adhesion along the falciform process of the dura mater, innumerable red points in the substance of the brain, a large quantity of water in the lateral ventricles and base of the cranium. *Thorax*. Viscera natural. *Abdomen*. Villous coat of the stomach is highly inflamed. Spleen is gangrenous.

Three rapid and fatal cases of surgical patients attacked in hospital with the epidemic are here detailed to show the violence of the disease.

Robert Hodges of the Royal York Rangers, *aetatis anno* twenty-seven of a full habit, about four months from Europe, was admitted to hospital at Orange Grove on 21 August 1818 with a slight ulcer on the foot. On 6 September, he was attacked with the following symptoms and had suffered some paroxysms of intermittent prior to his last admission. An unusual degree of stupor with an aversion to answer questions. Pulse full and about 90, skin hot and dry, bowels open, head painful.

> *Capiat Magnesiae sulphatis ʒfs statim*
> *Capili raso et postea habeat*
> *Affusio frigida*⁴⁸

Vespere. Has had no stool and is a little delirious, pulse and temperature as morning.

> *Habeat Magnesiae Sulphatis ʒi*
> *Statim et applicetur Empl: Lyttae*
> *Capiti.*⁴⁹

7th – Delirious through the night, pulse quick and feeble, skin cool, anxiety of countenance. He obstinately refused both medicines and comforts kept sinking gradually until 4 p.m., at which time he expired.

Sectio Cadaveris: External appearance of the body yellow. *Head* – the vessels of the pia mater turgid, the substance of the brain contained innumerable red points, the lateral ventricles contained about an ounce of serous fluid. *Thoracic* viscera natural. *Abdomen*. Liver of ordinary size, dark-brown colour and full of blood, stomach extremely vascular and containing a small quantity of black fluid, intestines generally black and in some parts gangrenous, spleen large and soft.

Aidan Burns of the Royal York Rangers, aetatis anno thirty-three, a strong, robust man but at present considerably reduced in the flesh. He has been in the West Indies for only four months. He was punished on the morning of 23 August and admitted into hospital in consequence. He speedily got well but was detained in hospital for a slight ulcer on the right leg. He was seized on 3 September with severe headache pains in his loins and extremities. Pulse 100, skin hot and dry, excessive thirst, tongue covered with thick fur, stomach irritable, bowels regular.

Capiat magnesiae sulphas et Hydrargyri submuriatis. Empl: Lyttae toto capitis et Scrobiculo cordis.[50]

The bowels were well opened, vomiting continued, and all the symptoms became aggravated, and in addition to their singultus,[51] became very distressing. Stimuli were given internally and applied to the surface of the body without benefit; he continued to vomit black matter until 4:00 p.m. of the 8th, when he expired.

Dissection: Fifteen hours after death, the fore part of the body is slightly yellow, and the back part purple. *Head* – vessels of the pia mater turgid and a quantity of jelly-like substance lodged between it and the membrane *Arachnoidea*.[52] The lateral ventricles contained about three fluid drachms of serum. *Thorax*. The left lung adhered firmly to *pleura costalis*.[53] *Abdomen* – Liver enlarged and of a dirty yellow colour; stomach large and contained about a quart of black fluid. Its villous coat is not as vascular as is usually found, the jejunum and ileum black as ink and perfectly rotten, and the spleen small and soft.

James Bond of the Royal York Rangers, *aetatis anno* seventeen of a delicate habit, about five months from Europe, was admitted to the surgical ward, a hired house about a quarter of a mile from the hospital, on 21 October 1818 with a large sloughing ulcer on the external malleolar process of the right leg. On the 30th, he was attacked by the following symptoms – severe headache, pulse small and quick, skin hot and dry, tongue furred and dry. Was brought to the medical ward at night. *Extracti Colocynthidis comp: gr xv combined with Hydrargyri submuriatis gr v*[54] was immediately given to him, and a blister was applied to the head.

31st – Headache relieved, pulse small and quick, skin natural, tongue mauvish, had three alvine dejections during the night.

Habeat sulphatis Sodoe ʒi statim.[55]

Vespere. Had an exacerbation of fever at noon. Cold affusion and *Liquoris Ammoniae Acetatis fl ʒi*[56] were administered, which relieved him considerably. Symptoms as at first.

R_x *Hydrargyri submuriatis Ɔi*
Pulveris Jacobi gr. Vi M[isce]f[ia] Pulvis
statim sumendus[57]

1 November – had some sleep in the night, pulse small and quick, skin cool, bowels open, says he has no pain, stomach irritable.

R_x *Hydrargyri submuriatis gr iii*
Camphorae gr ii Mucil: Acaciae
Gummi q: s: ad f[iat] Pil omni.
Hora sumendus appl[icetu]r
Empl: Lyttae regioni epigastrici[58]

At 3 p.m., the vomiting became black, pulse small and feeble, and skin cold. He had two fluid ounces of brandy every hour until sunset, when the symptoms continued. The surface was rubbed with bruised capsicum and spirits, and the stools which he provided during the day were quite black. The frictions were again repeated at nine o'clock when the stools became involuntary – the brandy to be repeated every fifteen minutes. *Applicetur Empl. Lyttae nuchae Capitis et Cruribus.*[59] He continued in nearly the same state until about 4:00 the ensuing morning when he expired.

Appearances post-mortem. Livid about the neck and shoulders. *Head.* Turgescence of the meningeal vessels, slight adhesion along the falciform process. Thoracic viscera natural. *Abdomen* – Liver exhibited no morbid appearance. The gall bladder was empty. The stomach contained a large quantity of black fluid similar to that thrown up – several gangrenous spots on the villous coat.

Sergeant Hutton of the Royal York Rangers, *aetatis anno* 36 of a full habit, about three months from Europe, was admitted to hospital at Orange Grove on 9 August 1818 with the usual symptoms of remittent fever, but in a very aggravated form which yielded to purgatives, bleeding, sudorifices and stimulants to a great extent but left him in a very weak state. The Cinchona bark and bitters with a nourishing diet were given. He continued in a prosperous state until 20 September when he was seized with the most alarming symptoms of the present epidemic – violent headache, pulse 120, intense heat of surface, dejection of countenance, incessant vomiting, bowels torpid. Calomel with Colocynth and purging enemas were given, cold affusion and vesicatories were applied to the epigastrium and nape of the neck. The vomiting ceased, the pulse became feeble, skin cool, and breathing laborious with every appearance of approaching dissolution. Blisters were applied to the head and breast, and Camphor, ammonia and *aristolochia serpentaria*[60] in combination with wine and brandy liberally were administered. He died at half past 9:00 a.m. of the 21st.

Dissection: External surface generally pale but livid about the neck and shoulders. *Head* – considerable serous effusion on the surface of the brain, strong adhesion along the falciform process[61] of the dura mater, a quantity of serum in the lateral ventricles and base of the cranium. *Thorax* – adhesion of the right lung to the *pleura costalis*.[62] Firm adhesion of the heart to the pericardium. *Abdomen* – liver natural, gall bladder full of thin, watery bile. Spleen of an immense size and sphacelated. Pancreas – stomach and intestines exhibited no morbid appearance.

The following cases of recovery are here detailed to point out the apparent salutary effects of bleeding.

Terence Smith of the Royal York Rangers, *aetatis anno* twenty-three of a full habit and sanguine temperament, five years in the country during which period he had two attacks of remittent fever. He was admitted to hospital at Orange Grove on 6 September 1818 at noon with the following symptoms: violent delirium, pulse 106 and feeble, heat ardent, surface covered with sweat, countenance agitated, strong pulsation of the carotids, appears to suffer pain on pressing the epigastrium, tongue foul.

> *Habeat Hydrargyri Submur: ℨfs et*
> *Extracti Colocynthidis Comp:gr v statim*
> *detratratur sanguis e brachio ad ℔ iii et*
> *Capiti prius raso app[licetu]r Empl: Lyttae*[63]

Vespere. He is sensible since the bleeding and expresses himself. Much relieved but states that the pain has been gradually returning this last hour.

> *Rep[etitu]r venesectionis ad libram cum semisse*[64]

Syncope[65] was produced, and he became covered with cold perspiration, pain of the head and epigastrium entirely removed bowels torpid.

Rep[etitu]r eadem Medicamenta et habeat Enemata Purgantes pro re nat[a].[66]

7th – Passed a good night, pulse and skin nearly natural, complains of a sense of constriction at the epigastrium.

> R_x *Hydrargyri submuriatis gr iv*
> *Pulveris Iacobi gr ii M[isce] tertius horis*
> *sumendus et habeat Haustus*
> *effervescens post singulis dosis*[67]

Vespere – Has a perfect apyrexia,[68] bowels rather torpid.

> *Capiat Ol: Ricini fl ʒi et enem[a]*
> *Purgans statim*[69]

8th – Continues his amendment; bowels opened. Bark was therefore administered; at noon, he had severe exacerbation of fever. The bark was therefore omitted and Calomel with James' Powder and effervescing draughts given. In the evening, he was perfectly free from fever and the bark was again given.

9th – Passed a good night – Pulse 90; heat natural.

Cont: Cinchona

Slight mercurial action took place. He continued gradually to improve and was dismissed from hospital on the 21st of the same month.

Francis Wilmore of the Royal York Rangers, *aetatis anno* 29 of plethoric habit, several years in the country, was admitted to hospital at Orange Grove on 11 September 1818. Symptoms seized the preceding evening with rigours, succeeded by heat and headache. Pain at the *praecordia* and across the loins with irritability of stomach. Pulse quick and moderately full, skin hot and dry, considerable thirst, tongue foul, bowels tolerably regular.

> *Capiat Hyd[rargyr]i: Submuriatis ∋i statim*
> *detrahatur sanguis e brachio ad*
> *℔ iiifs Capiti prius raso applicetur*
> *Emplastrium Lyttae*[70]

He became considerably exhausted immediately after the bleeding. Wine and brandy with *Liq. Ammonia comp:* were given frequently. *Vespere:* somewhat revived but still very low. Pulse quick and feeble. Skin cool and moist, stomach less irritable.

> R_x *Misturae Camphorae fl ʒifs*
> *Liquoris Ammoniae compositi fl ʒfs M[isce] f[iat]*
> *Haustus tertia quaque hora sumend[us]*
> *Applicetur Emplastrum Lyttae ventriculo*[71]

12th – Had some rest during the night, has no pain, vomiting restrained. Pulse quick and somewhat expanded, surface cool and moist, less thirst, tongue foul and moist, bowels open.

> *Eadem Medicamenta repetare*[72]

Vespere. Continues nearly in the state he was in at the morning visit.

Continuetur medicina ut supra[73]

13th – Rested well during the night but is extremely low this morning. He has no pain. Pulse quick and feeble, skin cool and moist, tongue cleaning, bowels open.

Rep[etitu]r Haustus ut hori[74]

Wine and brandy toddy to be given frequently.
Vespere: Feels himself better in every respect.

Cont[inuetu]r Medicamenta[75]

14th – Vomited considerably in the early part of the night but slept well towards the latter part and feels much better this morning. Pulse small, skin cool, stomach retentive, bowels regular.

Cont[inuetu]r Haustus ut supra[76]

15th – Had a good night and appears to have no other complaint than debility. The Cinchona bark and a nutritive diet were given and continued until the 21st at which period he was dismissed from hospital.

Meteorological observations from 21 September to 20 October – At the beginning of this period, occasional breezes occurred from the Southward and eastward, accompanied with showers of rain. About 3 October, a change took place, and the wind again became, as in the last month, variable with heavy falls of rain, much thunder and occasional calms. On the 15th, a complete change took place. The unwholesome westerly wind, so destructive to the residents of Port of Spain and Orange Grove, prevailed, and the exhalation of marsh miasmata from the neighbouring swamps and marshes were in full action. The weather was from this time, as in the previous month excessively sultry and oppressive.

The prevailing epidemic this month continued to extend to an alarming degree. Twenty-four cases of fever remained in the hospital on 20 September. Eighty were admitted, out of which number thirty-nine died. Also, two cases of dysentery, one old case of *Phthisis Pulmonalis*, and one of Pneumonia. Out of the number of fevers admitted, thirty-five were newcomers, including three of the battery. The other forty-five were men long in the country of the former. Twenty-two died, and of the latter seventeen.

The fevers until 3 October continued nearly of the same type as in the previous month, but after this, a complete change was evident, and the cases admitted, as well as those in hospital, assumed a most malignant and continued form, the despondency and prostration of strength was great. From the commencement, there was a peculiar anxiety about the patient not easily described. The eye in some was inflamed, and the face was flushed. More commonly, the eye had a glossy, watery appearance and appeared so prominent as if it had started from its socket, and the face was melancholy, ghastly and dejected. The tongue was parched and, at the edges, morbidly red. The temperature of the skin, as well as the state of the vascular system was in different cases very differently affected. In some, the pulse was full and rapid. In others, the circulation was languid and, during the whole progress of the disease, even in some cases, terminated fatally. The pulse never exceeded one hundred. In these, we observed little or no morbid heat, irritability of stomach with vomiting was constantly attendant and in some of the more malignant continued. Haemorrhage from the nose and gums occurred at a very early period, debility rapidly succeeded, and stimuli of the most powerful kind had no influence in checking its progress. Low-muttering delirium with *singultus*[77] and black vomiting gushing from the stomach in quarts full retained their senses to the last moment and expired when perfectly collected. In a few cases that recovered and in some that proved fatal, *Petechiae*[78] appeared all over the surface, particularly upon the face and extremities and generally appeared on the eighth or ninth day of the disease. In such till recovered it generally succeeded irritability of stomach. The patient kept unusually languid and, by those in attendance, was observed very averse to answer questions when spoken to.

The mode of treatment this month has consequently varied according to circumstances, such as appeared of a full habit and only a few months in the country, bleeding was tried with a very doubtful effect. The quantity taken was small, and the patient for a time, felt relieved by it, yet a state of debility rapidly succeeded. The stomach rejects almost everything offered, and the patient gradually sunk. The treatment in common adopted has been, in the first instance the administration of saline or mercurial purgatives and mercurial functions until ptyalism was produced, as irritability of the stomach and coma attended almost every case. Saline and Camphor Juleps with blisters to the epigastric region, head, neck and feet were had recourse to when the low stage succeeded, brandy, spirituous *ammonia compositus* into Camphor, ammonia, capsicum and others, in various forms and in large quantities were given, as well as the administration of stimulant enemas, and frictions with camphorated spirits were attentively persevered in.

When remission took place, it generally made its appearance by a gentle diaphoresis, diffused partially or generally over the surface of the body, with a natural and sound sleep. Bark at this time was used either in decoction substance or tincture with a moderate allowance of wine, porter or beer and nourishment. During this period, thirteen patients in a convalescent state from fever walking about the hospital using bark and nourishment in quantities and the animal functions appearing to be regularly carried on in every respect, relapsed, and not fewer than eight out of the number died, the whole of the hospital attendants were also attacked and two died. Two stewards employed in the hospital who had been both attacked the previous month also relapsed, and both were for days despaired; they, however, recovered.

A general panic prevailed at this time amongst the men of the corps at Orange Grove, and the idea of coming into hospital was considered by them as certain death. The generality of them, however, appeared very indifferent for existence, and the common call was "give me only rum, and I shall soon despatch myself". The old hospital attendants at this time were either dead or bed-ridden, and the very worse description of men for either morality or sobriety were now obliged to be employed in their stead for others of a better description could not be found, the medical officers fatigued by the pressure of sickness and the hospital attendants infamous conduct, had in consequence the most menial duties often to perform and one I was obliged to direct to be in constant attendance at the hospital, however notwithstanding every exertion on their part instances are numerous where the dying patient was robbed of his sick comforts not only by the unprincipled orderlies but by their more merciless comrades who only perhaps a few hours previously had escaped from the jaws of death, and scenes of irregularity and intoxication were witnessed which no ingenuity or exertion that I could devise or obtain could possibly prevent; as long as rum was in the island there was no possibility of preventing them from obtaining it at Orange Grove. One unfortunate man employed as a clerk in hospital at this time, for mutinous conduct to Assistant Surgeon O'Connor,[79] the steward and others in hospital has by the sentence of a court-martial paid the forfeit of his life.

Under all circumstances and seeing that the epidemic continued daily to spread with increased malignancy, I was induced to address the following letter to the officer commanding. I was happy and much gratified next day to see my suggestion carried into immediate effect.

Port of Spain, Trinidad, 16 October 1818
Sir,
I have the honour of stating to you that in consequence of the daily increasing sickness of the men of the Royal York Rangers at Orange Grove and the great mortality that is daily taking place amongst them, notwithstanding all the measures of precaution and means which have already been adopted to put a stop to it that it strikes me at this period of the season as the wind, in general, keeps steady from the east or south-east that they might benefit by a removal to Fort George if it was only for a period of two or three weeks. We have at this moment upwards of forty patients in hospital all in a most dangerous state from fever of a most malignant nature. The admissions are becoming daily more numerous, and the disease is at the same time assuming a more serious and aggravated type. Under these circumstances and as it is impossible they can become sicklier than they at present appear, I would certainly recommend to you most strongly and without loss of time to try the effect of a change of air to Fort George.

Signed
"James Sharp"
Lieutenant Col: Sonett
Commanding His Majesty's Troops, Trinidad

The irregularities of the men in the house were on a par with those in Orange Grove Hospital, and the admissions of fever from it were numerous; neither the fences nor palings at the gentlemen in the neighbourhood of it proved any obstacle for their obtaining rum and additional sentinels in getting it. I was, therefore, induced to run all hazards and to recommend their immediate return to Orange Grove Hospital and barracks, which took place on 23 October.

Detail of the Rapid Fatal Cases

James Tipton of the Royal York Rangers *aetatis anno* 26, five months from Europe of a robust constitution and intemperate habits, ill by his own account two days, was admitted to hospital at Orange Grove on the morning of 27 October 1818 with the following symptoms severe headache, great anxiety and prostration of strength, pulse 100 and feeble, heat of skin a little above the natural standard, tongue foul and tremulous bowels, constipated.

> R_x *Hydrargyri Submuriatis Ӡfs*
> *Extracti Colocynthidis Comp[ositae] Ʒfs in*
> *Pilulae vi distribuenda statim sumendus*[80]
> *Capiti raso et applicetur Empl:[astrum] Lyttae*
> *nuchae colli*[81]

2:00 p.m., became restless and uneasy, breathing laborious, bowels opened.

> R_x *Misturae Camphorae fl Ʒii*
> *Solucionis Ammoniae Comp[ositae]fl Ʒfs:*
> *M[isce f[ia]t Haustus*
> *Omni hora sumendus, applicetur*
> *Empl[astrum] Lyttae. Capiti et Pectori*
> *Brandy to be given freely*[82]

Vespere. Extremely restless pulse scarcely perceptible at the wrist, skin cold.

Cont[inuetu]r eadem Medicamenta[83] the surface to be frequently rubbed with camphorated spirits. This treatment was continued until one o'clock of the ensuing morning when death closed the scene.

Sectio Cadaveris. Eleven hours after death, skin of a purple colour and covered with numerous *petechiae*. Head – a quantity of bloody serum in the lateral ventricles and base of the cranium. *Thorax* – no morbid appearance. *Abdomen* – adhesion of the omentum to the gall bladder which contained a quantity of bile. Stomach contained a large quantity of black matter. Omentum much inflamed and, in some places, gangrenous, gangrenous spots on the intestines.

David Evans of the Royal York Rangers *aetatis* 19, of a delicate habit and about a year and a half in the country, was admitted to the hospital at Orange Grove on 6 October 1818. Symptoms on admission – slight pains of the head and back.

Prescription: Capiat Pilulae Purgantes sex statim[84]

7th was taken last night with great heat of skin, increased arterial action, hurried respiration and prostration of strength was bled to two pounds, and a scruple of submuriate of quicksilver[85] given is much better this morning, pulse soft, skin still hot, tongue foul, bowels open.

> R_x *Habeat Hydrargyri Submuriatis Ɜi statim*
> *Affusio frigida et Empl[astrum] Lyttae nuchae*
> *colli app[licetur]*[86]

Is much better, bowels well opened

> *Habeat Hydrargyri Submuriatis Ɜi Extempore*[87]

Vespere. Had an exacerbation of fever at noon.

> *Affusio frigida habeat et postea*[88]
> R_x *Solucionis Ammoniae Acetatis fl ℥i*
> *aetheris Nitrici fl ʒi M[isce] f[iat] Haustus*
> *omni hora capiendus*[89]

9th: Feels an internal sensation of cold, external temperature natural, pulse small and feeble. Tongue furred with fiery edges, bowels freely open.

> Rx Misturae Camphorae fl ʒi
> Solutionis Ammoniacae Comp[ositae] fl ʒi [:]
> M[isce] f[iat] Haustus, omni hora sumendus[90]

Brandy toddy to be given frequently
Vespere: pulse very low and feeble, skin hot, respiration hurried

> Cont[inuetu]r eadem Medicamenta
> Empl[astrum]: Lyttae cruribus applicetur[91]

Stimulants were given largely and unremittingly during the night. He died about 4 a.m. of the 10th.

Sectio Cadaveris[92]: Head – cerebral vessels turgid. A preternatural quantity of serous fluid in the ventricles and base of the cranium. *Thorax* – about two ounces of water in the pericardium. *Abdomen* – liver much enlarged. Gall bladder – empty. The stomach contained a quantity of black fluid, its villous coat highly inflamed.

The salutary effect of the removal of the corps from Orange Grove to Fort George soon became evident. For the seven or eight days after their arrival at that post, we had only three admissions of acute fever from it, and two of these, it was discovered, had been ill previously to their arrival.

A few men were left at Orange Grove as a guard over the regimented baggage and so on. They, with our hospital servants, afforded the greater proportion of the twenty-eight cases of fever admitted during the month. From 21 October to 28 October, there was little or no alteration in the state of the atmosphere, and the westerly wind continued to prevail. The cases of fever admitted, as well as those in hospital during this period, appeared, if possible, to assume a more malignant typhoid type, and relapses such as had recovered from the first attack became almost general and fatal.

About the beginning of November, the wind veered round to the north with strong breezes and heavy falls of rain. This change of the weather, however, had no evident effect in abating the malignant type of the fever in hospital. Doctors Menzies[93] and Bone[94] on 29 October arrived and the latter on 4 November took the medical charge of the men of the Royal York Rangers in hospital at Orange Grove. As the treatment he followed differed widely from what we had before adopted, I shall give in detail a few cases treated by him extracted from the medical register of the hospital.

13 November 1818: Detailed case of Private William Lee, Royal York Rangers, aged twenty-seven, a stout, muscular man, arrived in the West Indies from England in June last, was doing duty as a clerk in hospital when he was seized with fever which commenced yesterday at 4:00 p.m.

12 November: His first symptoms were giddiness, succeeded by trembling and pains in his loins, which continued for about three-quarters of an hour. These were followed by heat, perspiration and frequent vomiting. He had for some time back a foul inflamed ulcer below the inner ankle, which is at present black and bloody. His tongue is covered with a white crust, pulse 112.

> Hab[ea]t Balneum tepidum statim
> R_x Sulphat: Magnes: ʒii
> Aq[ua] Fontanae fl ʒviii omne horis quadra[tis]
> Radatur Caput[95]

14th: Has been extremely well purged, stools black and fetid, pulse 112, eye red and muddy, was very drowsy and stupid all yesterday and last night.

> R_x Tinct Sennae ʒi, Aq Menthae
> Syrup a[n]a ʒfs M[isce]
> Cap[ia]t ter quaterve die
> R_x Mist: Diaphoret ʒviii
> Solutio: Antim: Tart: ʒii
> Sp[iri]t[u]s aetheris Nitrici ʒii :
> Cap[ia]t ʒi 2dis horis
> et affusio frigida habeat[96]

15 November: Has been lying in a stupid comatose state during the night except when roused to take his medicine or drink, vomited and moaned frequently, is at present insensible to external objects, is throwing his legs about and groaning piteously, face, neck and breast yellow and covered with a greasy, clammy perspiration, hurried

respiration, he presents a shocking appearance, the black vomit is streaming out of his mouth faster than it can be wiped off; was directed to be taken out of the ward to prevent its having a bad effect on the other patients, died in the dead-house about one and a half hours after being moved at half past 9:00 a.m.

Detailed Case of Company Serjeant Major Kerns 3rd W.I. Regiment

11 November 1818: a native of Ireland aged about thirty-four years came from St Joseph on the fourth instant and went to reside into one of the huts or cabins to windward of the hospital, i.e., the eastward, was taken ill on Monday last 9 November about 4:00 p.m. he felt cold as if in an ague fit. He then became hot and perspired all the night. He reported himself sick the following morning but requested most earnestly that he should not be sent to hospital, saying, "If he was, he should be certain of dying". His request was acceded to by Assistant Surgeon Lenon[97,] and he had a dose of Calomel and Jalap, followed by a solution of Sulphate of Magnesia given him, which operated very briskly and which produced a perfect remission, but was at night seized with incessant vomiting. He was brought into hospital this morning (Wednesday, 11 November) at seven. His tongue is now covered with a white chalk-like crust, the tip and edges are of a scarlet red, his eyes duskish and muddy, abdomen not painful on pressure.

> *Radatur Caput et tegatur Empl[astrum]: Lyttae*
> *Imponetur Scrobiculo cordis Emplastrum Lyttae*
> R_x *Sulphat: Magnes: ʒi, Aq Fontanae ʒvi*
> *M[isce] [:] Cap[ia]t quadrante horis donec alvus*
> *plene solutus Erib[at?]*[98]

Vespere: Has been freely evacuated during the day having been at the night chair every ten minutes. His skin, though extremely hot, is covered with perspiration, moans frequently, heat of the body 103. His tongue is not so dry as in the morning, says he feels a sensation as if the bed were breaking under him and that he is afraid he shall fall through it. He expresses himself thus "that the heaviness is upon him". There is no tension of the abdomen, has vomited frequently during the day. It is always brought on by his attempting to move in his bed. His stools are watery and fetid with griping.

R$_x$ *Ag: Tepidae ʒ xii, Sulphat: Magnes ʒi*
Ol: Ricini ʒfs: M[isce] f[ia]t enema statim
Injiciendum. Habeat Aq[ua]: Hordei pro potu
Commune et : Solut sulph. magnesiae pro re nata
donec mane[99]

12th: His tongue is not so white as yesterday. Pulse 80 and small, eyes of dusky red colour, especially the left, heat under the tongue 100, was restless during the night ... fell asleep and slept till gunfire this morning.

R$_x$ *Potassae supertart[ratus] ʒi*
Aq Fontanae Oil M[isce], pro potu
commune, Balneum tepidum habeat[100]

13th: Pulse scarcely perceptible but is about 90. His tongue is of a blackish brown colour, his teeth are furred, has been very noisy and restless during the night, vomited frequently, feels cold to the touch, his eye is of a dusky yellow, and his skin is beginning to assume a yellow tinge.

Repet: Mist. cum supertart; potassae ut heri praescripta fuit, habeat balneum tepidum et lavatur corpus saepe in aq: tepid: cum aceto

Vespere: Has continued in a state of the most extreme debility since morning, requested the attendance of a clergyman who immediately waited on him, is perfectly composed, his intellects have never been disturbed during his illness, says that coming into hospital has been the cause of his death, that he is aware he is dying but that if he had been left in hut instead of being sent into the slaughterhouse of so many rangers (as he terms the hospital) he might had had a chance of recovery. He refuses all kind of medicine but is ordered to have any kind of beverage he wishes to take, continued gradually to get worse until 1:00 a.m. 14 November, and expired.

The following remarks were made by Assistant Surgeon O'Connor[101] of the Royal Artillery, under whose care the patient was placed on admission. Case of I. Kilmartin of the Royal York Rangers, aged thirty years of a robust habit much addicted to the use of ardent spirits during a service of several years in the West Indies, was admitted into hospital at Orange Grove on 23 October 1818 with the usual symptoms of the prevailing epidemic accompanied with great irritability of the nervous system and incessant vomiting. The bowels on admission were freely evacuated by Calomel with Jalap and other purgatives, and after the intestines were well cleaned out. Calomel and Opium in small doses frequently repeated until mercurial action took place. Debility was obviated by the free use of internal and external stimuli, and it is worthy of remark that brandy seemed to act as a charm in arresting the irritability of the stomach when everything else was rejected. The disease yielded to the above treatment and assumed a tertian type, which gave way to a few doses of bark. Although there was a slight irregularity and quickness of pulse, his appetite was tolerably good, and he laboured solely under debility. Doctor Bone, Physician to the Forces, having assumed the charge of the General Detachment Hospital on 5 November, prescribed the following medicine:

> R_x *Sulphatis Magnesiae ʒi*
> *Solutionis Antimonii Tartarizati fl ʒi*
> *Aqua Pura fl ʒviii secundis horis*
> *ad tertiam vicem*[102]

6th: Tongue was brown and foul and was marked to have the tumid cachectic habit; his stools were involuntary, and he soiled his bed, pulse 105.

> R_x *Pulvis Jalapae Comp: ʒi*
> *Mistura Diuretici habeat*[103]

The diuretic medicine consisted of the following:

> *Supertartratis Potassae ʒi*
> *Nitratis Potassae ʒi*
> *Pulveris Aromatici ʒi*
> *Syrupi fl ʒii – Aquae ʒii*
> *To have a pint of wine*[104]

7th: Vomited frequently. What he vomited was not black, face of a sallow, livid hue, pulse 100. Had nine stools since yesterday morning, which are of a dark colour.

R$_x$ Sulphatis Magnesiae ℥ii
Aquae Menthae piperatae fl ℥viii fiat
Haustus ad sextem vicem, Misturae
Diaphoretici ℥ii bibat de die[105]

8th: Vomited frequently since yesterday morning. A dose of bark that was administered was rejected shortly after.

R$_x$ Aquae tepidae fl ℥viii omni hora
Et Balneum tepidum[106]

9th: Began to turn quite yellow yesterday about noon. He is of a dirty yellow colour, makes a disturbing noise and is *in articulo mortis*. Died at 8:00 a.m.

In the dissection of these cases as well as in those that died the two previous months during the malignant and typhoid character of the disease. The body was, in general, of a livid purple or yellow colour and emitted an offensive smell. There was great vascularity of the vessels of the brain and considerable suffusion of lymph on the dura and pia mater and quantities of water were found in the ventricles and base of the cranium. The pericardium generally contained an unusual quantity of water. The villous coat of the stomach was in a corroded and sphacelated state and filled with black matter. The Pyloris and internal coat of the intestines generally presented the same appearances, often as black as ink, perfectly rotten and filled with similar black matter as was found in the stomach or with fetid faeces, although the bowels during the progress of the disease were freely evacuated. In the majority of them, and particularly those who had been addicted to rum drinking, the liver and spleen were large and indurated, and the former, but more particularly the latter, was commonly found perfectly rotten. The gall bladder was usually gorged with dark viscid bile. The kidneys were generally found natural, and the urinary bladder perfectly empty. The omentum and mesentery usually partook of the state of the intestines, perfectly black gangrenous and, in fact, rotten. The change of station but more particularly of the weather, which I have stated took place about the beginning of November, had the most happy effect, and the malignant fever amongst the men at Fort George ceased to appear about 8th of that month and only five cases of remittent fever from 21 November to 20 December were sent from that post, and two deaths alone occurred amongst the men of the rangers during the period in hospital at Orange Grove.

As the black house at Fort George was rather crowded, I suggested to the officer commanding the removal of one hundred and eighty men to Saint Joseph, and this was carried into effect on 3 November, and they now occupy the house, formerly the hospital, a well-constructed and well-ventilated barrack and which has lately had an addition of an excellent gallery upwards in breadth of 8 feet to the south side of it, it runs east and west and is completely protected from the bad effect of the foul air from the Maracas Valley which no doubt caused in a great degree such destruction amongst the men who formerly occupied the old barracks at this post, the present one is also completely sheltered from the north wind by a chain of hills which run parallel with it and at the same time is at such a distance that the free circulation of air though it is not obstructed. On 4 November, the hospital (formerly the mess room of this post) was established under the charge of Assistant Surgeon Cochrane[107] and during the first week they had thirteen admissions of fever and two deaths. There were also three admitted with acute dysentery. Mr Cochrane states that the irregularities of the men in drinking were great when they first went out.

In the cases of fever admitted the exacerbations and remissions were clearly marked. The former generally came on between the hours of 9:00 a.m. and 2:00 p.m. and continued until 9:00, 10:00 or 11:00 p.m., during which time the stomach generally became irritable, and the matter thrown up was of green colour, or the fluid which the patient had but a short time swallowed. The remission generally made its appearance by a gentle diaphoresis diffused partially or generally over the surface with an entire cessation of pain in every part except the back, which last in many continued for a day or two after. One of the fatal cases and one at present convalescent were bled, each to two pounds, on admission. Cold affusion, evacuants, sudorifices and blisters with Calomel in the primary stages, and bark in large and repeated doses in the remissions were administered. When the stomach became irritable, a blister to the epigastrium with capsicum and Camphor, effervescent draughts with tincture of Opium and purgative enemas were given until the irritability ceased, and the stomach became intensive.

The fatal case of acute dysentery William Ashcomb of the Royal York Rangers *aetatis anno*[108] 28 naturally of a strong habit but impaired by intemperance and effect of climate having been in the country upwards of seven years, recently discharged from hospital at Orange Grove where he had been eleven days with remittent fever, was admitted to hospital at St Joseph on 9 November 1818. Symptoms – frequent purging, griping and *tenesmus*,[109] pulse quick, full and hard, surface hot and dry, tongue clean, dejections slimy. He was bled to two pounds, neutral salts were given, and afterwards, submuriate of Quicksilver and Opium, the griping became excruciating. A blister was applied to the abdomen, small and repeated doses of neutral salts with mucilaginous enemas combined with Opium were administered and a tepid bath. Submuriate of Quicksilver and Opium were given until the mouth became affected. Compound powder of Ipecacuanha,[110] an infusion of Ipecacuanha in nauseating doses was exhibited with occasional benefit. The stools were exhibited with occasional benefit. The stools became black, watery and extremely fetid, and the patient considerably emaciated. A large portion of the villous coat of the rectum passed off by stool. He died at midnight on 5 December.

Sectio Cadaveris: Nothing extraordinary externally.

Abdomen: The whole of the intestinal canal gangrenous, particularly the colon and rectum. The villous coat of the latter had passed off per anno in a sphacelated state. Omentum in a state of incipient gangrene. Mesenteric Glands much enlarged and indurated.

At this post, from 21 November to 20 December, the wind was at the beginning North-East. Towards the latter part, it was South-East equally and accompanied with heavy falls of rain. The men here continued to indulge in their intemperate habits, and twenty-two cases of fever were admitted, out of which the seven that remained on the 20th died. Four cases of acute dysentery were also admitted, but they were soon discharged from adopting a similar practice as is detailed in the case of Ashcomb. The symptoms of those admitted with fever varied but little from what took place in the former month.

They were of the distinct remittent type of the West Indies in rather an aggravated form. In the advanced stage of the disease, the eyes and skin invariably became yellow, and *petechiae* commonly appeared over the body, especially on the face, neck and extremities. The treatment adopted and the appearances on dissection were in every case similar to what I have already endeavoured in this report to elucidate, and had we been fortunate enough to have seen the late work of Dr Jackson, I have no doubt, but we would have derived from it such useful instruction as would have guided and assisted us much during so long a period of sickness and labour.

The cases of catarrh pneumonia and *phthisis pulmonalis* which appear on the face of the half-yearly return affected chiefly the men of the 3rd West India Regiment and military labourers, with the exception of the cases of confirmed Phthisis which has carried off four of them. The two former were soon subdued by venesection, purging and an antiphlogistic regimen.

There has not been a case of *lues venerea* or chancre in the hospitals during the half year, and only one very slight case of Gonorrhoea has occurred. The four cases of ophthalmia[111] were also slight and generally cured by bleeding from the temporal artery, purging and a cooling regimen.

Several cases of Colica have also occurred. Evidently and decidedly the effect of drinking bad rum, but in no instance did it prove fatal, and opening the bowels freely with warm aromatic purgatives was the only remedy necessary for the accomplishment of a cure.

The men of the 3rd West India have for several months been much employed on fatigue and cutting down bush-wood. The consequence has been that the ulcer cases appear in great proportion on the face of the half-yearly return. Several have also occurred amongst the men of the Rangers. Some of them are constitutional; the generality, however, in both corps are slight and amounts only to fifteen, and the only application used is the adhesive strap. The vaccine has been here during the last half year in great abundance, but we have only had out of this garrison four or five children to inoculate with it. The whole, as well as the soldiers and others belonging to government, having previously been vaccinated or had the smallpox. Since the removal of the Rangers from the old barracks at Saint Joseph and their weakly men to Barbados and Europe, only seven cases of *Anasarca*[112] or Trinidad Cachexia have occurred during the last half year. The divided and sickly state of the Royal York Rangers during this period has not afforded me a sufficient opportunity of reporting on the interior economy of the corps in such a manner as can be satisfactory. As far as I have had an opportunity of seeing or learning their drills during this period have been but few.

The messing of the men appeared to me always tolerably regular and the regulations for a daily supply of vegetables were good. The system of keeping their canteen I conceive however, bad in this country. During my experience in the service, I have always seen it kept by the mess-man of the regiment, who was only allowed at certain hours to sell rum to the soldiers. The rum consumed in it is purchased by the officers themselves, and the profits arising from the retail of it goes towards defraying the expenses of their messing. It is open at all hours of the day which certainly will account for the scenes of irregularity and drunkenness which occurred and are stated in the body of this report. From a communication which I have had with the present commanding officer, this system he entirely disapproves of and intends immediately to put a stop to it and to place it on the same footing as is established in other corps.

The whole of the men in this garrison are daily inspected by a medical officer for the purpose of detecting sickness in its first stage or ulcers. This has been strictly attended to during the sickness and everything was tried to stop it but in vain. The barracks were repeatedly white-washed. The men in health were every morning at daylight marched to a distant river for bathing and washing their linen. Salts and other opening medicines were repeatedly given to them but to no purpose, and the removal of the corps to Fort George was therefore adopted and I hesitate not to say saved the lives of the greater proportion of them.

Signed
Dr Sharp
Surgeon to the Forces

Extract of Annual Report on Prevailing Diseases Treated in 59th Regimental Hospital and on the Principal Medical Occurrences for the Year Ending 31 March 1843, St James, Trinidad, by Surgeon T. Williams,[113] MD, 59th Regiment

Remittent Fever

I will here enumerate the numbers admitted and total treated for remittent during each quarter of the year at St James, with the deaths in each as follows:

Table 13.1: Quarterly Medical Statistics

Quarter Ending	Admitted	Treated	Died
30 June 1842	1	3	
30 September 1842	52	52	6
31 December 1842	31	33	
31 March 1843	57	63	13

Thus, it appears that the mortality by remittent fever during the last quarter (nine of which occurred in January and four in the first half of February) was more than double that of the whole.

In the first quarter of our residence here the troops were extremely healthy as regards fever and, I may add, as regards all other diseases. The weather at the time being variable as to moisture. During the second quarter to 30 September, a considerable number of fevers occurred with a mortality of six out of fifty-two treated, the weather being extremely wet accompanied with thunder and much lightning. In the third quarter to December, considerably fewer fevers occurred and were of a comparatively mild description up to the last four or five days, when several cases in a severe form appeared, which, of course, continued under treatment to the succeeding period. The weather during the early part of this quarter was wet, but towards the close, it became dry and cool. In the early part of the fourth or March quarter, this appearance of febrile disease (more particularly as regard severity) continued to increase until 13 February, when the troops were removed to encampment on the savannah at the recommendation of the P.M.O. The weather during the whole of this period here alluded to was dry and cool, indeed comparatively cold, more particularly of a morning and evening.

By a reference to the foregoing detail, it will be collected that an increase of fever and, more particularly, mortality has occurred at two periods differing materially as to the nature of the weather, that is, in the September quarter, which was very wet and in the March quarter which has been all through very dry and comparatively cool. With respect to any difference in the appearance of the fever at the two most unhealthy periods, I am inclined to think that during the last or dry period, the fever showed much less tendency to remission in its early stages and that there was much more speedy prostration of the powers of life, whereas, in the September quarter, remissions occurred earlier. The disease in many showed a disposition to assume the intermittent type of disease. I have heard the increase of fever in January ascribed by very old practitioners to dry weather and northerly winds and to the change from wet to dry weather. But it will be seen that an increase though not attended with so much mortality, occurred also at the wettest period of the year, when the winds were generally from south-east to west and under precisely similar circumstances as to duty and employment. I think it probable that the last increase of fever and mortality may have arisen in some respect from the coolness of the winds at this period rushing through the valley alluded to and acting on constitutions debilitated by the previous heat and moisture through a residence of nine months in this garrison.

This opinion may appear to be somewhat fortified by the fact that the fever and mortality almost wholly ceased upon removal of the troops to the little savannah, a dry spot near Port of Spain, where such influence does not appear to exist so forcibly. Malaria may, of course, and most probably did, influence its origin and progress from the quantity of wood on the uncultivated hills surrounding and from the uncultivated state of some of the surrounding grounds more particularly towards Cocorite. I have seldom, if ever, heard a satisfactory solution of these sudden burst[s] of fever at this or other stations in the West Indies during my long residence. Each individual has his peculiar views and looks with doubt upon those of others.

Under these circumstances, it is difficult, if not impossible, to come to a satisfactory conclusion upon so difficult a question.

With regard to the appearance of the fever usually met with at this place, the symptoms do not generally vary a great deal. The most prominent are intense headaches occipital or frontal, most generally the latter, pain of back, loins and lower extremities with cramps or spasms of the muscles of the legs, overwhelming nausea and frequent vomiting of bilious fluid, hot, dry skin, great thirst, quick pulse generally soft and compressible except in plethoric habits and recent arrivals. In some insidious cases, the pulse remains for some time at or below the natural standard. I have seen it as low as fifty and such cases, as far as I have been able to judge, are occasionally lingering and obstinate. The bowels are at first confined or irritable without effectual discharge, bilious and scalding dejections, great restlessness and inability to sleep. The illness is almost invariably described as having commenced with some rigour of intensity, but this is not often witnessed on admission, as it has generally passed off before the patient presents himself at the hospital. The headache generally continues for two or three days, even in the most favourable circumstances and in others, of course, for longer periods. But the pains of loins and lower extremities I have frequently found to disappear upon free evacuation of the bowels. A satisfactory remission is seldom obtained within two or three days from the commencement of treatment, although there may be, of a morning, some alleviation of the symptoms.

When such remission does occur at that period or sooner, I am inclined generally to consider the prognosis favourable. In more severe cases, the headache, nausea and heat of surface continued unabated if they do not increase. The bowels obstinate as regards effectual evacuation, the tongue coated of a greyish appearance or furred and streaked with yellow mucus, or dry and rough, the breathing becomes short and oppressed, the restlessness increases, and the mental faculties become more or less affected, the *scrobiculus* frequently becomes tender on pressure and thirst. However, pressing cannot be satisfactorily allayed in consequence of the irritability of stomach. Partial or even profuse general perspirations may appear without effectual relief and the eyes and skin not infrequently assume a yellowish tint. In cases of great prostration of strength, hiccough is not an uncommon symptom and tends materially to sink the patient still lower. The first symptoms of amendment in ordinary cases are the cessation of vomiting, the tongue becoming clean at the edges, a more satisfactory evacuation of the bowels, reduction of the pulse, a soft feel of the skin, and above all, the state of the countenance which is readily perceived but difficult to describe further than its exhibiting a degree of brightness and placidity so different from that of the same person a few hours previously. These symptoms frequently follow upon the patients obtaining some portion of sleep even of very short duration. In cases which proceed favourably the return of the exacerbation (if any) towards afternoon is not attended with such febrile excitement as before, the skin retaining a certain degree of softness and the pulse not rising to its former frequency. In the fever which occurred in January there was less tendency (as far as I could judge) to remission than at any former period and a greater tendency to disturbance of the mental faculties and to a state of coma. The prostration of strength also was greater and speedier.

On the whole, I think the fever appeared during that month in a severer form than previously, and as shown above, it was attended with much greater mortality. The duration, however, of this fever (stopped as it appears to have been by the encampment) was so short that it would be difficult to draw any general inferences. Whatever differences there may have been would appear to be caused by the state of the weather and this could lead one to suppose that the fever of the dry or spring season at St James is one of a worse description than at other times.

The post-mortem appearances have been usually as follows. There is some congestion of the vessels of the brain and membranes, but frequently to a slight extent. I have seen some perfectly normal in this respect. The thoracic viscera seldom exhibiting any appearances connected with this disease. The liver, particularly in drunkards, is large, sometimes pale, and at others dark coloured. Gall bladder, in almost every case, distended with black grumous bile. The inner coat of stomach and intestines almost uniformly more or less vascular and pulpy, in some to a very considerable degree. The pyloric end of the stomach and the duodenum being always chiefly so. The spleen large, generally soft, easily broken down and gorged with dark, grumous blood. One case opened presented as complete an exception from morbid appearances as could well be imagined. Head, thorax and abdomen were as healthy in this case as I had ever witnessed, yet the head had been much affected, and the disease terminated in convulsions in sixty hours.

Signed
T. Williams MD
Surgeon 59th Regiment

14. Reflections and Epilogue

The foregoing transcripts of reports written by several medical practitioners serving in the British military services during the eighteenth and nineteenth centuries offer several insights to our readers. In the first case, they provide first-hand accounts that substitute admirably for the medical commentary that we have grown accustomed to in this modern technological age. Today, at our fingertips, we can research the current medical debates in real time. We can scan millions of pages of data, and the advent of artificial intelligence even permits us to pose questions about that data and, possibly, to find answers to some of the most intractable issues. Secondly, these relatively unfiltered reports open to our view the competing medical philosophies that these practitioners and their contemporaries held. Here, in the various reports, we can follow the opposing complexities of confidence and despair, the assertiveness and the hesitancy of medical practitioners unsure of the origins of the deadly scourge of yellow fever. We follow this medical cohort from diagnosis to therapy. We look over their shoulders as they perform post-mortem examinations, all in search of answers to problems that they do not understand.

Additionally, as we read through their reports, we catch glimpses of the impact of the various prevailing debates that were circulating through the medical fraternity of their time. There is, for example, the question: does yellow fever reflect the operation of a contagion, or did the evidence dismiss that possibility? Questions, too, centred on the efficacy of the medicinal therapies – to bleed or not to bleed – were one of the preoccupations. This practice was based on the idea, dating back to the time of Aristotle, that all matter was essentially composed of four elements, namely, air, fire, earth and water. People assumed these elements had their parallel in the human body, in the four so-called humours: blood, phlegm, black bile and yellow bile. When these humours are balanced, the body experiences health. When ill health was apparent, it was felt that the underlying cause was an imbalance or over-accumulation of these humours. Thus, to restore balance, the physician had to get rid of the excess. The way doctors achieved this was through such supposed therapies as bleeding and purging, which involved inducing vomiting, diarrhoea, excessive sweating, excessive spitting, blistering, etc. At its least dangerous, bleeding might consist only of the application of leeches. However, at its extreme, there was the practice of venesection, which involved opening a vein and letting the blood pour out into a bowl. The risks were clear: death due to blood loss or infection, since there was little or no disinfecting of the instruments used.

However, most of the medical practitioners whom we encounter through their reports were wedded to a miasmatical regime which saw great efficacy in applying bleeding, blistering, vomiting, sweating and even spitting as counters to the causes they attributed to the disease. Few of them appeared to correlate the negative outcomes that many of their patients experienced to the very therapies that were employed. Instead, so wedded were most of these doctors to ancient theories of the cause of disease that they saw the death of their patients as being due to factors outside the treatment regime.

Notwithstanding the shortcomings of medical treatment at the time, the doctors that we are surveying must be commended for following up on all the available evidence. However, as we have seen, they missed the very signs that would have pointed them to the cause that they were looking for. Thus, one interesting aspect of the research carried out in many cases was the investigation of geographical and climatic conditions in various Caribbean locations. In such cases, minute details are recorded. What is not seen are the correlations that could have led to the discovery of the mosquito as the cause. Doctors recorded that moving some troops to higher locations, such as in Dominica, correlated to lower incidences of yellow fever.

Additionally, they saw some correlations between rainfall patterns and the outbreak of yellow fever in some locations. Yet, for all of this, they missed a correlation of these variables with mosquito infestation. In part, this failure is due to the philosophical blindness imposed by their adherence to miasmatic theory.

We cannot completely fault these doctors, given the prevailing medical knowledge of their time. However, evidence suggests that some publications from the late eighteenth century hinted at alternative explanations for the scourge they faced. Additionally, some voices from that period called into question aspects of their medicinal therapies. We note, for example, the work of Henry Warren.

In 1741, Warren, a medical practitioner who had worked in Barbados, published a work entitled "A Treatise Concerning the Malignant Fever in Barbados and the Neighbouring Islands, with an Account There from the Year 1733 to 1738". Warren begins his discussion by asserting that there was no "malignant distemper" indigenous to the island. Moreover, he observed that when the island was visited by what he termed variously "the Malignant and Ardent Fever of Barbados" and the *Febris Ardens Biliosa*, it was certain that "such have always been brought among us from some infected place". As far as Warren was concerned, yellow fever, which he noted the French had called *La Maladie de Siam* or *La Fievre Malchiltli*, and the Spanish, *Vomito Prieto* or the "Black Vomiting", was imported to Barbados from some "Asiatic" origin. Warren comes closer, perhaps than any of his medical contemporaries to touching on the real cause of yellow fever. It seems that he considered the possibility that yellow fever was caused not only by some "miasmatic influence" but by some more visible material cause. He observed that the bites of animals and some insects created "different distempers", but, unfortunately, he dismisses this possibility in the case of yellow fever.

It is noteworthy, however, that, unlike his contemporaries and certainly those who would follow them over the next hundred years or so, he was a moderate in advocating the traditional modes of treatment. He warns, "I do, in a great measure, forbid the ordinary evacuations, by bloodletting, emetics, vesicatories or purgatives in this pestilential fever, in which from long and attentive observation,

I declare them to be equally pernicious and destructive in their consequences..." Warren was equally appalled at the widespread use of Calomel (a mercury-based compound) by the local practitioners, whom he termed "plantation practitioners". If they understood "... the true nature of the use and inward operation of mercury, [he was] persuaded [that] they would be more cautious of playing with so dangerous a weapon...". In the place of these dangerous medicines, he advocated the use of "lenitive purges" such as "manna, cassia, lenitive electuary, or the like". Additionally, great care was to be taken to "keep up nature's strength and spirits by giving now and then a little warm Madeira wine, canary, or such cardiacs as are not too inflaming". In these prescriptions, Warren was way ahead of his contemporaries.

The medicines prescribed by Warren were generally mild compared to those that were often prescribed at that time. Manna refers to a secretion from flowering ash of Southern Europe. Sap-sucking insects feed on this plant and secrete a liquid, somewhat like honeydew. When dried, the secretion has a sweet taste. When eaten in large quantities, it is mildly laxative and was used as a medicine for that purpose. Lenitive purges were mild purges with a laxative action. Cassia was a plant related to cinnamon. Even in modern usage, it is known for its medicinal use in relieving nausea, flatulence and diarrhoea and in lowering the temperature of the body during a fever.

Unlike many of his contemporaries, and some of the doctors of later vintage, Warren had hit on a therapeutic regime that was significantly less harmful. Throughout the nineteenth century, doctors continued prescribing mercury-based compounds, which, if they did not kill the patient, either failed to relieve symptoms or made recovery more difficult. Certainly, Warren's patients would have been relieved of considerable agony by his decision to avoid totally the use of vesicatories. This term refers to the use of blistering agents, which were in common use at the time Warren wrote his treatise and, indeed, remained in common use throughout the eighteenth and nineteenth centuries.

By the 1880s, when Dr Carlos Finlay of Cuba connected yellow fever with the *Aedes aegypti* mosquito, medical science had advanced beyond the prevailing knowledge surrounding the practice of our

Reflections and Epilogue

medical reporters. Still, Finlay had his naysayers until his findings were later validated when American military doctors pursued his research in the late nineteenth and early twentieth centuries. However, our doctors in the British military services must not be left out of any history of the yellow fever virus and its ravages. In bringing some of these reports to light, I hope this publication advances historical knowledge on the journey toward resolving the problem.

Notes

Chapter 1

1. George Pinckard, *Notes on the West Indies*, vol. I (London: Baldwin, Cradock and Joy, 1806), 16.
2. Henry Rose Carter, *Yellow Fever: An Epidemiological and Historical Study of the Place of Origin* (Baltimore: The Williams and Wilkins Company, 1931), 180.
3. G.M. Findlay, "The First Recognized Epidemic of Yellow Fever," in *Transactions of the Royal Society of Tropical Medicine and Hygiene* XXXV, no. 3 (29 November 1941): 143–54.
4. Ibid.
5. Carter, *Yellow Fever*, 83.
6. Richard Ligon, *The True and Exact History of the Island of Barbadoes, 1657*, ed. J. Edward Hutson (Barbados: Barbados National Trust, 2000), 31.
7. Kenneth Kiple, *The Caribbean Slave: A Biological History* (Cambridge: Cambridge University Press, 1984), 165.
8. Ligon, *The True and Exact History of the Island of Barbadoes*.
9. Macfarlane Burnet and David White, *Natural History of Infectious Diseases* (New York: Cambridge University Press, 1972), 242.
10. Michael B. Oldstone, *Viruses, Plagues and History* (New York: Oxford University Press, 1998), 46.
11. David F. Clyde, *Two Centuries of Health Care in Dominica* (New Delhi: Sunshine Gopal, 1980), 24.
12. J. Edward Hutson, ed., *On the Treatment and Management of the More Common West-India Diseases* (Kingston: University of the West Indies Press, 2005), 31.
13. Sheldon Watts, "Yellow Fever Immunities in West Africa and the Americas in the Age of Slavery and Beyond: A Reappraisal," *Journal of Social History* (Summer 2001): 955–67.
14. Pinckard, *Notes on the West Indies*, vol. I, 212.

15. John Rollo, *Observations on the Diseases Which Appeared in the Army on St Lucia in 1778 and 1779, To Which Are Prefixed Remarks Calculated to Assist in Ascertaining the Causes; and in Explaining the Treatment of Those Diseases* (London: Charles Dilly, 1781). See also John Rollo, *Observations on the Means of Preserving and Restoring Health in the West Indies* (London: C. Dilly, 1783).
16. My assessment here is based on information on the area's ecology provided by Dr Karl Watson, a Barbadian historian with an extensive interest in Caribbean ecology.
17. Lana Hogarth, *Medicalizing Blackness* (Chapel Hill: University of North Carolina Press, 2017), 19.
18. Erica Charters, *Disease, War, and the Imperial State* (Chicago and London: University of Chicago Press, 2014), 59.
19. Ibid., 61 and 71.
20. Ibid., 82 and 83.
21. Billy G. Smith, *Ship of Death* (New Haven and London: Yale University Press, 2013), 157.
22. Ibid., 169–71.
23. Ibid, 169–71.
24. Ibid., 203–4.
25. Ibid., 204–5.
26. McNeill, John R., *Mosquito Empires: Ecology and War in the Greater Caribbean, 1620–1914* (New York: Cambridge University Press, 2010), 63.
27. Ibid., 68, 69.
28. Ibid, 69.
29. Ibid, 76.
30. Ibid, 66.
31. A. Peterkin (comp.), *Commissioned Officers in the Medical Services of the British Army: Charles II to the Accession of George II, 1660–1727*, vol. I (Aberdeen: Aberdeen University Press, 1925), xxi.
32. Roger Buckley, *The British Army in the West Indies: Society and the Military in the Revolutionary Age* (Gainseville: University Florida Press; Kingston: University of the West Indies Press, 1998), 274.
33. Letter from Admiral Cavendish to the Principal Officers and Commissioners of His Majesty's Navy, 10 August 1738 (ADM/106/86 PRO).
34. Letter from Admiral Cavendish to the Principal Officers and Commissioners of His Majesty's Navy, 31 August 1738 (ADM/106/86 PRO).

Notes

35. Affidavit of Henry Huntley 1 November 1739 (ADM/106/910/216 PRO).
36. Letter from Captain James Cornwall to the Principal Officers and Commissioners of His Majesty's Navy, 30 May 1738 (ADM/106/86 PRO).
37. A. Peterkin and W. Johnston, *Commissioned Officers in the Medical Services of the British Army, 1660–1960*, vol. I (London: Wellcome Historical Medical Library, 1968), xxiv–xxv.
38. Neil Cantlie, *A History of the Army Medical Department* (Edinburgh and London: Churchill Livingstone, 1974), 172.
39. Ibid.
40. Ibid., 173.
41. Ibid., 171.
42. Ibid., 181.
43. Ibid., xliv–xlvvi.
44. A reference to a theory of the causes of inflammation, common in the late eighteenth century.

Chapter 2

1. This report, located in the PRO file ADM/101 /83/3, relates to reports covering ships stationed off Jamaica. For some reason, Jamaica reports are not included in the file in which the reports from other BWI colonies are found.
2. Calomel is a compound of mercury, which is dealt with in greater detail later in this study.
3. The dried rhizome of a plant of the *Rubiceae* family, native to some South American countries, including Brazil. It is well known as an emetic. The indigenous peoples used it as a treatment for dysentery before the arrival of Europeans.
4. This is a reference to tincture of opium, which is an oral, liquid treatment for diarrhoea. It is a pain reliever as well, owing to its morphine content.
5. Tincture of opium.
6. This refers to a patent medicine produced by an English doctor, Robert James, about 1745. It consisted of a compound of arsenic and calcium phosphate and had no proven medicinal benefit. James touted it as a treatment for fevers in both humans and cattle.
7. Camphor is a waxy, colourless substance, made from the wood of the camphor laurel, common in East Asia. It was used in

managing symptoms of pain but was mildly poisonous.
8. Castile soap was developed, historically, following the discovery by European crusaders of the so-called Aleppo soap in the twelfth century. Eventually, the manufacture of Aleppo soap was taken up in the kingdom of Castile in Spain. Made using olive oil, which was abundant in Castile, it was a white soap that was in great demand throughout the twelfth to the nineteenth centuries. It is still manufactured.
9. Mixture including saline compounds as its base.
10. Thomas Young began his medical career as a hospital mate in 1776 and was appointed surgeon to the First Battalion of the First Regiment of Foot in 1780. He was posted to the Grenada Garrison on 1 August 1792 and then in 1795 to the Irish Guards. He was appointed principal medical officer in 1801. He died on 13 January 1836. His biographical details and those of all other medical practitioners in the British military are compiled from the listings provided in A. Peterkin and William Johnston, *Commissioned Officers in the Medical Services of the British Army 1660–1960*, vol. I and Robert Drew, *Commissioned Officers in the Medical Services of the British Army 1660–1960*, vol. II.
11. Most likely this is a reference to Andrew Gillespie, who began his career as a hospital mate until his later posting to the 2nd W.I. Regiment as assistant surgeon in 1803.
12. Calomel is a compound of mercury, which is dealt with in greater detail later in this study.
13. This is a reference to Colin Chisholm, who was surgeon to the 2nd Battalion of the 1st Regiment of Foot in 1775. He was commissioned as an officer of the Medical Department in the West Indies in 1796, having obtained his MD from King's College in 1793. He became a fellow of the Royal College of Surgeons in 1808. Chisholm was well known as the author of the medical book: *Diseases of Tropical Climates: Essay on the Malignant Pestilential Fever Introduced into the West Indian Islands etc.*, in 1794–1796. He died in London in 1825.
14. John Weir began his career as a surgeon in 1775 and on 28 May 1790 was appointed purveyor of hospital stores and medicines in Jamaica. He was appointed to the Medical Department of the Dragoon Guards on 24 February 1810 and subsequently became the first director general of the Army Medical Department. He died in London on 10 April 1819.

Notes

15. This remedy appears in the commentaries of other doctors whose reports I have transcribed.
16. A medicine made from the bark of a tree of the *Simaroubaceae* family. It causes irritation of the throat, the mouth and the digestive tract.
17. A powder made from the bark of the cinchona plant. Interestingly enough, quinine, which was later to be of great efficacy in the treatment of malaria, is one of the ingredients of this powdered bark.
18. This and the other following statements help to place Warner firmly in the miasma camp.

Chapter 3

1. The term loblolly boy was derived from an old English term for a thick gruel or soup. In Barbados, it was once used to refer to the local dish also known as cou cou, which consisted of a thick gooey meal made of boiled Indian corn. It probably came to be applied to the surgeon's assistants during the sixteenth century because these servants did the unpalatable tasks of removing amputated limbs, holding down patients for amputation, and the other messy tasks of cleaning up bloody and other discharges.
2. This was more than likely Robert Hartle, who began his medical career as a hospital mate in 1796. He is listed as attaining the rank of assistant surgeon by 1802 and surgeon to the 1st W.I. Regiment in February of 1804. He received his MD from St Andrew's in 1819 and was subsequently appointed deputy inspector of hospitals (D.I.H.) in 1823, and deputy inspector general in 1830. He died in Port of Spain, Trinidad, in 1860.
3. Edward Tegart started his medical career as a hospital mate in 1793. In 1794, he reached the rank of surgeon and by 25 March 1809, had been elevated to the rank of deputy inspector of hospitals. He served in the Caribbean theatre and in 1821 was appointed to the rank of inspector of hospitals (I.H.). He died in London in 1845.
4. The modern spelling is scrofula. This is an infection of the skin of the neck, caused by a bacterium associated with tuberculosis.
5. Alexander Menzies earned an MD from Edinburgh University in 1793 and was appointed hospital mate in the military service in 1801. He rose through the ranks of the medical service to the

position of assistant surgeon (1801) and to that of surgeon to the 3rd Battalion of the Light Infantry in 1803. His highest rank was that of D.I.H. in 1815. He died on a voyage from Barbados to England in 1822.
6. Dr Bone appears several times in the various reports and further details are found in other references.
7. The presence of coal tar in the hold of the ship would have been inimical to the growth of mosquito larvae, suggesting that the cause of yellow fever in this case was more likely to have been due to mosquito infestation in the vicinity of Bridgetown, or English Harbour, where the ship had spent some considerable time.
8. The lowest deck in a ship of three or more decks.
9. Brodie stoves were iron stoves that were introduced into wooden ships in the 1770s. The firebox in these stoves was enclosed, which made them safer to operate. In addition to the cooking meals or baking bread, these stoves kept the interior of the ship relatively warm.
10. See note 6 above.
11. Hugh Bone began his military medical service as a hospital mate in 1803 but later earned an MA and MD from Glasgow University in 1815. He was appointed successively assistant surgeon (1803), surgeon (1809), and physician to the forces (1815), possibly in consequence of his having obtained a university degree. He also served as D.I.H. (1825), deputy inspector general (1827) and later as inspector general (1840).
12. James Elliott began his medical military career as a hospital mate, continuing in that position until 1805. He was promoted successively assistant surgeon (Royal Corsican Rangers), in 1805, surgeon in 1809, and to a staff position in 1813. He attained the rank of D.I.H. in 1841.
13. Thomas Hall first appears in the military records as a hospital assistant in 1815. He was promoted to an assistant surgeon in 1825 and surgeon in 1840. He was listed deputy inspector general in 1855. At his retirement in 1857, he had reached the honorary rank of inspector general.
14. *Icterodes*, or *Febris Icterodes*, as it is described in William Aitken's 1864 book on medical treatment in the nineteenth century is a term used for yellow fever (See William Aitken, *The Science and Practice of Medicine*, 2 vols. (London: Charles Griffin and Company), vol. I, 481.

Notes

15. This reference to Dr Jackson is most certainly the eminent eighteenth-century, doctor whose book *A Treatise on the Fevers of Jamaica, with Observations on the Intermitting Fevers of America*, published in London in 1795, might be viewed as representing the conventional medical wisdom of the time on the matter of fevers.
16. Details on Hartle are found in other references in these reports.
17. Limber boards were movable planks that covered the bilge water passages that lay on each side of the keelson, which was a girder or timber placed above the keel, to give added strength to the vessel.
18. Not to be confused with the modern sense of the word. As used here, this most probably refers to the giving of an enema, using a type of syringe that antedated and prefigured the modern hypodermic syringe.
19. An exhaustive search has revealed that the individual who was mentioned in the document does not match any in the record of the medical officers of the British Army 1660–1960 (Drew). However, it is possible that this may be a reference to Charles McLean, who started his medical military career as a hospital assistant in general service on 8 July 1809. He later assumed the post of assistant surgeon to the 53rd Regiment of Foot on 27 December 1810. See note 26, p. 523.
20. Gastritis that is triggered by the gastric enzyme pepsin, sometimes exacerbated by stress.
21. Yellow fever.
22. Croton oil is a brownish-yellow oil that is expressed from the seeds of the *croton tiglium*. It is a very powerful purgative and can cause diarrhoea. Externally, it is an irritant to the skin, which might explain why it was so loved by medical practitioners of the time.
23. William Munro first appeared in the military records as a hospital mate in 1808, but by 16 February 1809, had been promoted assistant surgeon. He served as surgeon to the 8th West India Regiment from 1815 and was appointed staff surgeon on 5 January 1826. He was promoted to the position of deputy inspector general on 22 December 1848 and retired in 1855 with the rank of inspector general. His son, who carried the same name, became surgeon general. See also note 6, p. 530.
24. HM Brig *Ringdove* was a warship. This type of vessel was characterized by two squared-rigged masts; was highly

manoeuvrable and was capable of speeds of eleven knots. However, they were unable to sail into a head wind. She had sixteen guns.
25. HM Brig *Primrose* was also a naval warship similar to the *Ringdove*.
26. Alexander Cumming began his medical military career as a hospital assistant in 1814, after having gained an MA in King's College, Aberdeen, in 1812. He was promoted assistant surgeon on 23 December 1824. He was appointed surgeon to the 74th Regiment of Foot on 13 March 1835 and reached the rank of deputy inspector general in 1852, and that of inspector general in 1855. He died in 1858.
27. Richard Dowse started his medical military career as a hospital assistant 24 January 1814. He assumed the post of assistant surgeon to the 8th West India Regiment on 25 January 1815. He also served the 88th Regiment of Foot in this capacity from 10 March 1825. He subsequently assumed the post of surgeon to the 14th Regiment of Foot on 8 January 1836.
28. Delirium tremens is a severe, potentially life-threatening form of alcohol withdrawal marked by confusion, hallucinations, tremors and agitation.
29. Diaphoresis refers to excessive sweating.
30. *Subsultus tendinium* refers to a tremor of the limbs, caused by a twitching of the tendons. This is often brought on by a fever.
31. Loss of consciousness or fainting
32. Yellowish.
33. The act of swallowing.
34. An archaic medical term for the throat.
35. This is a historical or medical term referring to bowel movements or the discharge of fecal matter from the intestines. Alvine relates to the alvus, a Latin word for belly or abdomen.
36. Haematuria (blood in the urine) is caused by acute renal congestion.
37. Ptyalism refers to excessive salivation or hypersalivation.
38. Epistaxis is the medical term for nosebleed.
39. More likely this is a reference to *petechiae vibices*, which refers to reddish blotches of the skin, associated with haemorrhage.
40. Erysipelas is a skin infection that normally follows strep throat.
41. A thin membrane that lies between the dura mater and the pia mater, covering the brain. *Tunica* is an anatomical term derived from Latin that apparently refers to a fibrous system.

Notes

42. The pia mater is the innermost membrane covering the brain and spinal cord.
43. This term most likely refers to the ureters.
44. The upper part of the abdomen in the region of the lower ribs.
45. Thomas Draper began his career as a hospital mate in 1795. In April 1799, he was promoted to assistant surgeon in the 1st West India Regiment. His further promotion to surgeon to the 78th Regiment of Foot came in 1804. In 1816, he received successively the ranks of D.I.H., and deputy inspector general. He received the rank of I.H. in 1822, and the temporary or brevet rank of inspector general in 1825. Between 24 February 1837 and 23 February 1840, he had the local rank, in the West Indies, of inspector general, a post that was confirmed in Britain on 24 February 1840, just a few months before his retirement.
46. This was probably Henry Franklin, who is listed as a surgeon in the 3rd Dragoons in 1840. He died in Bermuda in 1864.
47. Thomas Spence started his medical military career as a hospital assistant on 3 August 1826. He was promoted to the rank of assistant surgeon to the 6th Regiment of Foot on 8 February 1827.
48. Such statistical representation offers some support for the view that, in general, Africans had some immunity to the disease, though this was a relative rather than an absolute immunity.
49. This was Adam Duncan, who was appointed to the staff position of assistant surgeon in 1835. He died at St Joseph in Trinidad, on 7 October 1838, just after he had been gazetted as assistant surgeon to the 67th Regiment of Foot.
50. Again, the observations of the doctors serving in the Caribbean sphere support a view that Africans were less susceptible than Europeans to yellow fever.
51. James Duncanson began his military career as a hospital mate in 1809. He was appointed assistant surgeon in 1811 but resigned on 25 July 1812. Perhaps this was to facilitate his pursuance of formal medical qualifications, for he is listed as having obtained an MD from Edinburgh in 1813. He re-joined the military service in 1815, when he was appointed as an hospital assistant. On 1 June, he was appointed as surgeon to the 1st West India Regiment and was still acting in that capacity when he died in Barbados on 17 April 1843.
52. This was Hugh Orr, who began his service as an hospital assistant in 1813. He was subsequently appointed assistant surgeon to the

89th Regiment of Foot in January 1822, and surgeon to the 1st West India Regiment on 30 December 1836. He died in Trinidad on 22 January 1839.

Chapter 4

1. Charles Ward began his military medical service as a hospital assistant on 1 February 1816. He died in Tobago on 14 April 1820. N.B.: Originally gazetted as "Wood".
2. William Donnelly started his military medical service career as an assistant surgeon on 10 July 1811. He died in Barbados on 8 November 1820.
3. Ralph Green started his medical military career as a surgeon's mate in regiment on 6 February 1787. He was later promoted to the rank of surgeon's mate on the hospital staff in October 1789. He was awarded the rank of surgeon to the 14th Regiment of Foot 26 September 1795. He later assumed the post inspector of field hospitals (I.F.H) on 8 January 1801. He subsequently assumed the post of deputy inspector of hospitals (D.I.H.) on 29 June 1802 and finally the post of inspector of hospitals (I.H.) on 26 August 1813.
4. This is most likely Nicholas Bradley, who had his first commission as assistant surgeon in the army on 1 August 1806, followed by a promotion to surgeon on 11 November 1811. He died on 5 May 1843 in England.
5. This is possibly a reference to Samuel Veitch, who began his military medical service as an assistant surgeon in 1801.
6. One of the racial classifications used in the Anglophone Caribbean at this time. A union between a European and an African produced a mulatto. A subsequent union between a mulatto and a European produced a mustee. In some cases, the complexion was the criterion used to classify such people.
7. Such comments appear to stamp the reporter as being a contagionist.
8. Calomel was a medicine widely used in the nineteenth century. It was a compound of Mercurous Chloride, which was used in cases that were considered bilious. It was also very toxic.
9. Robert Caverhill started his medical military career as a surgeon's mate on the hospital staff on 21 December 1811. He later became a hospital assistant to the Forces on 23 March 1815. He died in Barbados on 9 December 1820.

Notes

10. Henry McCreery started his medical military career as an assistant surgeon on 23 March 1809. He subsequently was conscripted into the West India Regiment on 3 June 1813. He was later promoted to the rank of surgeon with the West India Regiment on 26 October 1815.
11. Again, the matter of the relative immunity of blacks receives attention. And, yet again, the medical practitioners do report some deaths among this group.
12. See Report on Antigua.
13. William Forrester Bow started his military medical service career as an assistant surgeon on 28 January 1813 with the 27th Regiment of Foot. He also served as an assistant surgeon to the Lanark Militia.
14. George McDermott started his medical military career as a hospital mate for General Service on 25 August 1809. By 25 November 1815, he had been promoted to the rank of surgeon. He also served as surgeon in the 4th W.I. Regiment beginning on 10 December 1818.
15. Wormwood is a herb with the botanical name *Artemisia absinthium*. It has anti-inflammatory and pain-relieving qualities.
16. Such comments strongly suggest that there was a prevailing view that blacks, particularly those who had faced previous epidemics, were likely to have developed some immunity. There was less confidence that this also applied to whites.
17. Oxymuriatic acid gas, as it was commonly known in the nineteenth century, chlorine gas.
18. Charles Quartley Palmer started his medical military career as a surgeon's mate on the hospital staff from 10 October 1813 to 21 February 1816. He later assumed the post of hospital assistant to the forces on 22 February 1816. He was subsequently promoted to the post of assistant surgeon to the Royal York Rangers on 17 April 1817. He later served as assistant surgeon staff: f.p. from 25 June 1820.
19. This refers to coagulated blood or simply to the solid part of blood from which the serum has been removed.
20. A term used for a cutting instrument in surgery (scalpel).
21. Derivatives of opium generally used as a painkiller or sedative.
22. John Arthur started his medical military career as an assistant surgeon to the 4th Royal Veteran Battalion on 14 September 1804. He then moved to the rank of surgeon to the 60th Regiment of Foot on 5 September 1811. He attained the rank of physician

on 3 August 1815. He later assumed the post of D.I.H. on 27 May 1825.
23. Edward Tegart started his medical military career as a surgeon to the 30th Regiment of Foot. He later assumed the position of director inspector of hospitals (D.I.H.) on the 25 March 1809. He later held the post of inspector of hospitals (I.H.) on 25 March 1821 in the West Indies.
24. "Synocha", in William Cullen's nosology, refers to a continued inflammatory fever marked by a high temperature, a strong pulse and no evident local infection.
25. Stephen Panting started his medical military career as an assistant surgeon to the 6th W.I. Regiment on 31 May 1798. He assumed the post of surgeon to the 6th W.I. Regiment on 12 December 1798 and to the garrison of Tobago on 25 May 1804. He subsequently achieved the post of D.I.H. on 11 December 1823.
26. James Arthur started his medical military career as a hospital assistant to the forces on 7 March 1814. He died in Tobago on 22 September 1821.
27. George MacDermott started his medical military career as a hospital assistant to the General Service on 25 August 1809. He was later promoted to the post of assistant surgeon to the 60th Regiment of Foot on 30 November 1809. He assumed the post of surgeon to that regiment on 23 November 1815.
28. Latin term translated as "remittent fever". It was a diagnostic term in use by medical practitioners in the nineteenth century. In general, it refers to a fever in which there is varying temperature over a twenty-four-hour period, but it never becomes normal over that period.
29. Possibly a misspelling of *sinciput*, Latin for "half the head".
30. Yellow fever.
31. Hugh Bone started his medical military career as a hospital mate (surgeon's assistant on staff not attached to any regiment) 8 September 1803. He soon assumed the post of assistant surgeon to the 5th Regiment of Foot on 17 September 1803. He assumed the rank of surgeon to the 6th Regiment of Foot on 13 July 1809. He was promoted to the rank of physician on 7 September 1815. He also held the post of inspector general of hospitals in the West Indies from 2 October 1840.
32. George Home started his medical military career as a hospital assistant to the forces on 12 May 1815.

Notes

33. James Davidson started his medical military career as a hospital assistant to the forces on 24 June 1815.
34. This statement serves to identify this practitioner as being wedded to a miasmatic view of the cause of yellow fever.
35. Edward Doughty started his medical military career as an assistant surgeon on 30 October 1800. He then assumed the position of surgeon to the 85th Regiment of Foot on 25 November 1802.
36. John Rose Palmer started his medical military career as an assistant surgeon to the 11th Regiment of Foot on 26 November 1807.
37. Principal medical officer.
38. Alexander Menzies was first appointed as an assistant surgeon on 17 April 1801, after serving as hospital mate. He had earned his MD at Edinburgh in 1793. He was appointed as D.I.H. on 3 August 1815 and died on 16 March 1822, while en route from Barbados to England.
39. Hugh Bone began his military medical service as a hospital mate in 1803. He was appointed successively assistant surgeon (1803), surgeon (1809) and physician to the forces (1815). He also served as deputy inspector of hospitals (D.I.H.), 1825; deputy inspector general (D.I.G.), 1827; and later as inspector general (I.G.), 1840.
40. James Elliott began his medical military career as a hospital mate, continuing in that position until 1805. He was promoted successively to assistant surgeon (Royal Corsican Rangers), in 1805, surgeon in 1809 and to a staff position in 1813. He attained the rank of D.I.H. in 1841.
41. Edward Tegart started his medical military career as a surgeon to the 30th Regiment of Foot. He later assumed the position of D.I.H. on the 25 March 1809. He later held the post of inspector of hospitals (I.H.) on the 25 March 1821 in the West Indies.
42. The Brodie Stove was *en vogue* during the period of the mid-eighteenth century and the early nineteenth century with the Royal Navy.
43. An exhaustive search of the medical officers in the British Army 1660–1960 (Drew) has revealed that there were no officers by the name of Lainsworth. However, the name Loinsworth does appear. There is conclusive evidence which suggests that the staff surgeon mentioned in this report was, in fact, Augustus Lewis Loinsworth. He started his medical military career as an assistant

surgeon to the 1st Regiment of Foot on 7 May 1807. He was later appointed surgeon to the 4th West Indian Regiment on 26 September 1811. He served the 2nd Battalion, 60th Regiment of Foot, from 28 May 1812: half pay (h.p.)1818: full pay (f.p.), 9th Regiment of Foot, 30 September 1819. He was subsequently appointed staff surgeon on 28 December 1820.

44. William Bain started his medical military career as a hospital assistant on 24 June 1815. He graduated from Edinburgh as a doctor in 1817.
45. Most likely this was James Alexander Campbell, who began his career as regimental mate in 1796, advancing that same year to the rank of surgeon. He was appointed as D.I.H. in 1817.
46. "I had an attack of Gastric Disease on 20 September which confined me to my room five days. I was slightly yellow; the cause was the excessive heat of the weather and fatigue in Bridgetown," signed H. Bone.
47. This was more than likely Dr James Latham, a British military surgeon who is well known as a pioneer in the use of inoculation to reduce mortality from smallpox, between 1768 and 1786, while on service in Canada.
48. Robert Jackson was a British military surgeon whose first appointment was as surgeon to the 3rd Regiment of Foot in 1793. He served in Jamaica as an MD between 1774 and 1778 and is well known in the history of medicine as the author of several works, including *A Treatise on the Fevers of Jamaica* (1795), and *A Sketch of the History and Care of Febrile Diseases, More Particularly as They Appear in the West Indies among the Soldiers of the British Army* (1817).
49. Possibly a full-bodied person in the last stages of a debilitating illness.
50. Mephitic: Offensive to the smell, noxious, poisonous or pestilential. It was widely believed that "bad air", or as it was commonly termed, "malaire", was the cause of many local diseases.
51. Diseases that are associated with the lungs.
52. The trachea or windpipe is a tube that connects the pharynx and larynx to the lungs.
53. Rochelle Salts, also known as potassium sodium tartrate or potassium salts, were commonly used as a laxative.
54. Emetic tartar, also known as tartaric salts, was used as a mild laxative or an expectorant.

55. Sweating, most likely profusely.
56. Seidlitz Powders is the name given to a medication composed of a number of mixtures, namely, tartaric acid, sodium bicarbonate and potassium sodium tartrate. It was widely used as a mild laxative.
57. *Soda Tartarisata* or tartarite of soda was a compound of sodium bicarbonate and tartarite salt used as a mild laxative.
58. Cheltenham Salts was also known as Glauber's Salt, a hydrate of sodium sulphate that was also used as a mild laxative.
59. Cream of tartar, also known as potassium bitartrate, is a by-product of wine-making. It is used in cooking.
60. Cassia is known as a spice.
61. A saline diaphoretic medicine acts as a diuretic, i.e., helps to expel fluids from the body.
62. A cathartic extract was usually a medicine that helped to expel unwanted substances from the body.
63. Ptisans or tisanes were medicinal infusions of sweetened barley water.
64. The epigastrium is the upper central region of the abdomen.
65. Vitiated bile indicates bile of an impaired quality.
66. Waxy.
67. Dr Bone's entry in his report mentioned Mr Sproule – OMD. However, it would appear that the correct spelling of the name ought to be Mr Sproull, since he is the only individual who was gazetted as an OMD. Henry Sproull started his medical military career as assistant surgeon, OMD, on 1 August 1806. He was subsequently promoted to the position of surgeon, OMD, on 2 December 1812.
68. Minims were a unit measurement of fluid.
69. A diaphoretic medicine is one which is used to promote perspiration.
70. Paregoric or camphorated tincture of opium was used as a medication. It was widely used for its antidiarrhoeal, antitussive and analgesic properties.
71. Anodyne: a medicine used before the twentieth century to relieve or soothe pain by lessening the sensitivity of the brain or the nervous system.
72. Tincture of gential (gentian) is a bitter tonic. It stimulates the appetite and digestion and promotes the production of saliva, gastric juices and bile.

73. Spirit of lavender is a pleasant carminative and stimulant. Externally, it is used as a cooling lotion in headaches and febrile complaints.
74. A restless tossing or twitching back and forth of the body.
75. John Stuart started his medical military career as a hospital assistant on 19 May 1815.
76. The then governor of Barbados.
77. Henry McCreery started his medical military career as surgeon's mate on the hospital staff from 12 September 1807 to 22 March 1809. He later assumed the position of assistant surgeon to the 13th Regiment of Foot from 23 March 1809. He later served the 1st West India Regiment in the same capacity from 3 June 1813. He subsequently was promoted to the rank of surgeon and served in the 1st W.I. Regiment from 26 October 1815 and later the 9th Regiment of Foot from 28 December 1820.
78. This is in all probability Thomas Carey, who served as an assistant surgeon to the 20th Regiment of Foot in 1800, and later, on 30 April 1807, was appointed surgeon to the 21st Regiment of Foot. He is also listed as serving in Demerara on 22 June 1823.
79. Omitted section is illegible in the original document.
80. This paragraph is the source of the title of my publication.
81. In all likelihood, this is gastritis, centred in the stomach.
82. John Williams started his medical military career as a hospital mate for general service on 10 June 1812. He was subsequently appointed to the post of assistant surgeon to the 23rd Regiment of Foot on 13 May 1813.
83. John Erly started his medical military career as a surgeon's mate on the hospital staff on 4 December 1795. He ended this tenure on 24 June 1797. He later assumed the post of assistant surgeon to the 42nd Regiment of Foot on 25 June 1797. He subsequently was promoted to the rank of surgeon to the 42nd Regiment of Foot on 18 April 1800. He was next appointed to the post of physician on 3 September 1812. His next appointment was that of D.I.H./D.I.G. on 14 September 1815. His ultimate appointment was that of I.H./I.G. on 27 May 1827.
84. Sir James McGrigor had a long and outstanding medical military career. His achievements are many and well documented. Suffice to say he started his medical military career as a surgeon (by purchase) to the 88th Regiment of Foot on 25 September 1793 and to the Royal Horse Guards on 9 February 1804. He assumed the post of D.I.H. on 27 June 1805 and then D.I.G. on 25 August

Notes

1809. He subsequently assumed the rank of physician, Garrison of Plymouth (while I.G. Southern Command) on 13 June 1811. He finally was promoted to the post of director general of the Army Medical Department on 13 June 1815.

85. No listing for Mr Sermon A.S. in the medical officers in the British Army 1660–1960 (Drew) can be found.
86. Thomas Spence began his medical military career as a hospital assistant on 3 August 1826. He was later promoted to the rank of assistant surgeon to the 6th Regiment of Foot on 8 February 1827 and later to the 52nd Regiment of Foot on 26 October 1830. He was subsequently promoted to the rank of staff surgeon on 12 July 1839. He ultimately assumed the post of deputy inspector general of hospitals on 28 March 1854.
87. Phrenitis was an inflammation of the brain known today as meningitis..
88. Paroxysmal dyspnoea is a condition in which the individual suffers from short, sharp intervals of shortness of breath.
89. Possibly *chordae tendineae*, which is a reference to fibrous cords attached to the atrioventricular valves of the heart.
90. Henry Franklin started his medical military career as a surgeon's mate on hospital staff from 13 August 1808 to 28 June 1809. He later assumed the post of assistant surgeon to the 27th Regiment of Foot on 29 June 1809. He was subsequently promoted to the post of surgeon to the 27th Regiment of Foot on 26 May 1814. He was appointed surgeon on staff on 19 November 1830.
91. J.D. Gillkrest was the D.I.H. in London when he wrote an article on yellow fever in the *Cyclopaedia of Practical Medicine*, vol. II, published in 1833.
92. William Robinson started his medical military career as an assistant surgeon staff on 11 January 1839. He was later assigned to the 52nd Regiment of Foot on 12 July 1839. He assumed the post of surgeon staff to the 1st, 2nd and 3rd West India Regiments (as the exigencies of the service would have required) 23 August 1844. He died in Dominica on 19 December 1847.
93. Yellow fever.
94. An obsolete term referring to the intestines or the belly.
95. Post-mortem examination.
96. Ablutions here refers to special baths used in the treatment of the sick.
97. Laudanum, also known as tincture of opium, was used widely as a painkiller.

98. Edward Blakeney started his medical military career as an assistant surgeon staff on 17 October 1834. He later served in the same capacity to the 67th Regiment of Foot from 13 March 1835.
99. Omitted section is illegible in the original document.
100. Alexander Mackintosh started his medical military career as an assistant surgeon staff on 30 September 1836. He also served in this capacity to the 33rd Regiment of Foot from 18 February 1842. He drowned off the St Lucian coast on 25 May 1842.

Chapter 5

1. An exhaustive search of the medical officers in the British Army 1660–1960 (Drew) reveals that there was no medical officer by the name of R.G. Webb. However, the name Boleyne Gordon Webb appears. He started his medical military career as hospital assistant to the Forces on 28 December 1826. He was subsequently promoted to the post of assistant surgeon staff in July 1830.
2. The term "quotidian" is a reference to a fever that occurs daily.
3. Absence of fever.
4. Reference to the organs that produce chyle, a fluid formed in digesting fatty foods.
5. See report on Antigua.
6. A Mediterranean and African herbaceous vine related to the watermelon, which is used to prepare a powerful cathartic preparation.
7. Laudanum, also known as tincture of opium, was widely used as a painkiller.
8. A grain is a measurement used for weighing. One grain = 1/1000 part of one pound.
9. In medical terminology, *sensorium* refers to the state of a person's consciousness and awareness of their surroundings.
10. Post-mortem.
11. Coagulated.
12. See report on Barbados.
13. John Nicoll started his medical military career as an assistant surgeon staff on 11 August 1835. He subsequently served the 65th Regiment of Foot in the same capacity on 3 November 1837.
14. Daniel Scott started his medical military career as a hospital

Notes

assistant to the General Forces on 9 March 1815. He subsequently assumed the post of assistant surgeon to the 36th Regiment of Foot on 18 March 1824. He also served the same battalion as staff surgeon from 17 October 1834.

15. Robert Smith started his medical military career as an assistant surgeon staff on 26 October 1834.
16. John Riach started his medical military career as a hospital mate for general service on 18 May 1812. He was later promoted to the post of assistant surgeon to the 73rd Regiment of Foot on 2 July 1812. He also went on to serve as a surgeon to the 67th Regiment of Foot from 19 November 1930.
17. James Irwin started his medical military career as an assistant surgeon staff on 7 October 1836.
18. Post-mortem examination.
19. This refers to a structure or appearance that resembles the branching pattern of a tree.
20. Free from fever.
21. Jaundiced.
22. This is likely referring to jactitation or a twitching of the body.
23. Given the context, this possibly refers to a surgical incision into a vein.
24. William Birrell started his medical military career as a hospital assistant to the General Forces on 24 June 1815. He went on to gain his MD from Edinburgh 1817. He assumed the post of assistant surgeon to the 38th Regiment of Foot on 12 April 1821. He was later promoted to the rank of surgeon to the 77th Regiment of Foot on 5 May 1837.
25. A reference to an oil or ointment.
26. A reference to a footbath.
27. Possibly paroxysm, a reference to a sudden violent movement of the body.
28. The *timica arachnoid* and the pia mater are membranes covering the brain and spinal cord, forming two of the three layers of meninges, the other being the dura mater.
29. Lining of the thoracic cavity, including the diaphragm and also areas of the pleural cavity
30. John DeVerd Leigh started his medical military career as an assistant surgeon to the 76th Regiment of Foot on 18 May 1838.
31. A sudden muscular weakness.

32. Charles McLean began his career as hospital mate in 1809. He received an MD at Edinburgh in 1808 and was appointed assistant surgeon to the 53rd Regiment of Foot in 1810 and was promoted as surgeon to the same regiment in 1825. He reached the rank of inspector general in 1857. He died in 1864.
33. Alexander Melvin started his medical military career as hospital assistant in general service on 26 July 1810. He was later promoted to the rank of assistant surgeon to the 60th Regiment of Foot on 10 December 1811. He subsequently assumed the post of surgeon to the regiment on 10 December 1823.
34. Yellow fever.
35. An involuntary contraction of the diaphragm.
36. Charles McLean started his medical military career as a hospital assistant in general service 8 July 1809. He later served as an assistant surgeon to the 53rd Regiment of Foot from 27 December 1810. He was subsequently promoted to the rank of surgeon to the 53rd Regiment of Foot on 14 July 1825.
37. The only Beresford listed in the military medical service for this period is James Beresford, who began his career as an hospital mate on 1 February 1805. On 3 December that same year, he was appointed assistant surgeon to the 1st West India Regiment. By 23 November 1815, he was appointed to a senior position as a staff surgeon.
38. This is likely a reference to Frank Andrews, who was assistant surgeon to the 1st West India Regiment in August of 1842 and then to the 33rd Regiment of Foot in December of that year.
39. John Millar started his medical career as a hospital assistant on 21 May 1813: h.p., 25 July 1816: f.p., 25 March–September 1817. He subsequently assumed the post of assistant surgeon staff, 8 February 1821, and later the post of surgeon to the 43rd Regiment of Foot on 5 November 1829. He was promoted to staff, first class, on 16 December 1845.
40. Alexander Knox started his medical military career as an assistant surgeon staff, 12 April 1833: 62nd Regiment of Foot on 20 September 1833: Staff on 22 April 1836: 1st Regiment of Foot on 17 June 1836. He was promoted to the position of surgeon staff, second class, on 15 March 1844. He completed his MD at Edinburgh in 1832.
41. Paroxysm.

Notes 517

42. Listing of various medical authorities whose books were well known by practitioners of the late eighteenth into the mid-nineteenth centuries.

Chapter 6

1. See references in the Barbados Reports.
2. Robert Woulfe started his medical military career as an assistant surgeon to the 12th Regiment of Dragoons. He later assumed the post of surgeon to the 1st Regiment of Foot, on 26 November 1807. He also served the 4th W.I. Regiment as well as the 96th Regiment of Foot in the same capacity. He was promoted to staff surgeon on 4 July 1811. He died in Dominica on 13 November 1817.
3. Possibly this is Herman Storme May, who began his career as a hospital mate in 1810 and was appointed assistant surgeon in 1812.
4. We have encountered references to Dr Jackson in other reports in this compilation.
5. Robert Woulfe began his medical career as a hospital assistant in 1800. He was appointed assistant surgeon in 1801, and was promoted to surgeon to the First Regiment of Foot in 1807, and to the 4th W. I. Regiment in that same year. He died in Dominica on 13 November 1817.
6. Joseph Allen started his medical military career as a hospital mate for general service. He was soon afterwards promoted to hospital assistant on 6 January 1813. He was promoted to the position of assistant surgeon to the 8th W.I. Regiment on 27 January 1814.
7. Edward Oakley started his medical military career as a hospital assistant on 16 June 1815. He died in Dominica on 11 August 1817.
8. William Wilson started his medical military career as a hospital assistant on 9 August 1813.
9. See reference to Caverhill in the Reports on Barbados.
10. David Williams started his medical military career as a hospital assistant on 20 December 1813. He was subsequently promoted to the post of assistant surgeon to the 50th Regiment of Foot on 12 August 1819.
11. John Colville started his medical military career as a hospital assistant on 25 December 1815. He died in Barbados on 11 October 1816.

12. John Prendergast started his medical military career as a hospital mate to the general service on 3 May 1810. He was promoted to the post of assistant surgeon to the 82nd Regiment of Foot on 16 April 1812. He died in the W.I. on 5 December 1816.
13. John Wales started his medical military career as a temp. assistant surgeon, OMD, on 30 January 1813. He was subsequently promoted to the post of 2nd assistant surgeon, OMD, on 20 November 1813. He died in Barbados on 4 December 1816.
14. John William Payne started his medical military career as a hospital mate in general service on 21 November 1811. He later served as an assistant surgeon to the 3rd W.I. Regiment from 3 June 1813. He died in Barbados on 19 February 1817.
15. William Birmingham started his medical military career as a hospital assistant on 25 December 1815. He died in Dominica on 6 November 1817.
16. Information on this doctor appears in the Reports from Antigua.
17. David Williams started his medical military career as a hospital assistant on 20 December 1813; he received h.p. on 25 July 1816; f.p. on 12 February 1818.
18. Alexander Ralph started his medical military career as an assistant surgeon to the 12th Regiment of Foot on 31 March 1814.
19. Off the island of Trinidad.
20. This most likely refers to Edward Bancroft, who published a pamphlet in 1811 entitled "An Essay on the Disease Called Yellow Fever". Bancroft studied medicine at Cambridge and between 1795 and 1799 was a doctor in the British military service. He eventually settled in Jamaica, where he died in 1842.
21. If anything, this doctor was quite familiar with the works published by the medical experts. His reference here shows his familiarity with the work of Dr Robert Jackson, who published a pamphlet in 1791 entitled "A treatise on the fevers of Jamaica, with some observations on the intermitting fever of America, and an appendix containing some hints on the means and of preserving the health of soldiers in hot climates".
22. Edward Dow started his medical military career as an assistant surgeon to Royal Corsican Rangers from 28 January 1808. He served the 20th Regiment of Dragoons on 7 December 1809; also, the 33rd Regiment of Foot from 19 December 1811: Staff, 12 November 1812. He was later promoted to the rank of surgeon to the 37th Regiment of Foot on 25 December 1812. He

Notes

was subsequently promoted to the post of D.I.H. on 5 November 1829.
23. *Petechiae* are small red or purple spots on the skin due to haemorrhage of the capillaries
24. The diaphragm.
25. Spitting.
26. Painful, frequent urination.
27. William Lyons started his medical military career as a hospital mate for general service on 27 June 1811. He subsequently served as apothecary to the forces on 9 September 1813. He was promoted to the post of surgeon staff on 11 June 1818. He gained his MD from Edinburgh in 1827.
28. Possibly meant overweight.
29. Bloodletting.
30. The area between the stomach and the duodenum.
31. The membrane that lines the inner surface of the ribs.
32. While his report lists him as N. Birrell, it is likely that this refers to William Birrell, who began his career as hospital assistant in 1815. He earned his MD from Edinburgh in 1814 and was promoted to assistant surgeon in 1821. His promotion to surgeon of the 76th Regiment of Foot came in 1837. He died in 1849.
33. John Glasco started his medical military career as an assistant surgeon to the 83rd Regiment of Foot on 21 April 1808. He subsequently was promoted to the rank of surgeon to the 59th Regiment of Foot on 8 February 1816: h.p. 25 May 1816: f.p. 60th Regiment of Foot on 19 September 1822. Staff, 20 April 1826.
34. Discoloured by bloody discharges.
35. Twitching of the body.
36. An exhaustive search in the *Commissioned Officers in the Medical Services of the British Army 1660–1960* (Drew) for F. Macaw has proved fruitless.
37. James Connell started his medical military career as a hospital assistant on 16 June 1825. He was later promoted to the rank of assistant surgeon to the 53rd Regiment of Foot on 10 November 1825: 3rd Regiment of Dragoons on 19 November 1830. Superseded on 15 August 1837. He was reinstated as assistant surgeon of the 23rd Regiment of Foot on 30 March 1838. He was promoted to the rank of staff surgeon second class on 2 July 1841.

38. John Crespigny Millingen started his medical military career as an assistant surgeon to the 92nd Regiment of Foot in 1839.
39. Robert Smith started his medical military career as an assistant surgeon on 26 September 1834. He served the 21st Regiment of Foot on 21 November 1834, then 19th Regiment of Foot from 26 January 1841. He was subsequently promoted to staff surgeon second class from 8 December 1845.
40. *Oleum terebinth*, also known as oil of turpentine, was used primarily as an external stimulant.
41. *Mistura camphorae*, also known as camphor water, was used primarily as an external stimulant but was also used internally in small amounts.

Chapter 7

1. Frederick Albert Loinsworth started his medical military career as a surgeon's assistant on the hospital staff from 18 February 1803 to 22 July 1804. He was subsequently appointed assistant surgeon to the 85th Regiment of Foot on 23 July 1804; and to the 14th Regiment of Foot on 15 May 1806. He was promoted to the rank of surgeon, 96th Regiment of Foot, on 8 June 1809.
2. Yellow fever.
3. Involuntary contraction of the diaphragm.
4. His preceding comments clearly show that he tended towards a miasmatic cause of the disease, but he also believed that it was spread by contagion.
5. Alexander John Ralph started his medical military career as an assistant surgeon to the 12th Regiment of Foot on 31 March 1814; 2nd Regiment of Foot on 29 September 1814.
6. See earlier reference to John Glasco in the Dominica reports.
7. Patrick O'Callaghan started his medical military career as a hospital assistant on 18 July 1826. He was subsequently promoted to the position of assistant surgeon to the 27th Regiment of Foot in 1828.
8. Part of the thin tissue that lines the abdomen, surrounding the stomach and other organs.
9. Anthony Cuddy started his medical military career as a hospital assistant on 18 July 1826. He subsequently was promoted to the post of assistant surgeon staff on 25 June 1828.
10. The information entered on the commissioned officers in the Medical Services of the British Army 1660–1960 is inconclusive

Notes 521

as to who this officer is. There are two entries as hospital assistants: William Campbell Robertson and William Robertson. Both were commissioned in 1828 and there is no mention of the regiment they served in that capacity.
11. Bleeding.

Chapter 8

1. A clear reference to the influence of miasmatic theories on his thinking.
2. William Parry started his medical military career as a hospital assistant on 20 December 1813. He was promoted to the position of assistant surgeon to the 4th Regiment of Foot in 1822, and received a staff appointment on 19 January 1838. On 17 April 1838, he was appointed surgeon in a regiment of the Dragoon Guards, and to the 4th Regiment of Foot on 6 December 1839. He retired in 1856, with the honorary rank of deputy inspector general.
3. Twitching of the limbs.
4. Extensive patches of subcutaneous blood.
5. A clear reference to the influence of miasmatic theories on his thinking.
6. The view was widely held that the working classes in the military were more susceptible to illness than their superiors due to a greater tendency to drunkenness and other excesses.
7. Andrew Tonnere started his medical military career as a hospital mate in general service. He subsequently was promoted to the post of hospital assistant on 12 July 1810. He was later promoted to the post of assistant surgeon to the 83rd Regiment of Foot on 28 October 1813. Subsequently, he was appointed staff assistant surgeon on 20 March 1823.
8. William Cullen was a celebrated eighteenth-century physician and author of medical texts, in particular on the classification of fevers.
9. Dr John Mason Goode was an English physician of the nineteenth century who authored several medical treatises between 1800 and 1830. His titles included *Book of Nature, System of Nosology* and *Study of Medicine.*
10. An inflammatory condition, often characterized by the development of a solid inflammatory mass.

11. Tuberculosis.
12. The common cold.
13. Gonorrhoea.
14. The area of the diaphragm.

Chapter 9

1. James Patterson's military career began in 1810, when he was appointed a hospital mate. In 1811, he was promoted to the position of assistant surgeon. He obtained his MD from Glasgow in 1818. On May 1826, he was appointed to the position of surgeon to the 13th Regiment of Foot. He died in Edinburgh in 1866.
2. An archaic rendering of defecation or of faeces.
3. Spitting.
4. Abdomen.
5. This term was used in the eighteenth and nineteenth century to denote a continuous fever.
6. Antiphlogistic was a term used to describe a substance that was anti-inflammatory or reduced fever.
7. There were at least two William Munros who served in the British medical service between 1800 and 1837. However, this was most likely the William Munro who began become deputy inspector general in 1848 and inspector general in 1852.
8. This possibly refers to a study of the course of action that led to the fever.
9. Literally translates from the Latin as "first force". More than likely, it refers here to the purging of the assumed miasmatic influences or first causes of the illness from the patient.
10. Yellow fever.
11. Fainting or dizziness.
12. Richard Dowse began his medical career as a hospital assistant on 24 January 1814. A year later, he was appointed assistant surgeon to the 8th West India Regiment. He is listed in the military records as having served in the Guadeloupe and Martinique campaigns of 1815. He was promoted to the rank of surgeon to the 14th Regiment of Foot in 1836, and to the staff in 1842. After a long career in the military medical service, he reached the rank of deputy inspector general in 1855 and retired with the honorary rank of inspector general in 1857.

Notes

13. A bacterial infection of outer layers of the skin.
14. Whatever fluid had been taken by the patient.
15. The pouch at the head or beginning of the large intestine.
16. Richard Thompson Telfer was born on 21 February 1814. At the age of twenty-one, on 17 July 1835, he received his first appointment to the military medical service as assistant surgeon (staff). It is not clear where he received his medical training, but this first appointment suggests previous service, possibly as a surgeon's assistant. It appears that he received an appointment to the 14th Regiment on 8 September 1835.
17. Daniel Scott's military career began in 1813, when he was appointed as an hospital mate. In 1815, he was appointed to a hospital assistant. He was promoted to assistant surgeon in 1824 and staff surgeon in 1834. On 2 August 1850, he was appointed deputy inspector general. He obtained the MD from Marischal College, Aberdeen, in 1851, and subsequently, on 25 September 1857, received the rank of inspector general. He received the high honour of being named as the Queen's Hospital physician in 1870. Scott died in Edinburgh in 1873.
18. Six-monthly/biannually.
19. A twitching of the joints.
20. Hiccoughs.
21. Faecal discharges or other discharges from the intestine.
22. *Epistaxis* is a medical term for nosebleed.
23. Food or drink previously taken.
24. Subsultus tendinum is an archaic medical term for twitching of the joints.
25. Strangury is the slow and painful discharge of the urine, due to spasm of the urethra and bladder.
26. At the point of death.
27. Twitching of the limbs, previously referenced in this publication.
28. *Sinapisms* is a medical term used to refer to blisters or poultices.
29. *Pediluvia* is an archaic medical term for a foot bath.
30. The gall bladder.
31. Hiccoughs.

Chapter 10

1. John Pullein Hawkey started his medical military career as a hospital assistant on 23 December 1824. He was subsequently promoted to the post of assistant surgeon to the 4th Regiment

of Foot on 16 June 1825; on 29th Regiment of Foot on 27 April 1826. He was later promoted to the rank of surgeon staff on 20 September 1839.
2. Richard Dowse began his career as a hospital assistant in 1814, followed by an appointment as assistant surgeon to the 8th W.I. Regiment in 1815. He was appointed surgeon to the 14th Regiment of Foot on 8 January 1836. He was appointed deputy inspector general in 1855, and inspector general on 7 January 1857. He died on March 21, 1873.
3. Possibly the reporter's term might be better read as aetiology.

Chapter 11

1. George Whitfield Cockell started his medical military career as a surgeon's mate on the hospital staff on 19 August 1799. He was appointed assistant surgeon to the 54th Regiment of Foot on 9 May 1800. He assumed the post of surgeon to the 79th Regiment of Foot on 25 June 1801.
2. Thomas Mostyn started his medical military career as a surgeon's mate on the hospital staff from 7 November 1810 to 18 December 1811. He later assumed the post of assistant surgeon to the 27th Regiment of Foot on 19 December 1811. He subsequently assumed the post of surgeon to the regiment on 6 October 1825.
3. Alexander Melville started his medical military career as an assistant surgeon to the 46th Regiment of Foot on 10 September 1807. He later assumed the post of surgeon to the 3rd West India Regiment on 26 September 1811. He subsequently rose to the rank of staff surgeon, West Indies, on 3 August 1826.
4. Alexander Stewart started his medical military career as an assistant surgeon to the 6th Garrison Battalion on 25 November 1813. He later assumed the post of surgeon staff on 15 May 1818.
5. Francis Arthur McCann started his medical military career as an assistant surgeon to the 101st Regiment of Foot on 11 September 1806. He was later promoted to the post of surgeon to the same Regiment on 13 January 1814. He subsequently assumed the post of staff surgeon on 19 November 1830. He gained his MD from Edinburgh in 1818.
6. Sir John Hall started his medical military career as a hospital assistant on 24 June 1815: h.p. 25 February 1816: f.p. 25 September 1817. He assumed the post of assistant surgeon staff on 12 September 1822 and surgeon staff in 1827.

Notes 525

7. See reference in the Barbados Reports re Dr Hugh Bone.
8. See note on Barbados re Dr Charles Palmer.
9. James Murray Drysdale started his medical military career as a hospital assistant on 19 February 1824. He was subsequently promoted to the post of assistant surgeon to the 16th Regiment of Foot on 10 November 1825. He later assumed the post of surgeon to the 33rd Regiment of Foot on 26 February 1841.

Chapter 12

1. John Arthur started his medical military career as an assistant surgeon to the Royal Veteran Battalion on 14 September 1804. He was subsequently promoted to the post of surgeon to the 60th Regiment of Foot on 5 September 1811. He later received his accreditation as a physician on 3 August 1815.
2. Stephen Panting started his medical military career as an assistant surgeon to the 6th West India Regiment on 31 May 1798. He was later promoted to the rank of surgeon to the 6th West India Regiment on 12 December 1798. He was later transferred to the garrison at Tobago on 25 May 1804. He was elevated to the position of staff surgeon on 3 March 1809. He became deputy inspector of hospitals (D.I.H.) (brevet) on 11 December 1823.
3. An exhaustive search in the *Medical Officers in the British Army 1660–1960* (Drew) for A.S. McAvoy has proved unfruitful.
4. This is possibly a reference to Dr William Samuel Johnson, who had authored the publication, "An Essay on the Yellow Fever" in 1795.
5. It is possible that the reporter is using this term as a synonym for the term exacerbations.
6. James Safe started his medical military career as surgeon's mate on hospital staff on 19 October 1798. He was subsequently promoted to the post of assistant surgeon to the 15th Regiment of Dragoons on 30 August 1799. He later assumed the post of surgeon to the 14th Regiment of Foot on 20 March 1806 and later to the post of staff surgeon on 20 May 1813.
7. Most likely this is an archaic rendering of paroxysms.
8. Thomas Morgan started his medical military career as an assistant surgeon to the 22nd Dragoons on 1 August 1807. He died circa 1810.
9. Patrick Hughes started his medical military career as an assistant surgeon of the 1st Battalion, Light Infantry of Militia, Ireland, on

25 September 1803. He was subsequently promoted to surgeon staff (Portugal) under the command of Gen. Sir W. Carr Beresford on 10 October 1811, and surgeon staff, permanent rank, on 25 September 1814.
10. Here again is evidence that the doctors in the British military and naval services were, at this time, quite familiar with the published medical texts on the treatment of yellow fever.
11. Yellow fever.
12. Reference to a disease in which the skin presents with raised red patches.
13. This and all similar following references are to yellow fever.
14. Andrew Colvin started his medical military career as hospital mate for general service, He soon thereafter was appointed to the post of hospital assistant on 25 June 1812. He was subsequently promoted to the post of assistant surgeon to the 59th Regiment of Foot on 9 September 1813. He died in Tobago on 22 October 1820.
15. Charles Stewart started his medical military career as an assistant surgeon on 7 July 1837. He then served in this capacity to the 86th Regiment of Foot from 5 October 1841. He gained his MD from St Andrew's University in 1836.
16. The slight depression found just below the sternum, in the area of the solar plexus.
17. Swollen.
18. Characterized by red blotches.
19. The general mental health.
20. The white fibrous tissue covering the eyeball.
21. A deep infection of the hair follicles, characterized by abscess formation, pus and necrotic tissue.
22. The top part of the skull.
23. In the area of the neck.
24. The tissues associated with the capillaries and connective membranes that line the ventricles of the brain.
25. Erysipelas is a skin condition characterized by a reddish rash. It was sometimes referred to as St Anthony's Fire.
26. Simeon Henry Hardy started his medical military career as an assistant surgeon staff, on 2 November 1838. He had graduated from Trinity College, Dublin, with a BA in 1834 and an MB in 1837.
27. Smallpox.

Notes

28. Possibly "asthenic" which term describes general disability, lack of physical strength or weakness.
29. Refers to a condition in which the skin is covered with reddish spots, caused by the rupture of capillaries.
30. This refers to weals on the skin, associated with subcutaneous bleeding.
31. Medical term for the nostrils.
32. Thick or clotted.
33. Oily or greasy.
34. Discoloration due to underlying bleeding.
35. The term *febris cont: communis* is of Latin origin, *febris* being the Latin for "fever", and *communis* the Latin for "common". The abbreviation *cont.* is most likely an abbreviation of the Latin *continuans*, which in this context means "continuing". A likely translation is thus "a common continuing fever".

Chapter 13

1. James Sharp started his medical military career as an assistant surgeon to the 68th Regiment of Foot on 16 October 1800. He also served the 87th Regiment of Foot in the same capacity, starting on 25 January 1802. He later assumed the post of surgeon to the 6th West India Regiment on 25 May 1804, then the 16th Regiment of Foot on 7 May 1807. He was subsequently promoted to the post of staff surgeon on 26 September 1811. He died at Demerara on 9 October 1825.
2. Ipecacuanha is a drug made from the dried root of the plant *Cephaelis ipecacuanha*. This plant is found in Brazil and Peru and several other regions of South America.
3. Dover's Powder is a reference to the medicinal compound first prepared by Dr Thomas Dover of Britain, sometime in the eighteenth century. As first formulated, this powder was made of ipcacuanha, opium and potassium sulphate. It was a sudorific that induced sweating, which to eighteenth-century medical thought made it ideal for the treatment of fevers.
4. Red-faced, with a tendency towards puffiness of the face.
5. The area of the solar plexus (or pit of the stomach).
6. The pubic region.
7. Sweat.
8. Let him take mercurous chloride [Calomel] fifteen grains immediately.

9. Let him take powdered jalap root, half a drachm immediately.
10. Let him take mercurous chloride (Calomel) one scruple immediately and effervescent draughts as required. Apply cantharides plaster to the stomach.
11. Repeat the mercurous chloride as above.
12. Let him take an infusion of calumba [root] two fluid ounces, four times a day. (Calumba root is obtained from the plant *Jateorhiza calumba*, a native of Mozambique and is bitter to the taste.)
13. Recipe/Prescription: mercurous chloride one scruple, James's powder half a scruple. Gum acacia mucilage [a thin solution of the gum] a sufficient quantity to make a [pill] mass. Make into six pills to be given immediately. Apply cantharides plaster to the nape of the neck. (Cantharides plaster was a blistering agent.)
14. Continue the infusion of Calumba as before.
15. Recipe/prescription: Rectified ether half a fluid drachm. Tincture of opium twenty minims. Pure water one [fluid] ounce. Mix to make a draught. To be taken as required. Let him have a purging enema immediately and apply cantharides plaster liberally to the chest.
16. Continue the same medicines, and to have stimulating enemas.
17. Let him take compound extract of colocynth one scruple immediately. And then magnesium sulphate solution until it has had [a laxative effect]. Take blood from the arm to two and a half pounds.
18. Let him take mercurous chloride one scruple, and James's powder half a scruple immediately.
19. Let him have mercuric chloride half a scruple, and James's powder eight grains immediately.
20. Recipe/prescription: Camphor mixture one and a half fluid ounces. Rectified ether [and] compound ammonia solution, of each half a fluid drachm: mix to make a draught, and let him take it every two hours. Apply cantharides plaster between the shoulder blades and to the inner parts. And a [Guinea pepper/bird pepper/cayenne pepper] poultice to the soles of the feet. Wine and brandy freely.
21. Continue the same medicines and add tincture of opium forty minims.
22. Recipe/prescription: Camphor, ammonium carbonate [guinea pepper/bird pepper] berries, of each five grains. Extract of opium one grain, syrup a sufficient quantity to make a bolus [large pill],

Notes 529

and give it every three hours. Apply cantharides plaster to the head and the pit of the stomach. Wine and brandy continued.
23. Autopsy.
24. Let him take a scruple [twenty grains] of compound gamboge pills [normal dose five to ten grains].
25. Shower?
26. Mercurous chloride and James's powder.
27. In the process of becoming gangrenous.
28. Mercurous chloride and James's powder.
29. Magnesium sulphate.
30. Compound gamboge pills a scruple and then magnesium sulphate solution.
31. A scruple of compound gamboge pills.
32. Blistering plaster.
33. Camphor mixture combined with compound ammonia solution.
34. Mustard plasters.
35. Ammonium acetate.
36. Syrup made of salt of tartar and lemon juice, possibly used as an antacid.
37. Silver nitrate.
38. Compound of mercury and ammonia.
39. James Cochrane started his medical military career as a hospital assistant on 9 August 1813. He was subsequently promoted to the post of assistant surgeon to the Royal York Rangers on 7 July 1814. He retired h.p. on 8 November 1819.
40. Peter Stewart started his medical military career as hospital assistant on 19 May 1815: h.p. 25 February 1816: f.p. 20 December 1821.
41. Let him take compound gamboge pills one scruple immediately and after two hours magnesium sulphate one and a half ounces [presumably in water: the usual dose is given as two to four drachms, a quarter to half an ounce].
42. Let him take mercurous chloride one scruple immediately. Cold shower, shave his head. Apply cantharides plaster and to have immediately after his bath the following draught: Recipe/ prescription: Solution of ammonium acetate [mindererus spirit], peppermint water, of each one fluid ounce, mix.
43. Let him have compound gamboge pill one scruple immediately. Take blood from the arm one pound and from the temporal artery half a pound.

44. Recipe/prescription: Camphor mixture. Ammonium acetate solution [Mindererus spirit] of each two fluid ounces. Rectified ether, of each half a fluid drachm, mix to make a draught to be taken at bedtime.
45. Let him take camphor mixture one fluid ounce every hour with tincture of opium twenty minims [as a] single dose. Apply cantharides plaster to the stomach and to have two fluid ounces of wine every hour.
46. Repeat the camphor mixture as above.
47. Recipe/prescription: Camphor mixture one fluid ounce. Compound ammonia solution one fluid drachm, mix to make a draught to be given every hour. Apply cantharides plaster to the nape of the neck.
48. Let him take magnesium sulphate half an ounce immediately. Shave his head and then let him have a cold shower.
49. Let him have magnesium sulphate one ounce immediately and apply cantharides plaster to his head.
50. Let him take magnesium sulphate and mercurous chloride. Apply cantharides plaster to the whole head and to the pit of the stomach.
51. Hiccoughs.
52. Protective membrane that covers the brain and spinal cord.
53. Membrane lining the thoracic cavity and the lungs.
54. Compound extract of colocynth fifteen grains combined with mercurous chloride five grains.
55. Let him have sodium sulphate (Glauber's Salt) one ounce immediately.
56. Cold shower and ammonium acetate solution [Mindererus spirit] one fluid ounce.
57. Recipe/prescription: Mercurous chloride one scruple. James's Powder six grains, mix to make a powder [specific dose form, usually tipped down the throat from a folded piece of paper] and give immediately.
58. Recipe/prescription: Mercurous chloride three grains. Camphor two grains. Gum acacia mucilage, a sufficient quantity to make a pill to be given every hour. Apply cantharides plaster to the stomach area.
59. Apply cantharides plaster to the nape of the neck, the head and the legs.
60. Preparation made from a plant commonly known as Virginia snakeroot.

Notes

61. A projection or prominence that is often seen on the skull.
62. The portion of the thorax that lines the ribs and the region of the intercostal muscles.
63. Let him have mercurous chloride half a scruple and compound extract of colocynth fifteen grains immediately. Take blood from the arm to three pounds and the head being previously shaved, apply cantharides plaster.
64. Repeat the bloodletting to a pound and a half.
65. Fainting.
66. Repeat the same medicines and let him have purging enemas as required.
67. Recipe/prescription: Mercurous chloride four grains. James's Powder two grains. Mix, give every three hours and let him have effervescent draughts after each dose.
68. Absence of fever.
69. Let him take castor oil one fluid ounce and a purging enema immediately.
70. Let him take mercurous chloride one scruple immediately. Take blood from his arm to three and a half pounds. His head being first shaved, apply cantharides plaster.
71. Recipe/prescription: Camphor mixture one and a half fluid ounces. Compound ammonia solution half a fluid ounce, mix to make a draught, to be given every three hours. Apply cantharides plaster to the stomach.
72. The same medicine to be repeated.
73. Continue the medicine as above.
74. Repeat the draught as yesterday.
75. Continue the medicine.
76. Continue the draught as above.
77. Involuntary contractions of the diaphragm.
78. Spots of bleeding under the skin.
79. James Lynch O'Connor started his medical military career as a temporary assistant surgeon, OMD, on 10 November 1813. He later assumed the post of second assistant surgeon, OMD, on 28 May 1814.
80. Recipe/prescription: Mercurous chloride (calomel) half a scruple [ten grains]. Compound extract of colocynth half a drachm. Make into six pills and give immediately.
81. Shave his head and apply cantharides plaster [blistering plaster] to the nape of the neck.

82. Recipe/prescription: Camphor mixture two fluid ounces. Compound ammonia solution half a fluid drachm. Mix to make a draught to be given every hour. Apply cantharides plaster to head and chest.
83. Continue the same medicines.
84. Let him take six purging pills immediately.
85. Twenty grains of mercurous chloride (calomel).
86. To have one scruple of mercurous chloride immediately. Give a cold affusion. and apply cantharides plaster to the nape of the neck. ([Affusions could be lotions (washing with a sponge or rag soaked in the liquid), aspersions (shaking drops of the liquid onto the body) or shower baths: the latter is probably the most likely here.]
87. To have one scruple of mercurous chloride quickly.
88. To have a cold-water shower (see note 76) and then:
89. Recipe/prescription: Solution of ammonium acetate one fluid ounce. Nitric ether [spirit of nitric ether, sweet spirit of nitre] one fluid drachm. Mix to make a draught to be taken every hour.
90. Recipe/prescription: camphor mixture one fluid ounce. Compound ammonia solution one fluid drachm. Mix to make a draught to be taken every hour.
91. Continue the same medication. Apply the cantharides plaster to the legs.
92. Post-mortem examination.
93. See Report on Barbados.
94. See Report on Barbados.
95. To have a warm bath immediately: Recipe/prescription: Magnesium sulphate two drachms [in] eight fluid ounces of spring water every quarter of an hour. Shave his head.
96. Recipe/prescription: Tincture of senna, one ounce; mint water and syrup, half an ounce each: Mix, to be taken three or four times a day. Recipe/prescription: diaphoretic [sweating] mixture eight ounces. Antimony tartrate solution three drachms. Spirit of nitric ether two drachms, give one ounce every two hours, and to have a cold shower.
97. James Browne Lenon started his medical military career as a hospital mate for general service; he became a hospital assistant on 25 March 1813. He assumed the post of assistant surgeon to the 8th West India Regiment on 9 June 1814. He was later assigned to the 3rd West India Regiment on 8 August 1816.

Notes

98. Shave his head and cover it with cantharides plaster. Put cantharides plaster on the pit of his stomach. Recipe/prescription: Magnesium sulphate one drachm, spring water six ounces. Mix and let him take it every four hours until the bowels are completely emptied.
99. Recipe/prescription: Warm water twelve ounces, magnesium sulphate one ounce, castor oil half an ounce. Mix to make an enema and inject immediately. To have barley water as his normal drink and repeat the magnesium sulphate solution [enema] as needed until morning.
100. Recipe/prescription: Potassium bitartrate [cream of tartar] one ounce, spring water two pints, mix for his normal drink. To have a warm bath.
101. Previously referenced.
102. Recipe/prescription: Magnesium sulphate one drachm. Ammonium tartrate solution one fluid drachm, eight ounces of pure water. [Give] every two hours, repeat three times.
103. Recipe/prescription: Compound powder of jalap one drachm. To have a diuretic mixture.
104. Recipe/prescription: Potassium nitrate one drachm, aromatic powder one drachm, syrup two fluid ounces – water two pints. To have one pint of wine.
105. Recipe/prescription: magnesium sulphate two drachms, peppermint water eight fluid ounces. Make into a draught [and] repeat six times, two pints of diaphoretic mixture to be drunk in the day.
106. Recipe/prescription: eight fluid ounces of warm water every hour and warm baths.
107. James Cochrane started his medical military career as a hospital assistant on 9 August 1813. He was subsequently promoted to the post of assistant surgeon to the Royal York Rangers on 7 July 1814.
108. Age.
109. Tenesmus is a term used to describe straining, especially ineffective and painful straining during a bowel movement or urination.
110. Ipecacuanha is a plant found in Brazil which was used primarily as a diaphoretic, an expectorant and also as a stimulant to the digestive system.
111. Ophthalmia is a reference to the inflammation of the eye.

112. Anasarca is a medical condition characterized by widespread swelling of the body due to fluid accumulation in the tissues.
113. Thomas Williams started his medical military career as a hospital assistant on 3 November 1825. He subsequently assumed the post of assistant surgeon to the 19th Regiment of Foot on 28 September 1826. He also served as surgeon to the 59th Regiment of Foot from 27 January 1841. He obtained his MD from Edinburgh in 1824.

Bibliography

Primary Sources

"Journal of His Majesty's Ship *Alfred*. W. J. Warner Surgeon, 1 October 1797–31 March 1798 (ADM 101/83/3)." London, National Archives.

"Returns and Reports Concerning Yellow Fever; Report on Yellow Fever: Barbados, Antigua, Demerara, Berbice, Dominica, Grenada, Montserrat, St Kitts, St Lucia, St Vincent, Tobago, and Trinidad (1818 Dec–1840 Apr) WO334/165." London, National Archives.

Affidavit of Henry Huntley 1 November 1739 (ADM/106/910/216. London, National Archives.

Aitken, William. *The Science and Practice of Medicine*. 2 vols. London: Charles Griffin and Company, 1764.

Carter, Henry Rose. *Yellow Fever: An Epidemiological and Historical Study of the Place of Origin*. Baltimore: Williams and Wilkins Company, 1931.

Chisholm, Colin. *Diseases of Tropical Climates: Essay on the Malignant Pestilential Fever Introduced into the West Indian Islands etc., in 1794–1796*. Philadelphia: Thomas Dobson, 1796.

Drew, Robert. *Commissioned Officers in the Medical Services of the British Army, 1660–1960: Roll of Officers in the Royal Army Medical Corps*, vol. II. London, Wellcome Historical Medical Library, 1968.

Findlay, G.M. "The First Recognized Epidemic of Yellow Fever." In *Transactions of the Royal Society of Tropical Medicine and Hygiene* XXXV, no. 3, 29 November 1941.

Hillary, William. *Observations on the Changes of the Air and the Concomitant Epidemical Diseases in the Island of Barbados*.

Edited by J. Edward Hutson, and Henry S. Fraser. Kingston, Jamaica: University of the West Indies Press, 2011.
Letter of Admiral Cavendish to the Principal Officers and Commissioners of His Majesty's Navy, 10 August 1738 (ADM/106/86 PRO).
Letter of Admiral Cavendish to the Principal Officers and Commissioners of His Majesty's Navy, 31 August 1738 (ADM/106/86 PRO).
Letter of Captain James Cornwall to the Principal Officers and Commissioners of His Majesty's Navy, 30 May 1738 (ADM/106/86 PRO).
Ligon, Richard. *The True and Exact History of the Island of Barbadoes, 1657*. Edited by J. Edward Hutson. Barbados: Barbados National Trust, 2000.
Peterkin, A., and W. Johnston. *Commissioned Officers in the Medical Services of the British Army, 1660–1960*, vol. 1. London: Wellcome Historical Medical Library, 1968.
Pinckard, George. *Notes on the West Indies*, vol. 1. London: Baldwin, Cradock, and Joy, 1816.
Rollo, John. Observations *on the Diseases Which Appeared in the Army on St Lucia in 1778 and 1779, To Which are Prefixed Remarks Calculated to Assist in Ascertaining the Causes; and in Explaining the Treatment of Those Diseases*. London: Charles Dilly, 1781.
———. *Observations on the Means of Preserving and Restoring Health in the West-Indies*. London: C. Dilly, 1783.
Warren, Henry. "A Treatise Concerning the Malignant Fever in Barbados and the Neighbouring Islands, with an Account There from the year 1733 to 1738." London: n.p., 1741.

Secondary Sources

Buckley, Roger N. *The British Army in the West Indies: Society and the Military in the Revolutionary Age*. Gainesville: University of Florida Press; Kingston: University of the West Indies Press, 1998.
Cantlie, Neil. *A History of the Army Medical Department*. London: Churchill Livingstone, 1974.
Charters, Erica. *Disease, War, and the Imperial State*. Chicago: University of Chicago Press, 2014.
Clyde, David, F. *Two Centuries of Health Care in Dominica*. New Delhi: Sushima Gopal, 1980.

Bibliography

Cook, Gordon C. *Disease in the Merchant Navy: A History of the Seamen's Hospital Society.* London: Radcliffe Publishing, 2007.

Downs, Jim, *Maladies of Empire: How Colonialism, Slavery, and War Transformed Medicine.* Cambridge, Massachusetts: Belknap Press at Harvard University Press, 2021.

Fitzharris, Lindsey. *The Butchering Art: Joseph Lister's Quest to Transform the Great World of Victorian Medicine.* New York: Scientific American, 2017.

Hempel, Sandra. *The Medical Detective: John Snow, Cholera and the Mystery of the Broad Street Pump.* London: Granta Books, 2006.

Hogarth, Lana. *Medicalizing Blackness.* Chapel Hill: University of North Carolina Press, 2017.

Hutson, J. Edward, ed. *On the Treatment and Management of the More Common West-India Diseases, 1750–1802.* Kingston: University of the West Indies Press, 2005.

Kiple, Kenneth F. *The Caribbean Slave: A Biological History.* Cambridge: Cambridge University Press, 2002.

———, ed. *Plague, Pox and Pestilence.* London: Wiedenfeld and Nicolson, 1997.

Macfarlane, Burnet and David White. *Natural History of Infectious Disease.* Cambridge: Cambridge University Press, 1972.

McNeill, John R. *Mosquito Empires: Ecology and War in the Greater Caribbean, 1620–1914.* Cambridge: Cambridge University Press, 2010.

Murphy, Jim. *An American Plague: The True and Terrifying Story of the Yellow Fever Epidemic of 1793.* New York: Clarion Books, 2003.

Oldstone, Michael B. *Viruses, Plagues, and History.* Oxford: Oxford University Press, 1998.

Porter, Roy. *Blood and Guts: A Short History of Medicine.* London: Penguin Books, 2002.

Richardson, Bonham C. *The Caribbean in the Wider World 1492–1992: A Regional Geography.* Cambridge: Cambridge University Press, 1992.

Sheridan, Richard B. *Sugar and Slavery: An Economic History of the West Indies, 1623–1775.* Kingston: Canoe Press, University of the West Indies, 1994.

Smith, Billy G. *Ship of Death.* New Haven: Yale University Press, 2013.

Snowden, Frank M. *Epidemics and Society: From the Black Death to the Present.* New Haven: Yale University Press, 2019.

Watts, Sheldon. "Yellow fever Immunities in West Africa and the Americas in the Age of Slavery and beyond: A Reappraisal," *Journal of Social History* (Summer 2001): 955–67.

Weaver, Karol K. *Medical Revolutionaries: The Enslaved Healers of Eighteenth-Century Saint Domingue.* Champaign: University of Illinois Press, 2006.

Index

n indicates "note"

acclimatization to disease, 14–15, 228–29; *Extract of Annual Report on the Prevailing Diseases among the Troops Stationed at St Christopher* (1840–41), 323, 323t9.5

admissions and mortality from the disease category among white troops (1840–41), (*Extract of Annual Report on the Prevailing Diseases among the Troops Stationed at St Christopher*), 322t9.3

admissions of cases at Brimstone Hill, each month, noting weather conditions (*Extract of Annual Report of Medical Transactions and Prevailing Diseases at St Christophers, Nevis and Tortola, Jan. 1836–Feb. 1837*), 311t9.1

African enslaved militia, 14

African Black population: immunity of, 6–7, 25, 68, 124, 136, 505n48, 505n50; death from disease, 89; increase in Barbados of, 6–7. *See also* coloured inhabitants

Afro-Caribbean women, nursing care by, 17

ages of fatal cases (*Extract of Annual Report of the Medical Occurrences of the 67th Regiment, April 1838–March 1839, Stationed at George Town, Demerara*), 208t5.2

Alfred, HMS, report on yellow fever aboard the (1796), 27–37

Allenby, Dr (St Pierre, Martinique), 32

Amerindian labour, 6

Antigua, yellow fever reports filed in (1820–1840s), 38–67; preview of, 38. *See also* reports from Antigua

Arthur, Dr John (surgeon): reports from Barbados made by, 68–112; travel to Tobago, 124

atmosphere of ships (as contributing to sickness), 41, 43, 129, 345. *See also* mephitic air

attacks with fever and deaths in the Queens, June–Aug. 1816 (*Remarks on the Lately Prevailing Fever at Dominica*), 226t6.1
Aux Cayes prison, Saint Domingo, 28

Barbados, yellow fever reports filed in (1821–1840s): arrangements to ensure health, 127–28; barracks and sickness, 131–33; black servants ordered to attend to yellow fever patients, 125; building inspections, 130–31; by Dr Arthur, 68–112; by Dr MacDermott, 115–18; by Dr Green, 123–24; by Dr Tegart, 112–15, 124–28; family living arrangements, 153–65; preventive measures taken by N. Pierce, 132–36; preview of, 68; repair of Naval Hospital, 136
Barbados, yellow fever outbreaks: arrival, sickness, deaths and recoveries (1820–21), 119–20t4.1; between 1647 and 1649, 4–5; connected to the sugar revolution, 6; of 1647, 4, 5, 7; of 1648, 3; of 1691, 7
Barbados climate, 8
"Barbados Distemper", 5
bark (prescribed for yellow fever symptoms), 31, 292, 378, 467. *See also* chinchona
Barrack Department (non-military personnel), 69
Black immunity. *See* African Black population: immunity of
Black Invalid Garrison Company (Grenada), 272
Black personnel, *fatality rate in coloured personnel employed at Naval Hospital,* 137t4.4
Black servants ordered to attend to yellow fever patients, 98–99, 125
Black troops, 25
black vomit, 2; *el vómito prieto,* 3; and recovery, 143–49, 372
bleeding (as symptom), 2, 31, 89, 267, 320, 335, 360, 372–73, 409; incident report on cases and outcomes, 1816, (*Remarks on the Lately Prevailing Fever at Dominica*), 227t6.2; subcutaneous type, 527n30, 527n34, 531n78; types of, 492
bleeding (as a remedy), 11, 13, 18, 25, 28, 31, 189, 227t6.2, 271, 308–9, 310, 315, 321, 326, 371, 394, 395, 402, 408, 419, 452, 460, 463, 467–69, 484; ineffectiveness of, 110–11, 197, 198, 225, 248, 275–76, 472; with leeches, 492
Bone, Hugh, 40, 42, 502n6, 502n11
Brazil, tick and horsefly as vector in, 2
British Guiana, yellow

Index

fever reports filed in (1830s–1840s), 195–223; black troops, 210; climate as contributing factor, 221; deaths reported, 200–1, 205; preview of, 195; symptoms, 200–5, 205–6, 209, 211–13, 218; white troops, 210, 220; yellow fever discounted as cause of outbreak, 222–23

British military doctors, 19–24; treatment by seen as certain death, 17–18; recruitment of, 20–21; shortage of, 21–22; standards for, 23; structural changes concerning, 24; treatment of yellow fever in the Caribbean by, 25–26

Brodie stoves, 42, 43, 129, 509n42; description of, 502n9

Buckley, Roger, study of medicine in eighteenth century British Army and Navy in the W.I., 19

Burnet, Sir Macfarlane, and David White, study of diseases, 5

calomel (as treatment), 9–10, 32, 86, 111, 180; 205; 250, 254, 268, 307–8, 351, 362, 404, 443, 469, 482, 494; and ammonia, 248; a compound of mercury, 499n2, 500n12, 506n8, 527n8, 528n10, 531n80, 532n85; ineffectiveness of, 40; and Jalap, 285, 289, 335, 478, 480; and Opium, 452; questioning of use as treatment, 33, 494; to produce salivation, 28–29, 277; prophylactic use of, 30; as a purgative, 198, 260, 262, 276, 352–54, 405, 467; and quinine, 199; side effects of, 138; with Castile Soap and rhubarb *puls gr*, 33

camphor, 32, 35, 268, 457–9, 460, 463–5, 467, 469, 472, 474–5 482, 499–500n7, 528n20, 528n22, 528n33, 530n44–47, 530n58, 531n71, 532n82, 532n90; with Opium, 405

camphor water, 520n41

camphorated tincture of opium, 511,70

Cantlie, Neil (*A History of the Army Medical Department*), 22

Carlisle Bay, Barbados, 42

Carter, Henry Rose, 4

cassia (medicinal plant), 10, 142, 494, 511n60

Castile soap, 32, 500n8

causes of yellow fever, 8–11, 41, 43, 103–7, 141–43; intemperance, 38–39

Cavendish, Admiral, 1738 request for surgeon, 20

Charters, Erica (*Disease, War, and the Imperial State: The Welfare of the British Armed Forces During the Seven Years'*

War), 15
children. *See* women and children
chinchona *(Pulv Cort)*, 35, 467, 501n17. *See also* bark
chirurgery, 10
Chisholm, Colin, *(Diseases of Tropical climates: Essay on the Malignant Pestilential Fever Introduced into the West Indian Islands etc., in 1794–1796)*, 500n13
Clark, James (Caribbean physician, 1790s), 14
class specific, yellow fever attacks as, 307
climate (as cause of disease), 57, 62, 66, 104, 113, 118, 185, 211, 291, 304–5, 352, 412, 460, 492. *See also* miasma as cause of disease
Clyde, David, 6
coal tar, 502n7; and lack of ventilation in ships, 41–43
coloured inhabitants, 300, 301
colours of diseases, 5
commerce affected by disease, 103
"Congo", referenced as link between yellow fever and the West Indies, 68
contagion, 68, 102, 149, 154, 229–32, 244–47, 250, 288, 386, 390–93, 401, 412–14, 417, 425, 436–37, 424, 506n7, 520n4; exposure and, 104, 125–26; not found, 45, 56–57, 127, 153–54, 191, 302, 344, 345, 393, 409, 424; of the plague discussed, 133–34; on St Kitts (1818), 309–10; theory of, 113, 132, 137–38, 158–61, 171–73, 176, 240, 462, 491; on Tobago (1805), 386
Cornwall, Capt. James, 21
croton oil *(croton tiglium)*, as treatment, 25, 47, 307, 308, 353, 503n22
Cumming, Alexander, 504n26

dampness, 36
deaths, accounts of by yellow fever, 4–5, 29, 53–58; 126–27, 70–98; 149–53; ages, 64; after bleeding, 31–32; in Barbados, 73–74, 88–89, 92–99; in Dominica, 266–67; in St Vincent, 63. *See also* symptoms; yellow fever
deaths in British Guiana, 210, 213; *ages of the fatal cases*, 208t5.2; *cases of yellow fever and fatalities among military units*, 209t5.3; *incidence and mortality of yellow fever by military unit strength*, 219t5.4; *summary of strength, admissions, and deaths of military ranks by period of residence*, 208t5.1
deaths of non-commissioned officers and privates in the army serving in the Windward and Leeward Colonies, Jan. 1796–Dec. 1807, 396–

Index

98t12.3
delirium tremens, 504n28
Demerara, 91–92; cases of fever compared between Berbice and, 214–18
dengue fever, 16
diaphoresis (excessive sweating), 504n29
Disease, War, and the Imperial State: The Welfare of the British Armed Forces During the Seven Years' War (Erica Charters), 15
diseases treated during the year (1843–44), St Christopher (*Extract of Annual Report on the Prevailing Diseases, St Christopher, April 1843–March 1844*), 338t9.6
disposal of deceased's belongings, 125
doctors in the British military. *See* British military doctors
Dominica, 492; 1817 outbreak in, 101, 394
Dominica, yellow fever reports filed in (1810s–1840s), 224–69; preview of, 224
Downing, Lucy, 4
Dowse, Richard, 504n27
Dr James's Fever Powder, 31–32, 35, 499n6
Draper, Thomas, 505n45
drunkenness. *See* inebriety; intemperance
Du Tertre, Père Jean-Baptiste, 3
Duncan, Adam, 505n49
Duncanson, James, 505n51

dysentery, 88, 231–34, 237, 238, 265, 292, 320, 452, 455, 462, 482–3; indigenous treatment for, 499n3

Elliot, James, 42, 502n12
emetic tartar, 510n54
emetics, 9, 13, 30–31, 35, 196, 493, 499n3, 503n18; unpopular, 30
enslaved Africans, importation of, 6–7; as militia, 14
environmental factors, yellow fever outbreaks and, 224
epidemics, yellow fever, 4. *See also* outbreaks
Epidemics and Society: From the Black Death to the Present (Frank M. Snowden), 16–17
erysipelas (skin infection), 504n40
"Essay on Disease Incidental to Europeans in Hot Climates" (James Lind), 15
Europeans, 3, 201, 300, 394–95, 452

fatality rate in coloured personnel employed at Naval Hospital, Barbados, 137t4.4
fear of yellow fever, 2
Febris Ardens Biliosa, 8
Febris Continua Icterodes, 192–93
Febris Icterodes (yellow fever), 406, 415, 421–22, 502n14
Febris Quot: Intern, 202
Febris Remittens, 202, 267–69, 331–37, 447–48

fevers (as symptom), 195–200, 229–31, 232t6.3, 339, 448–50, 487–90; intermittent nature of, 196–97; post-mortem, 199–200; remedies employed, 198–99, 399–405
Fièvre Malchiltli, 8
Finlay, Dr Carlos, connected yellow fever with the *Aedes aegypti* mosquito, 494–95
Findlay, G.M., 3–4
Firefly, H.M.S., 191
first-person narratives on yellow fever, 38, 491
foul air aboard ships. *See* atmosphere of ships
Franklin, Henry, 505n46
freshwater on board ships, 42–43

gangrene, 138–39
gastric disease, 136, 138–43, 153–54
gastritis, 503n20
geography and climate of the Caribbean, 492
germ theory, 9
Gillespie, Andrew, 33, 500n11
Grenada, introduction of yellow fever to, 16, 381; at fish market bog, 277
Grenada, yellow fever reports filed in (1816–1840s), 270–98; climate, 271–72, 273, 287, 291–92; preview, 270
Guadeloupe, 1648 outbreak, 3

Haitian Revolution, and L'Ouverture's knowledge of yellow fever, 16–17
Hall, Thomas (Hospital Assistant), 44–47; 502n13
Hankey (ship of death), 15–16
Hartle, Robert, 501n2, 503n16
Heela, H.M.S., 191
higher elevations, and lower incidences of yellow fever, 305, 346, 492
historical debate over causes of yellow fever, 3–7
historical literature on yellow fever, 1
history of yellow fever in the Caribbean, 13–19
Hogarth, Lana (*Medicalizing Blackness: Making Racial Difference in the Atlantic World, 1780–1840*), 14
Hunter, John (surgeon general, 1790s), 23
Huntley, Henry (military surgeon), 20–21
Hutson, J. Edward, 5
hypersalivation (ptyalism), 504n37

immunity to yellow fever: as an acquired trait, 14, 507n16; Africans and, 6–7, 9, 14, 25, 68, 136, 505n48, 507n11; and dengue fever, 16; Europeans lacking, 5, 248
incidence and mortality of yellow fever by military unit strength (*Extract of Annual Report on the Diseases of the Troops in British Guiana, April 1846–*

Index

March 1847 by J. Millar), 219t5.4
inebriety, 72, 84, 521n6; death by, 114
infection aboard ships, 91–92
intemperance, 270; as cause of yellow fever, 38–39, 282, 474, 482
intoxication, 473
Ipecacuahana (an emetic), 30–31

Jackson, Dr (*A Treatise on the Fevers of Jamaica, with Observations on the Intermitting Fevers of America*), 503n15
Jamaica: sickness in, 191; reports from, 27, 499n1
Jamaica, Newcastle military post, 347
Jamaican Blacks, song about yellow fever by, 18
James's Powder. See Dr James's Fever Powder
jaundice, 2, 5, 32–33, 139, 142, 145, 146, 320
jungle yellow fever, 2

Kiple, Kenneth, 4–5

Latham, Dr (pres. of the Royal College of Physicians London), questioned on disease, 133–34
laundry, unhealthy nature of, 162
Le Boeuf (French ship), and 1648 epidemic in Guadeloupe, 3
Ligon, Richard, 4–5; *A True and Exact History of the Island of Barbadoes*, 5
lime juice rub, 35
liver: enlarged, 205; failure, 2
loblolly boy, 39, 501n1
L'Ouverture, Toussaint, awareness of yellow fever used in military strategy, 16–17

Madeira wine, as a remedy, 33, 494
Maegaera, H.M.S., 191–92
Maladie de Siam, 8
manna, 494
Massachusetts, 1648 ordinance blocking ships from the W.I., 3–4
matter, four elements of, 491–92
McNeill, John R. (*Mosquito Empires, Ecology and War in the Greater Caribbean, 1620–1914*), 17–18
medical developments, 195
medical philosophies, 15, 491
medical practitioners, recruitment by military of, 21–24
medical treatises on practicing Caribbean medicine, 7
medical treatment of yellow fever, doctors' views from the Eighteenth Century on, 8–13
Medicalizing Blackness: Making Racial Difference in the Atlantic World, 1780–1840 (Lana Hogarth), 14
medicinal therapies: questioning

of, 493; efficacy of, 491
melena (black tarry stools), 2
Menzies, Alexander, 40, 42, 501–2n5
mephitic air, 141–42, 510n50. *See also* atmosphere of ships
mercurial fumigation, 310
mercury (as treatment), 9–10, 18, 25, 40, 158, 189, 209, 232, 315, 318, 372, 405, 432–33, 435, 460, 494, 529n38; ineffectiveness of, 343; as injurious, 145, 403, 404; and ptyalism, 55, 308. *See also* calomel
miasma (as cause of disease), 124, 281, 303, 316, 340, 345, 367, 376–82, 521n1; miasmic school, 8, 501n18. *See also* climate; swamps
military medicine. *See* British military doctors
monkeys, jungle yellow fever and, 2
Montserrat, yellow fever reports filed in (1820s), 299–306; climate and disease, 304–5; preview, 299; swamp (miasma), 299, 300–1, 303–4
Morn Bruce hospital diaries, 242
mortality rate in the Caribbean, 2; for British troops 1778–1789, 12t1.1, 12–13; for British troops, 1796–1802, 6; for black troops in 1804, 6
Mosquito Empires, Ecology and War in the Greater Caribbean, 1620–1914 (John R. McNeill), 17–18
mosquito larvae, suppressed by coal tar, 502n7
mosquitos, 12; *Aedes aegypti*, 2, 6, 494; correlation with yellow fever missed, 11, 492–93; importation of, 3, 7, 15
Munro, William (Staff Surgeon), 47–48; 503n23

National Archives (Kew, London), 27, 38
native Caribbeans, yellow fever susceptibility of, 5–6
naval surgeon, *Pyramus* seeking an experienced and active, 130

onset of yellow fever among military personnel by age, rank and arrival date, 165–66t4.6
opium, tincture of *(Tinct Opii)*, 31, 499n4
origins of yellow fever epidemics, historical discussion of, 8–13
Orr, Hugh, 505–6n52
outbreaks of yellow fever: factors in, 2–3; Guadeloupe, 1648, 3; Yucatan Peninsula, 1648, 3

phlogistic theory of disease, 25
Pinckard, Dr, 10–11; account of voyage to W.I. in 1795, 3
Pontrefid, HMS, introduction of yellow fever at Port Royal through the, 28

Index 547

Port Royal, Jamaica, yellow fever at, 27–29; Naval Hospital at, 29
post-mortem examinations: Barbados, 88, 107–9; British Guiana, 207, 213; Dominica, 267; Grenada, 288, 295–96; St Christopher, 307, 322, 329–30; Tobago, 366, 374–76, 444–45; Trinidad, 464, 465, 467, 481
precautions taken against disease, 98–102
pre-Columbian New World, 5–6
ptyalism (hypersalivation), 55, 504n37
Pulv Cort (chinchona derivative), 35, 501n17
Pyramus, HMS: accounts of sickness on, 38–44; examined by inspector of hospitals, 128–30

quarantine of ships from W.I., 4
Quassia (stomach tonic), 35
quinine, 196, 199, 202, 203, 204, 206, 263, 268, 297, 308, 352, 353, 354, 501n17

racial differences in immunity, 68
rainfall patterns, outbreaks correlated with, 493
remittent type, 201
reports from Antigua: *Abstract of Annual report to Accompany the Annual Return of Sick and Wounded Troops in the Windward and Leeward Islands Command, April 1838–March 1839 by T. Draper*, 59–64; *Extract of Annual Report on Diseases Treated...April 1838–March 1839, by Surgeon J. Duncanson*, 65–67; *Extract of Annual Report...from Antigua by William Munro* (Dec. 1825–Dec. 1826, 47–48; *Extract of Half-Yearly Report of the Detachment Hospital 35th Reg. Monks Hill, 1821. Also Remarks*, 38–44; *Extract of Report of Medical Transactions and Prevailing Diseases in the 14th Regiment of Foot from 1 Jan. 1836–31March 1837 by R. Dowse*, 49–58; *Extract of Report of Antigua, Dated 10 Jan. 1836 by A. Cumming*, 49; *Half-Yearly Report Dated Shirley Heights 20 Dec. 1821 by Thomas Hall*, 44–47
reports from Barbados: *Bone's letter to M. Chevrin dated 14 June 1822, Naval Hospital Barbados*, 167–73; *Extract of Annual report of the Medical Occurrences...April 1842–March1843 by C.J. Palmer*, 192–94; *Extract of Annual Report of Sickness and Mortality...April 1839–Feb. 1840 by Mr W. Robinson*, 181–85; *Extract of Annual Report of* Steamers, Royal

Navy at Barbados 31 March 1842 by A. Mackintosh MD, 190–92; *Extract of the Half-Yearly Report from Barbados, Dec. 1821 by G. MacDermott*, 115–18; *Extract of Half-Yearly Medical report by Dr Bone*, 20 Feb. 1822, 149–51; *Half-Yearly Remarks on Diseases from July to Dec. 1821 by E. Tegart*, 112–15; *Report of Observations to Accompany the Annual Report of the Sick... Nov.1838–March 1839 by T. Spence*, 174–81; *Report of Observations...April 1839–40 by T. Spence*, 185–90; *Report of the Storekeeper General's Department showing the dates of their arrival at Barbados, sickness deaths, recoveries, etc.*, 165–66; *Return of the storekeeper general's arrival at Barbados*, 166–67

reports from British Guiana: *Extract of Annual Medical Report of the Diseases of the Troops, etc., April 1841–March 1842 by A. Melvin*, 210–14; *Extract of Annual Medical Report of the Service Company's 67th Regiment for the Year Ending 31 March 1838 by E.H. Blakeney*, 200–5; *Extract of Annual Report and Observations on the Diseases, etc.,...April 1842–March 1843 by A. Melvin*, 214–16; *Extract of Annual Report of Diseases Prevailed at Detachment Hospital 69th and 1st West India Regiments of Capory, Jan.–Dec. 1835 by Assistant Staff Surgeon R.G. Webb*, 195–200; *Extract of Annual Report of Medical Occurrences in the 76th Regiment Hospital, April 1839–March 1840 by Leigh MD*, 209–10; *Extract of Annual Report of the Medical Occurrences of the 67th Regiment, April 1838–March 1839, Stationed at George Town, Demerara by E.H. Blakeney*, 207–8, 208t5.1, 208t5.2; *Extract of Annual Report on the Diseases... April 1846–March 1847 by J. Millar*, 219–23; *Extract of Annual Report on the Diseases That were Treated in the Hospital of 76th Regiment at Demerara, April–Nov. 1838 by W. Birrell*, 205–7; *Extract of Annual Report with Observations...April 1843–March 1844 by Staff Surgeon C. Maclean, MD and Letter to him by J.B. Beresford, Jan. 1844*, 216–19

reports from Dominica: *Extract of Annual Medical Report of the Garrison of Dominica, March 1839, by F. Macaw MD*, 263–65; *Extract of Annual Medical*

Index

Report of the Garrison of Dominica, April 1841–March 1842, by James Connell, 265–67; Extract of Annual Medical Report of the Garrison of Dominica, April 1845–March 1846, by Robert Smith, 267–69; Extract of Half-Yearly Report of Prevailing Diseases in the Detachment Hospital on Morne Bruce Dominica, June–Dec. 1821, by Edward Dow, 251–54; Extract of Yearly Report of Disease and Medical Occurrences at Dominica, Dec. 1826, by John Glasco, 259–63; Extracts of Letters from Major Cassidy (1817), 239–51; Extracts of Observations on the Diseases That Occurred in the Detachment of Royal Artillery 35th Regiment Stationed in Dominica, Dec. 1825–Dec. 1826, 255–59; Ordnance Hospital, St Ann's Barbados, May 1817, 227–39; Remarks on the Lately Prevailing Fever at Dominica by John Arthur, MD, (1818), 224–27

reports from Grenada: Copy of Remarks, Dec. 1815–June 1816, by F.A. Loinsworth, Surgeon to the Forces at Grenada, 270–72; Extract from Half-Yearly Report, Dec. 1817, by A.J. Ralph, Assistant Surgeon, 278–82; Extract of Annual Report of the Diseases and Medical Occurrences of the Troops at Grenada, Dec. 1828–Dec. 1829, by John Glasco, 290–98; Extract of Annual Report of the Diseases of the Troops Serving at Grenada, Dec. 1827–Dec. 1828, by John Glasco, 283–86; Extract of Annual Report on the Diseases at the Garrison at Grenada, Dec. 1827–Dec. 1828, by P. O'Callaghan, 287–90; Half-Yearly Medical Report of Diseases, June 1816–Dec. 1816, by Frederick A. Loinsworth, Surgeon to the Forces, 272–78

reports from Montserrat: Extract of Annual Summary Report of Diseases Treated in the Detachment Hospital and Prevailing on the Island of Montserrat, Dec. 1826–Dec. 1827 by A. Tonnere, Assistant Staff Surgeon, 303–7; Extract of Half-Yearly Report Dec. 1820–June 1821 from Montserrat by William Parry, Hospital Assistant, 299–302

reports from St Christopher (St Kitts): Extract of Annual Report of Medical Transactions and Prevailing Diseases at St Christophers, Nevis and Tortola, Jan. 1836–Feb. 1837 by Staff Surgeon W. Munro, 311–20; Extract of Annual

Report of the Prevailing Diseases among the Troops, April 1839–March 1840, Staff Surgeon D. Scott, 321–22; Extract of Annual Report on the Prevailing Diseases among the Troops Stationed at St Christopher, April 1840–March 1841 by D. Scott, 322–30; Extract of Annual Report on the Prevailing Diseases among the Troops, April 1842–March 1843 by Staff Surgeon D. Scott, 331–37; Extract of Annual Report on the Prevailing Diseases, April 1843–March 1844 by Staff Surgeon D. Scott, 337–43; Extract of Observations on the Yearly Return of Diseases That Were Treated in Her Majesty's Military Hospital at St Christopher, Dec 1826–Dec. 1827 by J.B. Patterson, 307–10

reports from St Lucia: *Extract of Annual Report on Medicine Transactions and of the Diseases Prevailing among the Troops in St Lucia, April 1846–March 1847* by J.P. Hawkey, MD and Staff Surgeon 1st Class, 344–47; *Extract of Report (Annual) of Medical Transactions and Prevailing Diseases in the Island of St Lucia and Its Dependencies, April 1839–March 1840* by Richard Dowse, Surgeon 14th Foot, 348–50

reports from St Vincent: *Extract from Remarks on the Half-Yearly Return of the Sick, Dec. 1819* by G.W. Cockell, Surgeon to the Forces, 351–52; *Extract of Annual Report of Medical Occurrences, during the Year Ending March 1843*, by Staff Surgeon John Hall, 364–65; *Extract of Annual Medical Report, March 1840* by F. McCann, MD, Staff Surgeon, 356–57; *Extract of Annual Report of Medical Transactions in the Garrison Hospital at St Vincent, March 1842*, by Staff Surgeon John Hall, 357–64; *Extract of Annual Report of the Prevailing Diseases, Jan.–Dec. 1835* by Alexander Stewart, MD, Surgeon to the Forces, 355–56; *Extract of Annual Report on the Prevailing Diseases, Dec. 1828–Dec. 1829, by Alex Melville Jr*, Staff Surgeon, 354–55; *Extract of Report on the Diseases Treated in the Left Wing of the 27th Regiment, Dec. 1828–Dec. 1829* by Thomas Mostyn, Surgeon, 27th Regiment, 352–54

reports from Tobago: *Extract of Annual Report of Prevailing*

Index

Diseases in the Garrison of Fort King George, Tobago, April 1841–March 1842, by S.H. Hardy, Staff Assistant Surgeon, 445–48; *Extract of Annual Report of the Medical Occurrences in the 92nd Highlanders at Tobago, April 1842–March1843* by C.J. Palmer, Surgeon, 448–50; *Extract of Annual Report on the Diseases Which Prevailed in the Garrison of Fort King George, Tobago, April 1839–March 1840*, by Charles Stewart, MD, Assistant Staff Surgeon, 437–45; *Extract of Half-Yearly Report from Tobago to 20 Dec. 1819* by Staff Surgeon, S. Panting, 421–22; *Half-Yearly Report of Sick of the Troops at Tobago to 15 Dec. 1818*, by Staff Surgeon S. Panting, 406–14; *Half-Yearly Report of Sick of the Troops at Tobago to 20 June 1819*, by Staff Surgeon S. Panting, 415–20; *Return of Officers' Servants, Hospital Orderlies and Patients Admitted into Hospital with Other Diseases Who were Subsequently Attacked with Yellow Fever at Tobago from March 1820*, 427–31; *Sketch of Such Cases of* Febris Icterodes *as Occurred among the Officers of the 9th and 21st Regiments and their Servants While at Tobago in 1820* by S. Panting, 431–37; *Special Report on Fever from Tobago* by Dr John Arthur, Physician to the Forces, 367–406; *Supplementary Report to 20 June 1820 Follows Mr Arthur's for Dec. 1820* by Ralph Green Inspector of Army Hospitals, 423–27

reports from Trinidad: *Extract of Annual Report on Prevailing Diseases Treated in 59th Regimental Hospital and on the Principal Medical Occurrences for the Year Ending March 1843, St James, Trinidad,* by Surgeon T. Williams, 486–90; Quarterly Medical Statistics, 486t13.1; *Staff Surgeon Sharp's Half Yearly Medical Report from Trinidad, June–Dec. 1818,* 451–86

resistance to yellow fever, 7

return of convalescents of fever treated in the Naval Hospital, Barbados (20 Oct. – 18 Dec 1821), 121–22t4.2

rhubarb, 32, 33

Rollo, John, commentary from 1781 and 1783 on treatment of yellow fever by, 11–12; figures on mortality rates among troops, 12t1.1, 12–13

Saint Domingue, deaths by

yellow fever, 16–17
salin (stomach remedy), 32
saline mode of treatment, 361t11.3, 362t11.3
salt of tartar, 31, 529n36
schedule for Horatio Warder and John Calometi, 152t4.5
Scottish medical schools, 23
scrofula, 40, 501n4
Sectio Cadaveris, 202
ship environment, 43, 189
Ship of Death: A Voyage that Changed the Atlantic World (Billy G. Smith), 15–16
Smith, Billy G. (*Ship of Death: A Voyage that Changed the Atlantic World*), 15–16
snake root (Seneca), 11
Snowden, Frank M. (*Epidemics and Society: From the Black Death to the Present*), 16–17
soldier's wife, account of, 157
spleen, enlarged, 205
spruce beer, 30
St Christopher (St Kitts), yellow fever reports filed in (1821–1840s), 307–43; *cases of yellow fever: number treated between 1 May and 18 Dec. 1836, exclusive of Blacks,* 316t9.2; *deaths of races by month* (1843–44) 339–40t9.7; epidemic outbreak, 312–16, 323–30; *mortality by age, strength and service duration, 1840–41,* 323t9.4; nature and causes of the disease, 341–43; preview, 307; weather conditions, 311–12, 311t9.1
St Christopher (St Kitts), 3; yellow fever on, 49–50
St Kitts, 1648 outbreak, 3
St Lucia, yellow fever reports filed in (1839, 1846), 344–50; preview, 344; remittent fever, 348–50
St Lucia, yellow fever outbreak of 1778–1789, 11–12
St Vincent, yellow fever reports filed in (1819–1840s), 351–65; *attacks and deaths, 1831–43,* 358t11.2; *cases of fever treated by two doctors, 1841–42,* 361–62t11.3; *fatality, prevalence of, from epidemic fever in the garrison of St Vincent,* April–Sept. 1839, 357t11.1; preview, 351
St Vincent, 16, 197
Storekeeper General's Dept. showing the dates of arrival at Barbados, sickness, deaths, recoveries, etc, 165t4.6, 166t4.7
stranger's fever, 5
strength alterations, 337–41
strength, cases, and mortality report, May–Sept. 1838, (*Extract of Annual Medical Report of the Garrison of Dominica*), 264t6.4
strengths, admissions, and deaths of military ranks by period of residence (*Extract of Annual Report of the Medical*

Occurrences of the 67th Regiment, April 1838–March 1839, Stationed at George Town, Demerara), 208t5.1
subsultus tendinium (tremor of the limbs), 504n30
surgeons, ship's request for, 20
swamps, 36–37, 380. *See also* miasma
symptoms (of yellow fever), 2–3, 28, 40, 176–81, 183–85, 187–88, 202–5, 205–6, 209, 211–13, 218, 283–86, 289–90, 293–98, 306, 317–20, 321–22, 325–29, 370–74, 431–37, 439–4; 452–84; as indication for hospitalization, 125; remission and relapse, 471–72

tartar emetic, 13, 307
Tegart, Edward (inspector of hospitals), 38, 39, 40, 42, 501n3
Tennent, Dr John, treatment of yellow fever symptoms, 11
theories of disease, 492
Tobago, yellow fever reports filed in (1820s, 1840s), 366–450; miasma, 376–82; *cases and deaths from the epidemic remittent fever at Tobago, April–July 1841,* 445–46t12.5; *employed persons about the sick in the garrison or hospital, Tobago, Nov. 1818–March 1819, list of,* 388–90t12.2; *mortality report by age, military unit strength, at Tobago, April–July 1841,* 446t12.6; *mortality report by period of residence, military unit strength, at Tobago, April–July 1841,* 447t12.7; *return of a detachment of the 4th regiment stationed in the island of Tobago, Deaths, April 1819 to Sept. 1820,* 426t12.4; *sick at Tobago, 1806–17,* 383–85t12.1; sickness, 415–20, 423–26
treatments for yellow fever, 11–12, 13, 28–33, 39, 110–11, 205–7
Trinidad, yellow fever reports filed in (1818, 1840s), 451–90; living quarters, 455, 485; preview, 451; weather, 470
tuberculosis, 501n4
typhus, 29

urban yellow fever, 2

vaccination, 47, 420, 447, 484–85
venesection, 18, 362. *See also* bleeding
venesection, modern discussion of, 492
vesicatories (blistering agents), 9, 10, 494
Vine, Richard, 4
vinegar rub, 35
vomit, taste and chemical makeup of, 109–10. *See also* black vomit

vómito prieto, 3, 8. *See also* black vomit

Warner, W. J. (ship's surgeon on *HSM Alfred*), report on experiences in the Caribbean in the 1790s by, 27–37, 501n18

Warren, Henry (medical practitioner in Barbados), 8–11; on causes and treatment of disease, 493–94; *Treatise Concerning the Malignant Fever in Barbados and the Neighbouring Islands, with an Account There from the Year 1733 to 1738,* 8

Watson, Dr Karl, 498n16

weather conditions. *See* admissions of cases at Brimstone Hill, each month, noting weather conditions

Weir, John (first director general of the Army Medical Dept.), 34, 500n14

white employees at Naval Hospital who escaped sickness, 20 June 1821–20 Feb. 1822, 134–35t4.3

white orderlies and sickness, 124, 125–26

women and children: accounts of disease among, 47, 60, 65–66, 85, 88, 136, 148, 157, 172, 300, 424–25; disease in Dominica among, 233—34; fatalities in Antigua among, 65–66; fatalities in Barbados among, 69, 76–77, 79–80, 81, 82–83, 96–97, 159, 170–71, 182t4.8

yellow fever, 358–59; attacks of in Barbados, 153–60, 168–73, 175, 193–94; description of as gastric disease, 137–43; in Granada, 273–82; in Montserrat, 299–302; in St Lucia, 344–46; in St Vincent, 359–64; terms for, 502n14; in Tobago, 367–70, 422, 423–26, 427–31, 437–39; transmission of two kinds of, 2. *See also* symptoms

yellow fever admissions and deaths by period of residence and class strength (Barbados, 1840s), 190t4.9

yellow fever cases and fatalities among military units (*Extract of Annual Report of Medical Occurrences in the 76th Regiment Hospital, April 1839–March 1840 by Leigh MD*), 209t5.3

yellowing of skin (as symptom), 126–27

Young, Thomas (surgeon), 33, 500n10

Yucatan Peninsula, 1648 outbreak in, 3

www.ingramcontent.com/pod-product-compliance
Lightning Source LLC
Chambersburg PA
CBHW021413300426
44114CB00010B/478